Psychiatric Genetics

Psychiatric genetics has become 'Big Biology'. This may come as a surprising development to those familiar with its controversial history. From eugenic origins and contentious twin studies to a global network of laboratories employing high-throughput genetic and genomic technologies, biological research on psychiatric disorders has become an international, multidisciplinary assemblage of massive data resources. How did psychiatric genetics achieve this scale? How is it socially and epistemically organized? And how do scientists experience this politics of scale?

Psychiatric Genetics: From Hereditary Madness to Big Biology develops a sociological approach of exploring the origins of psychiatric genetics by tracing several distinct styles of scientific reasoning that coalesced at the beginning of the twentieth century. These styles of reasoning reveal, among other things, a range of practices that maintain an extraordinary stability in the face of radical criticism, internal tensions and scientific disappointments.

The book draws on a variety of methods and materials to explore these claims. Combining genealogical analysis of historical literature, rhetorical analysis of scientific review articles, interviews with scientists, ethnographic observations of laboratory practices and international conferences, this book offers a comprehensive and detailed exploration of both local and global changes in the field of psychiatric genetics.

Michael Arribas-Ayllon is a senior lecturer in the School of Social Sciences at Cardiff University. His research interests are in the sociology of genetic knowledge, histories of biomedicine, applications of genetic testing, medical communication and professional decision-making.

Andrew Bartlett is a sociologist working at the University of York and the University of Sheffield. He has a long-standing interest in the sociology of 'Big Biology' and has written papers on a range of topics in the sociology of science, including the interdisciplinarity of bioinformatics, the organization and publics of psychiatric genetics, and social issues with regard to genome editing.

Jamie Lewis is a lecturer in Sociology in the School of Social Sciences at Cardiff University. His research interests coalesce around the sociology of science and technology studies (STS), public understanding of science (PUS) and medical sociology. He has published papers on bioinformatics, psychiatric genetics, stem cell research and public engagement.

Genetics and Society

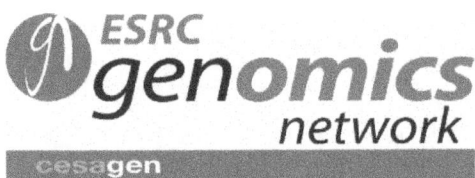

The books in this series, all based on original research, explore the social, economic and ethical consequences of the new genetic sciences. The series is based in the Cesagene, one of the centres forming the ESRC's Genomics Network (EGN), the largest UK investment in social-science research on the implications of these innovations. With a mix of research monographs, edited collections, textbooks and a major new handbook, the series is a valuable contribution to the social analysis of developing and emergent bio-technologies.

Series Editors:

Ruth Chadwick, *former Director of Cesagene, Cardiff University*
John Dupré, *Director of Egenis, Exeter University*
David Wield, *Director of Innogen, Edinburgh University*
Steve Yearley, *former Director of the Genomics Forum, Edinburgh University.*

Science and Democracy
Making Knowledge and Making Power in the Biosciences and Beyond
Edited by Stephen Hilgartner, Clark A. Miller and Rob Hagendijk

Knowing New Biotechnologies
Social Aspects of Technological Convergence
Edited by Matthias Wienroth and Eugenia Rodrigues

Cybergenetics
Health Genetics and New Media
Susan Kelly, Anna Harris and Sally Wyatt

Psychiatric Genetics
From Hereditary Madness to Big Biology
Michael Arribas-Ayllon, Andrew Bartlett and Jamie Lewis

For more information about this series, please visit www.routledge.com/Genetics-and-Society/book-series/GANDS.

In this detailed and wide-ranging ethnographic study, Arribas-Ayllon *et al.* provide an insightful exploration of the reorganization of infrastructures and expertise in psychiatric genetics. Their analysis of the distribution of value and emotional, boundary and engagement work across scientific hierarchies is particularly rich. Demonstrating how the relative immobility of more marginalised actors functions as a necessary condition for scaled up biology, this important book invites the scientific and academic community to look again at how reward should be distributed in the era of Big Biology.

Anne Kerr, Professor of Sociology, University of Leeds

Arribas-Ayllon, Bartlett, and Lewis's book invites us to follow them through the revolving doors and glassy atriums of a new science centre to consider the changing ways in which psychiatric genetics is taking place. Their work is a rich introduction to the spaces this discipline now occupies within the epistemologies of medical psychiatry, the interdisciplinary university campus, and the genetic infrastructures of global science. It both situates psychiatric genetics as particular form of inquiry, assembled from genealogies of clinical, statistical, and laboratory reasoning, as well as demonstrating how this is articulated through a wider network of affective relations and imaginaries circulating within research publications, patient involvement activities, and public engagement events. The effect is to render the complex processes that constitute the contemporary geographies of big biology visible, with all of its promises and compromises. The book demonstrates the value of thinking about science through questions of space, scale, and speed. It is also timely too, as the unresolved tensions at the heart of psychiatric genetics continue to generate new scientific inquiry and social controversy in the search for the biological causes of psychiatric disorders.

Gail Davies, Professor in Human Geography, University of Exeter

This book eloquently chronicles how the merger of mental health and heredity aligned itself with existing big biologies. As a consequence, the organisation of its consortia, the scale of its inquiries and the governance of its knowledge-making became increasingly relevant for understanding the development of Psychiatric Genetics, something Arribas-Ayllon, Bartlett and Lewis have understood very well. This book makes for great reading, especially for those interested in the intersections of the governance of science and critical sociology.

Bart Penders, Assistant Professor in Biomedicine and Society,
Maastricht University

Against the background of the historic Human Genome Project and the contemporary Human Brain Project, this fascinating book turns to the scaling-up of psychiatric genetics. Opening the door to one of the UK's largest research centres in this field, the authors show us the new state-of-the-art building and its scientists, attending to its history, the labour and infrastructuring involved, including interactions with patients and publics. Together they tell a comprehensive, multifaceted story of the emergence of a specific type of Big Biology, emphasising how the organisation of research is key to what we know and how we understand ourselves.

Niki Vermeulen, Senior Lecturer in History/Sociology of Science,
The University of Edinburgh

What does the reconfiguration of psychiatric genetics into 'Big Biology' mean for scientists, knowledge-production, and the circulation of substances, data, and capital? Arribas-Ayllon, Bartlett, and Lewis investigate these issues (and more) through close genealogical, rhetorical, and ethnographic research, exploring the styles of scientific reasoning underpinning psychiatric genetics. They brightly illuminate the challenges and opportunities that come with new kinds of collaboration, technological processing, and epistemic imaginaries – and the wider consequences of these for biomedicine and society.

Martyn Pickersgill, Wellcome Trust Reader in Social Studies of Biomedicine,
The University of Edinburgh

Psychiatric Genetics

From Hereditary Madness to Big Biology

Michael Arribas-Ayllon, Andrew Bartlett and Jamie Lewis

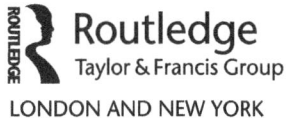

Routledge
Taylor & Francis Group

LONDON AND NEW YORK

First published 2019 by Routledge

2 Park Square, Milton Park, Abingdon, Oxfordshire OX14 4RN

52 Vanderbilt Avenue, New York, NY 10017

Routledge is an imprint of the Taylor & Francis Group, an informa business

First issued in paperback 2020

British Library Cataloguing-in-Publication Data
A catalogue record for this book is available from the British Library

Library of Congress Cataloging-in-Publication Data
Names: Arribas-Ayllon, Michael, author. | Bartlett, Andrew (Andrew James), 1977- author. | Lewis, Jamie, 1979- author.
Title: Psychiatric genetics : from hereditary madness to big biology / Michael Arribas-Ayllon, Andrew Bartlett and Jamie Lewis.
Description: Milton Park, Abingdon, Oxon ; New York, NY : Routledge, 2019. | Includes bibliographical references.
Identifiers: LCCN 2018051627| ISBN 9781138999985 (hardcover) | ISBN 9781315657967 (ebook)
Subjects: LCSH: Mental illness–Genetic aspects. | Behavior genetics.
Classification: LCC RC455.4.G4 A77 2019 | DDC 616.89/042–dc23
LC record available at https://lccn.loc.gov/2018051627

ISBN: 978-1-138-99998-5 (hbk)
ISBN: 978-0-367-66142-7 (pbk)

Typeset in Times New Roman
by Wearset Ltd, Boldon, Tyne and Wear

Contents

Tables

Acknowledgements

This book has been ten years in the making. The fieldwork commenced in 2008 when Michael Arribas-Ayllon and Andrew Bartlett were researchers at Cesagen (the ESRC Research Centre for Economic and Social Aspects of Genomics). It is only appropriate that we gratefully acknowledge the Economic and Social Research Council (ESRC) for funding which essentially kick-started our careers. Jamie Lewis re-joined Cesagen as an associate member in 2009 and was also supported by core funding from the ESRC as well as the Medical Research Council. We wish to extend a warm thanks to our old colleagues at Cesagen for creating a collegial and intellectually rich environment, which has left a lasting impression on our careers. Thanks also to Dr Katie Featherstone and Professor Paul Atkinson who have been involved in various stages of this project. We would also like to thank Professor Adam Hedgecoe for his useful insights and his moral support over the years. Cardiff University has also been generous in granting a year-long period of research leave for Michael Arribas-Ayllon to write up substantial portions of the book. Without this support the book would have taken considerably longer to complete. Very special thanks go to all the scientists, researchers and technicians who participated in and supported this work. Some of the scientists who generously gave their time over the years are now colleagues. In many ways, this book has been much more than an ethnographic study of scientific work – it has also established meaningful relationships across the social and life sciences.

Several chapters in this book draw on some previous material by authors. Chapter 3 is a revised version of 'Complexity and accountability: The witches brew of psychiatric genetics', first published 14 May 2010 in *Social Studies of Science*, 40(4): 499–524 by Michael Arribas-Ayllon, Andrew Bartlett and Katie Featherstone with permission from Sage. Chapter 4 draws on material from 'Sociological ambivalence and the order of scientific knowledge' first published 18 November 2013 in *Sociology*, 48(2): 335–351 by Michael Arribas-Ayllon and Andrew Bartlett, with permission from Sage. Chapter 5 draws on material from two papers 'Inscribing a discipline: Tensions in the field of bioinformatics', first published 13 May 2013 in *New Genetics and Society*, 32(3): 243–263 by Jamie Lewis and Andrew Bartlett, with permission from Taylor & Francis; and 'Hidden in the middle: Culture, value and reward in bioinformatics' first published 11 July 2016 in *Minerva* 54: 471–490 by Jamie Lewis, Andrew Bartlett and Paul Atkinson with permission from Springer. Material appearing in Chapter 7 draws on the paper 'How UK psychiatric geneticists understand and talk about engaging the public', first published 22 January 2015 in *New Genetics and Society* 34(1): 89–111 by Jamie Lewis and Andrew Bartlett with permission from Taylor & Francis.

We wish to thank Gerhard Boomgaarden, Senior Publisher at Routledge, for his incredible patience and for granting several extensions for the completion of the manuscript. Mihaela Diana Ciobotea, Editorial Assistant, was generous in offering assistance during the final stages of completion.

As anyone who has written a book will know, it is our families who also live with this strain. Michael Arribas-Ayllon would like to dedicate this book to his wife Turid for her marathon patience and support. Andrew Bartlett would like to dedicate this book to Anna, Rosa and Jasmine. Jamie Lewis would like to dedicate this book to Rachael.

Introduction

Entering 'Big Biology'

Psychiatric genetics has become 'Big Biology'. The implied prestige of this statement will perhaps be surprising to some given that modern genetics studies have not enjoyed the success of locating 'genes for' mental illnesses. Indeed, the eugenic origins of the field, the failure of previous research programmes, and a cultural uneasiness towards a disease model of mental disorders have left their mark on the field. Certainly, the success of the Human Genome Project (HGP) has provided an infrastructure for psychiatric genetics to become large-scale *in spite* of its controversial history. The buildings that it now occupies say a great deal about the 'stability' of this science and the 'durability' of its social networks (Gieryn 2002). But this has not always been the case.

In the UK, the physical origins of psychiatric genetics were humble to say the least. Peter McGuffin (2017: 124) describes the first dedicated unit as 'a make-shift post-war prefabricated building, affectionately known by staff as the "the hut", on the fringe of the campus of the Maudsley hospital in Camberwell'. It was here that the German-trained psychiatrist, Eliot Slater, established the first Medical Research Council (MRC) Psychiatric Genetics Unit in 1959. What attracted intellectual capital to the unit was not the physical resources of the building, but a different form of scientific capital – the acclaimed Maudsley Twin Register. When the American psychologist, Irving Gottesman, joined the unit in 1963, it sparked one of the most productive intellectual collaborations in the early history of the field. Working with James Shields, Gottesman developed a model of 'polygenic' inheritance for schizophrenia that eventually gained ascendency.

Today, biological research on psychiatric disorders is more likely to be found in 'centres of excellence' than cramped facilities buried in medical departments and research hospitals. These new buildings reflect the rise of the biosciences more generally with psychiatric genetics now housed in veritable machines of innovation (Thrift 2006). In these spaces, Big Biology is now beginning to confirm the theoretical models it developed in the 1960s. In one of the largest genome-wide molecular studies of its kind, a consortium of over 200 international research groups assembled nearly 37,000 cases and 113,000 controls.

The results are said to not only confirm a polygenic architecture of common disease but many other 'biological insights' too, the most prominent of which support the speculated link between immunity and schizophrenia (Schizophrenia Working Group of the Psychiatric Genomics Consortium 2014). As we entered Big Biology, we looked around and asked: what do these spaces do?

The site of most of our qualitative sociological research is one of the largest psychiatric genetics groups in the UK. In 2013, the group (we call the 'Centre' hereafter) moved to a new state-of-the-art building having won, a few years earlier, a significant research council grant. Described at the time as being the 'gateway to the university', the home of the Centre is representative of a new generation of bioscience buildings that hope to deliver a new generation of therapies. Contemporary bioscience buildings such as these are both functional and symbolic. As you approach from the outside of the Centre, you are greeted with green spaces, a line of trees and a path that directs you towards a large cathedral-like atrium. The sharp edges of the building's exterior are devised with environmental sustainability in mind, but they also connote the 'cutting-edge' research being conducted inside. The large glass panes that form the walled exterior capture light but they also enact transparency (see Stephens and Lewis 2017). In contrast to what some may see as the field's 'dark' and controversial history, the buildings that house psychiatric genetics research – in this case the building that is now home to the Centre – are grand, open, ambitious and inclusive.

The entrance to the building is accessed by two large revolving doors. Gieryn (1999: 431) remarks that 'doors say much about a building' because they give a sense of those for whom they were built. Upon entering the building, its implied constituencies are greeted by the semi-public space of the central court. Austere and spacious, the high ceilings of the white-painted atrium and the glass planes exaggerate its physical dimensions. Save for a few red sofas scattered about, the space is uncluttered, the exhibitory qualities of which are intended to foster closer relations between science and the public. Indeed, the central court and the modern lecture theatre are designed to hold public events and exhibitions. However, this is a tightly controlled openness. For all the design cues suggestive of inclusion, visibility and transparency, the building and, in particular, the research facilities are still carefully managed and centrally controlled. Visitors are not necessarily required to sign in, but security and building supervisors *are* located in a central booth in full view of all who enter. Openness is reserved for the ground floor, while the laboratories themselves on the upper floors are restricted, with staff requiring a security card to activate the doors.

The new building is a far cry from that which the Centre had once occupied. Its previous home, although certainly not old, was cramped and deemed no longer fit for purpose. Located on a hospital campus, it was hidden away behind the main hospital building. Visitors had to be 'buzzed' into the building by security. Once inside, they were required to sign in and wait beside a small security booth in a corridor, with the laboratories and offices only accessible with a security card. In the small area available to visitors, there was no place to sit and wait to be collected. It had none of the inclusivity and transparency built into the new building. Many of those involved in psychiatric genetics worked in laboratories and offices in the basement level. The tunnel-like corridors of the basement – known colloquially as the 'rat maze' – were dark and unwelcoming, and the limited space meant that some of the scientists attached to the Centre were dispersed across the hospital campus. The move to the new, purpose-built building was intended to accommodate an ever-expanding group working in a field that was growing in scale and prestige.

More than just symbolizing the elevated status of psychiatric genetics, the new building also reveals a purposeful architecture designed to encourage interaction and sociability. There is a coffee shop downstairs, 'break out' rooms and other spaces for meetings on several floors, as well as glassless windows between the upper levels to allow conversations to flow between researchers. The large open-plan offices on each floor are consistent with the 'decentralization' of the laboratory (Galison and Jones 1999). The dispersion of physical and managerial structures is shaped by the latent architecture of information networks. The connectivity and portability of hardware and software have transformed the positioning of workers in relation to physical space. Freed from the industrial base of 'mechanical architectures', social and electronic architectures are marked by closer relations between business and research, with laboratory designs looking more like an office environment. This 'decloistering of science' (Galison and Jones 1999) not only produces greater flexibility, but the mobility required for teamwork and collaboration is built into the fabric of the building. In the new structure, 'wet lab' and 'dry lab' workers are located on the same floor, sometimes in the same office. Locating the Centre in a single building establishes a critical mass (and mix) of expertise, as those with different skills, knowledge and sensibilities are co-located to stimulate interdisciplinarity (Thrift 2006). But, while horizontal mobility is encouraged in the new building, vertical hierarchies are maintained. Senior researchers have their own offices, while mid-career academics share offices, and the junior researchers are located among the hectic business of the open-plan area. Hierarchy is built into the use and distribution of space (Stephens and Lewis 2017).

Another aspect of design enhancing the performance of biological research is the electronic infrastructure that fuses adjoining work spaces, local laboratories, international collaborators and remote servers into a single network of interoperability. Connectivity, the capacity for data and information to move between laboratories, is a key property of decentralized Big Biology projects. In the new ensembles of collaborating consortia and coordinating committees, it makes little sense to think of the 'experiment' as a specific event or a single location. Galison and Jones (1999) observe similar arrangements among laboratories involved in particle physics during the 1980s and 1990s. The dissolution of central hierarchies in favour of dispersed committee-based tasks, lateral affiliations of university groups, and electronic networks of information, has rendered the fixed identity of a single 'experimenter', or even a single 'experimental group', obsolete in these Big Science formations. Just as 'electronic architecture fundamentally reshapes the physical architecture' (Galison and Jones 1999: 529) of large-scale physics, so too the social and electronic architectures of post-HGP biology have produced new geographic and spatial arrangements (see Chapter 4). The biological experiment is dispersed among multiple locations within a global network of software and hardware.

The building that houses the psychiatric genetics research of the Centre is similar to many other temples of contemporary, interdisciplinary bioscience. Their common architectural features are statements of the kinds of activities they seek to maximize – sociability, flexibility, mobility, connectivity, transparency, co-extensiveness, etc. Perhaps, we could attribute this genre of scientific architecture to a logic of interdisciplinarity (Barry *et al.* 2008) or to some kind of 'epistemic ecology' of innovation (Thrift 2006). And yet, underpinning this regime is another dimension that eludes a spatial analytics of buildings. The distributed nature of contemporary bioscience is also a response to the increasing 'scale' of knowledge production. What these buildings can only imply are the ways in which they are already linked to a much larger, and in many ways, virtual domain of 'mass inscription'. Especially in biology, seeing and inscribing the properties of life at the molecular scale is creating new assemblages of biological research dedicated to extracting its value. In the case of psychiatric genetics, we seek to understand the ways in which the increasing scale of production governs contemporary biological research. Throughout this book a key question we ask is: how does a politics of scale operate in contemporary psychiatric genetics? No matter how dispersed the biological experiment has become, the focus of our ethnographic study explores how Big Biology is experienced by members in a single location.

Psychiatric genetics as 'Big Biology'

In recent years, there have been initiatives within sociology to describe and analyse the practices of large-scale research in biology. In an obvious sense, projects using genotyping and sequencing technologies require an infrastructure that is qualitatively different to, and produce data at a far greater rate than, previous scales of biological research. What is less obvious, however, is the visibility of this scale, the manner of its integration and interaction, and its reshaping of what epistemically counts as 'biology' in large-scale research. In line with recent scholarship, we contend that the rhetoric of scale in contemporary bioscience deserves careful scrutiny (Davies *et al.* 2013). We argue that psychiatric genetics – a field that has adopted high-throughput technologies and techniques – can be conceptualized as 'Big Biology'. We use this category to critically distinguish 'genomics' from previous organizational and methodological approaches to genetics research, but we also use this term to emphasize the differences and the overlaps between large-scale biological research and the objects of study in previous sociological work on 'Big Science' (Weinberg 1961).

The parallels between the classic examples of Big Science found in physics and large-scale biology are clearest when the instantiations of scale focus on massive centralized budgets and concentrations of expensive equipment, as was to some degree the case with the HGP, despite its essentially 'federalized' form of organization. The centralized facilities of twentieth-century physics attracted much academic interest as sites involving larger aggregations of scientists (Capshew and Rader 1992; Collins 2003, 2004; Galison and Hevly 1992; Hilgartner 2013; Knorr-Cetina 1999; Traweek 1992). In 'Big Physics', scale emerges from funding priorities, geopolitical ambitions, global governance, international collaborations and specific sets of expertise (Kriege 1996; Knorr-Cetina 1999). In these studies, the centralization of technical infrastructure becomes a visible marker of scale.

By contrast, scale does not operate along the same dimensions of centralization and visibility in much post-HGP large-scale biology, and the same is true of the large-scale psychiatric genetics being conducted at the Centre. Big Biology has come to denote the *distributed management* of scientific sites, the outsourcing of key components of production, and their less visible research practices that include a wide variety of expertise (Davies *et al.* 2013; Hilgartner 2013; Lezaun 2013). In the contemporary biosciences, scale increases horizontally with 'the experiment' distributed widely across different spatial and temporal domains. This means that the constituent research components can be kept manageably small, allowing the overall scale to be partially 'hidden', or at least one step removed from the everyday laboratory lives of its contributors. In these large-scale 'ensembles of research technologies' (Hackett 2005), the labours of those at work in Big Biology can be invisible to each other; the work of fieldworkers collecting material may be invisible to laboratory biologists, who outsource work to unseen subcontracted technicians, who produce data that are collected and analysed by bioinformaticians in the 'dry lab' whose expertise is obscure to laboratory biologists, and so on. As an analytical category, Big Biology captures the fluid relations of knowledge and scale which are oriented towards managing the multifaceted complexity of biological objects.

In studying a field that seeks to genetically dissect psychiatric disorders, the concept of Big Biology matters because contemporary psychiatric genetics is 'large-scale' without resembling the archetypal Big Science of physics. For instance, when we first visited the previous site of the Centre on the hospital campus, in 2008, there was no highly visible apparatus, no warehouses of sequencing machines, no material sign that these laboratories exceeded the scale of 'ordinary' biology. As we learned, the work necessary for the production, circulation and analysis of data was not centralized in one physical location, but distributed between collaborators, outsourced to technicians in service laboratories, and accommodated in the vast increase in productive power engendered by the miniaturization and automation of laboratory processes. The scale of psychiatric genetics did not impress upon our senses in the manner of, say 'Big Physics' (for example, CERN or LIGO), because many of its processes have been dispersed and distributed, allowing individual laboratories to retain the superficial characteristics of 'small biology'.

Styles of reasoning

The recent appearance of Big Biology in psychiatric genetics is an interesting sociological story in itself, but without a strong historical perspective we risk having only a fleeting understanding of its epistemic organization. For instance, we might assume that the so-called 'omics' revolution of high-throughput technologies has ushered in a new 'paradigm' of molecular genetics. The shift from single-gene determinism to probabilistic models of systems biology may appear to be a decisive break from the past. Depending on one's historical perspective, or lack of it, we might see more discontinuity and revolution than accumulation in the life sciences. But there are still other reasons why the sociology of scientific knowledge needs a historical perspective. Without a historical understanding of psychiatric genetics, we would fail to recognize the ways in which distant problems and controversies have shaped its social and epistemic organization. We would fail to appreciate the field's remarkable stability and resilience in spite of its failures and criticism. In short, we need the past as a way to understand the present.

This book explores the conditions of possibility of psychiatric genetics using Hacking's framework of 'styles of scientific reasoning' (1982, 1992, 2002). Originally adapted from Alastair Crombie's (1981, 1994) historical work on 'styles of scientific thinking', Hacking (1982) takes an explicitly relativist stance to ask how reasoning is *possible* in science. Styles of reasoning are systems of possibility that come into existence by introducing their own candidates of truth and falsehood. The standards of objectivity for arriving at the truth 'have no existence independent of the styles of reasoning that settle what is to be true or false in their domain' (Hacking 2002: 161). The truth of facts, observations and explanations is what we arrive at by reasoning in that style. The relativism of scientific reasoning explains why there is no obvious vantage point to judge their rationality or irrationality, and thus why they are curiously immune to independent criticism. Hacking shows that there is more continuity in scientific reasoning than what is allowed for by revolutions in the history of science. In contrast to Kuhnian paradigms (Kuhn 1962), styles of reasoning are more durable and widespread, and tend to accumulate over time.

Styles of reasoning offer a more precise tool for thinking about different forms of scientific inquiry. Unlike Crombie's styles, where 'thinking is too much in the head' (Hacking 1992: 3), Hacking's emphasis on *reasoning* is meant to give priority to social practices. Styles of reasoning are thus practical as well as theoretical; they are impersonal and collective activities rather than 'research mentalities' (Crombie 1981). They have more in common with Fleck's (1979/1935) 'thought collective', or Foucault's (1972) notion of 'episteme'. As practical and theoretical activities of getting at the truth, different styles of reasoning can coexist as complementary modes of inquiry; they can be fused together to form a 'compound ... a new intellectual substance' (Hacking 1992: 182–183); indeed, several styles can occupy one and the same field. When Crombie originally produced his list of six styles, he 'offered a sensible template of modes of investigation in the sciences' (Hacking 2012: 600). We can crudely summarize these styles as (a) *mathematical*, (b) *experimental exploration*, (c) *hypothetical modelling*, (d) *probability*, (e) *taxonomy*, and (f) *historico-genetic explanations*.[1] But, like any list, it is not intended to be exhaustive or reified. There are most likely many more styles of reasoning but Crombie's six are sufficient in stating those which have become 'our standards of good reason' (Hacking 2012: 601).

Styles of reasoning are conditions of possibility for new kinds of science. In the historical chapters that follow (Chapters 1 and 2), we argue that the *clinical*, *statistical* and *laboratory* styles of reasoning made psychiatric genetics possible in the early twentieth century. But as Elwick (2012) has recently explained, to say that modes of scientific inquiry are conditions that make science possible is not a statement of causality – styles of reasoning do not cause new sciences, but are 'circumstances that are necessary for other phenomena to occur' (Elwick 2012: 619). Styles of reasoning form in relation to other conditions such as contingent historical events, social institutions, economic circumstances, etc. For instance, in Shapin's and Schaffer's (1985) work on the history of experiments, Hacking cites the 'custom of trust among the gentry who formed the Royal Society' (Hacking 2009: 44) as a condition that made the laboratory style possible. As for psychiatric genetics, we must turn our attention to the domain of medical knowledge in which styles of reasoning about 'hereditary madness' appear and disappear in specific institutions.

Jewson (1976) gives prominence to institutionalized relationships in his description of 'medical cosmologies'. He argues that different modes of production in the domain of medical knowledge can be associated with a distinct gestalt of medical discourse. Similar to Kuhn's 'paradigm' and Foucault's 'discursive formation', medical cosmologies are structured relationships that surround the production of medical knowledge; they 'are not only statements about the world but are also ways of relating to others in the world' (Jewson 1976: 623). The distinct cosmologies of Bedside Medicine, Hospital Medicine and Laboratory Medicine (Ackerknecht (1967) also includes Library Medicine) are institutional arrangements in which styles of reasoning come to be established.

Jewson's (1976) and Ackerknecht's (1967) nomenclature provides a useful way of showing how transformations in the discourse of 'hereditary madness' were linked to a distinct *apparatus* of medical interactions, modes of production and practices of reasoning. Psychiatric genetics emerges from the interplay and convergence of clinical, statistical and laboratory styles of reasoning in the early twentieth century when Emil Kraepelin became the director of the German Institute for Psychiatric Research in Munich. The Institute itself was a clinic, hospital and laboratory, which established the conditions for Ernst Rüdin to conduct the first family study of schizophrenia in 1916. Referring back to Crombie's template of styles, we are not proposing that the *clinical* and *laboratory* styles of psychiatric genetics were new; rather, they were a fusion of existing styles on Crombie's list.[2] In early biological psychiatry, Kraepelin's clinical style was a new way of ordering and standardizing symptoms by means of *taxonomy* as well as *statistical* analysis of patient populations. The laboratory style of *experimental* exploration had already established the principles of recessive inheritance among certain categories of species or traits. But for psychiatric genetics to become a coherent science of human heredity, the clinical style of ordering symptoms and the laboratory style of imputing principles of inheritance had to align with a mathematical description of populations. Indeed, it was a *statistical* style of reasoning that permitted the extension of clinical observation to the analysis of regularities of populations. Only then was it possible to claim that psychiatric disorders aggregate in families because they are quantitative traits with real, biological properties.

Lastly, styles of reasoning offer a plausible explanation of the *durability* of psychiatric genetics. This is an important factor given its controversial history. Styles of reasoning are characterized by their 'self-authenticating nature' (Hacking 1992: 191) – the more a style is used the more convinced we become that it gets at the truth. Each style has its own 'self-stabilizing techniques' (Hacking 1992: 193) that enables us to understand the stability of the sciences. For psychiatric genetics, the recent incarnation of Big Biology signifies a stunning transformation of its public visibility, scales of production and global organization. Though it might be tempting to say that genomics 'saved' the field from controversy and obscurity, we argue that there has been no fundamental change in its core styles of reasoning. The rapid growth of *-omic* technologies is not a gestalt switch to a new paradigm of 'molecular psychiatry' but a reorganization of its styles of reasoning. The ability to genotype thousands of cases and controls is only a technical 'revolution' insofar as it provides an infrastructure for stabilizing the *clinical, statistical* and *laboratory* styles of psychiatric genetics.

Networks of production

Since 2005, a central method of psychiatric genetics[3] has been Genome-Wide Association Studies (GWAS). Described as a 'brute force' approach of testing thousands of common variants, GWAS are essentially a distributed network of production. The candidates of truth and falsehood they produce – statistically significant associations between genotype and phenotype – are the product of a whole chain of 'inscriptions' (Latour 1987, 1999). DNA is genotyped on machines, transformed into annotated data, downloaded on computer hard drives or remote servers, analysed using bioinformatic software, producing statistical descriptions of the imagined qualities of living bodies. Along this chain of inscriptions, descriptions of bodies and illness are rendered amenable to computational devices which are now central to reasoning in a clinical, statistical and laboratory style.

The mobility of genome data is a distinguishing feature of large-scale biology. In the open data practices of post-HGP *-omic* sciences, there is an expectation that data will be made available to other laboratories. In acquiring the attributes of 'usability', living structures *in vivo* are abstracted to create readable inscriptions, allowing information *in silico* to circulate as a medium of exchange across different spaces and different styles of reasoning. Data mobility also shapes the arrangement of expertise within Big Biology. The work of verifying new candidates of objectivity involves new forms of expertise suited to a scientific landscape awash with genomic data. As we will show, the hybrid field of 'bioinformatics' has become an essential component of large-scale psychiatric genetics. Big Biology requires not only multidisciplinary cooperation, but the involvement of liminal, interdisciplinary domains (see Chapter 5).

The relatively concentrated, more archetypical Big Science of the HGP laid the foundations for increasingly distributed post-HGP Big Biology (Collins *et al.* 2003). In addition to investing in new technologies and techniques, the main concern for research managers in the post-HGP life sciences is arranging different forms of expertise into an efficient assembly of production. During the first phase of GWAS at the Centre (2005–2010), as scientists began forming their own networks of collaboration both locally and globally, the transition to large-scale research was experienced as being difficult. Beyond the managerial rhetoric of investing in people and skills, we found a contradictory and fluid arrangement at work. In the empirical chapters that follow (Chapters 4–8), we show how the clinical, statistical and laboratory styles of psychiatric genetics are either remotely concealed among distributed processes or organized around 'trading zones' (Galison 1999). This 'horizontal' expansion and reorganization of expertise is, of course, consistent with multidisciplinary collaboration. But in the networks of large-scale biology, the mobility and visibility of actors is organized 'vertically'. By this we mean that the opportunities to accumulate value by being seen and recognized are distributed hierarchically. In ways that may be unique to large-scale biology, the circulation of 'data' is granted more mobility and visibility than some of those who are charged with extracting its value.

The empirical story that unfolds from our interviews and observations highlights the tensions endemic to the decentralized laboratory. Like other programmes that employ *-omic* technologies, the field of genomic psychiatry is a 'network of consortia'. The scale of research conducted by the Centre is rendered stable and manageable by virtue of its partnership with multinational consortia of cooperating (and competing) laboratories. The imperative to share resources, especially data, between laboratories involves a 'dance of enemies' as one scientist put it. While those leading the Centre have to contend with the sacrifice of autonomy that comes from being a partner in such a dance, those further down the hierarchy have watched as the scale of production has outrun the distribution of reward and recognition.

Argument and methods

The arguments developed in this book are the product of several different methods or 'research styles' for investigating science. Broadly speaking, the chapters set out to reconstruct psychiatric genetics in a manner that might be described as genealogical, rhetorical and ethnographic. These methods are not discrete nor separate modes of inquiry but invariably overlap throughout the book.

The genealogical style refers to a process of historical reconstruction. In the broadest sense, it refers to an 'epistemological history' (Lecourt 1969; Canguilhem 1991) of relevant practices, discourses, institutions, methods and techniques that form the condition of possibility of a genetic thought style within biological psychiatry. We prefer to group these conditions of possibility under the term 'apparatus' (Foucault 1975)[4] to show how transformations in the discourse of hereditary transmission come to be established in different formations of medical knowledge. Knowledge is treated as a collective phenomenon – a system of possibilities and regulated practices for testing truth or falsity. However, in ways that may be construed as a departure from traditions of focusing on 'epistemological rupture' (Bachelard 1938/2002) or 'paradigm shifts' (Kuhn 1962), we find much less evidence of discontinuity in the history of psychiatric genetics (see Chapter 2).

Starting with the writings of physicians in the Renaissance, we apply a genealogical style in Chapter 1 to trace the rise of hereditarian explanations of insanity. The task is to explain how transformations in 'Hospital Medicine' (Jewson 1976) gradually clarify and differentiate the domain of irregular transmission of disease. By the early nineteenth century, classical notions of 'hereditary disease' are swept aside in favour of *heredity* (see Lopez-Beltrán 1992, 2004, 2007). The concept of heredity introduces a new distinction between 'natural' (physiological) variation and 'accidental' (pathological) variation of the species. Especially in the Parisian hospitals, a new type of medicine is practised where large-scale examination of 'cases' are correlated with organic lesions. The popularity of hereditarian themes in early psychiatry coincides with a failure to establish an organic lesion responsible for mental illness (Dowbiggin 1991; Foucault 2008). Techniques of psychiatric questioning about family history are linked to the systematic collection of asylum statistics, after which an increasingly divergent explanation appears whereby any oddity or eccentricity in the family is interpreted as a sign of progressive pathological heredity.

By the mid-nineteenth century, heredity becomes a sophisticated science as the organization of 'transmission stories' lose their individuality and begin to refer to abstract properties of a population (Hacking 1990). The first step towards a science of heredity involves the systematic collection of positive *and* negative cases among stable populations. For psychiatrists, this involves the collection of cases in the asylum, and for Galton (1869), the collection of genealogical and biographical data of talented individuals. Galton's contribution to a science of heredity forms part of a general stabilization of a domain of production where the scope of biological heredity is gradually disciplined by a statistical style of reasoning. Galton offers a coherent methodology with which to mathematize genealogy and to demonstrate the 'blending' of inheritance through ancestral influences.

With the rediscovery of Mendel's laws, the bitter controversy between the Galtonian and Mendelian schools highlight enduring tensions between statistical and biological approaches to heredity. These tensions are not only constitutive of psychiatric genetics but continue to have a lasting influence on its research programmes. For instance, the ambivalence of Mendelian and quantitative models are instrumental in explaining the failure of linkage studies in the 1980s as well as the recent success of GWAS. The search for 'common genes' in the population demonstrates the collapse of a categorical model of psychiatric disease since many genes of small effect are likely to be continuously distributed in the population as quantitative traits. Although modern GWAS claim to dissolve the epistemic boundaries of a biological and statistical science of heredity (Kendler 2015), in later chapters we show how a statistical style of reasoning has become epistemically central but remains institutionally peripheral to contemporary psychiatric genetics (see Chapter 5).

Chapter 2 traces the birth of psychiatric genetics to a small but diverse network that took shape in Germany at the beginning of the twentieth century. The landmark publication of Ernst Rüdin's family study of schizophrenia in 1916 is considered a major improvement on early applications of Mendelism in neuropsychiatry. The break with neuropsychiatry comes from a biologically informed psychiatry that begins to orient its gaze towards the clinical course and outcome of disease. In particular, it was the German apparatus of the university hospital and the research institute that brings 'Hospital Medicine' into alignment with 'Laboratory Medicine' (Jewson 1976). Emile Kraepelin is the principal figure of this new alignment who stabilizes psychiatric nosology and sets the foundations for a science of heredity. When Kraepelin famously split psychosis into its affective and non-affective features, Rüdin selected the stable clinical features of 'schizophrenia' as the object of his family study.

Other networks of production also intersect with a mature science of heredity. The transformation of (ancestral) genealogy according to biological principles of heredity substantially alter the way family pedigrees are collected and ordered. The application of Weinberg's 'Mendelian statistics' introduce changes in the way samples of probands are ascertained and measured. In fact, all the methodological innovations of Rüdin's study belong to a network of production that formed around Kraepelin's 'research institute'. Not unlike the methodological diversity of contemporary 'multidisciplinary' research centres, the Munich Institute assembled *clinical*, *statistical* and *laboratory* styles of reasoning around large patient populations.

The remainder of Chapter 2 explores the disturbing legacy of German psychiatric genetics and the role that controversy has played in the discipline. A rhetorical approach considers the ways in which scientists reconstruct their own history by rebuilding a narrative of continuity and progress. Given the controversies surrounding twin and adoption studies, we examine some of the strategies by which scientists seek to 'authenticate' their statistical style of genetic epidemiology. Growing awareness of bias and error leads to decisive improvements in methodological design and execution. Various practices of 'curating' discordant findings show that the literature of twin and adoption studies is a pliable resource rather than a static canon of universal validity. Unlike some of its critics, we do not treat the genetics of psychiatric disorders as something inherently false and unsavoury. The place of this book is *not* to critique the knowledge claims of contemporary psychiatric genetics, but to understand the ways in which critique has shaped the discipline.

Following the failure of linkage studies in the 1980s, in Chapter 3 we consider the rhetorical aspects of a particular genre of scientific writing. The 'review article' has become an important form of writing that offers an official description of scientific activity and a stable genre for giving these descriptions a narrative form. A feature of these papers are the ways in which key events and controversies are reconstructed to bridge disciplinary boundaries, gather allies or reshape the past. Not only are they official statements of the field but review articles also engage in multiple activities such as popularization (Hilgartner 1990), fact construction (Myers 1992) and narrative reconstruction (Hedgecoe 2001). It is precisely the action-orientation of speculative and programmatic claims in science that forms a clearly emerging genre of scientific accountability. Analysis of a selection of articles reveals an emerging view of 'complexity' in psychiatric genetics (Arribas-Ayllon *et al.* 2010). Accounts of complexity appear to engage in the management of intellectual responsibility for past failures as well as speculative promises about the future. More than just descriptions of the natural world, the rhetoric of complexity seeks to assemble a multidisciplinary domain of tractable problems, which have important implications for orienting the field to GWAS.

In Chapters 1 to 3, the work of reassembling psychiatric genetics situates the present formation of Big Biology within a history of recurrent controversy and epistemic reconstruction. The remainder of the book (Chapters 4 to 8) presents our ethnographic fieldwork in and around a UK research centre. The fieldwork was conducted in four phases over a nine-year period. The first project was conducted by Arribas-Ayllon, Bartlett and Featherstone (2008–2010), which focused on the reorganization of large-scale biological research at the Centre. The second project conducted by Lewis (2009–2014) focused on the public understanding and public engagement of the Centre's activities; the third project, conducted by Bartlett and Lewis (2008–2011), examined the stabilization of bioinformatics in UK institutions including at the Centre; and the final project, which was led by Arribas-Ayllon (2016–2017), involved follow-up observations and interviews at the new Centre building. Together, the fieldwork combines multiple local observations of scientists working on large-scale biological research projects across a range of psychiatric disorders. The empirical components of our fieldwork included observations of laboratory work, international conferences, staff away days, training events, workshops and over 70 public lectures. We also include data from a UK-wide survey of bioinformaticians and over 60 interviews with scientists at, or attached to, the Centre.

The ethnographic style that informs these chapters is concerned with the conduct and management of Big Biology in psychiatric genetics. We prefer to describe this style of research as 'ethnographic' rather than 'ethnography' because the former implies intermittent access to cultural domains of science through observation, description and interviews, rather than a sustained period of immersion. Having said this, two of the authors (Arribas-Ayllon and Lewis) have maintained long-lasting relationships with scientists at the Centre. Arribas-Ayllon continues to contribute to 'social and ethical issues' at scientists' conferences and summer schools, while Lewis was employed at the Centre as a social scientist to research, organize and manage public engagement activities. In fact, Lewis combines both ethnographic and participatory research to understand how scientists imagine and engage their publics (see Chapter 7).

In addition to the sustained duration of fieldwork, another strength of the study is the mutually reinforcing relationship between genealogical, rhetorical and ethnographic styles of research. For instance, a genealogical style offers a broad temporal and epistemological context to understand the social and political origins of psychiatric genetics, the conditions out of which controversies arise, and the ongoing reconstruction of its narrative. Rhetorical analysis provides an in-depth understanding of the construction of scientific literature, but it also offers a method of interpreting scientists' *accounts* as descriptive, explanatory and performative activities (Scott and Lyman 1968). In this book, research interviews are treated as both situated accounts *and* evidence of scientific practice.

Several important arguments emerge from the empirical components of our study. When we commenced our fieldwork in 2008, the Centre was already undergoing considerable change adapting to a large-scale approach. In Chapter 4, we explain how consortium-based GWAS operates along a continuum of collaboration–competition that intensifies processes of production. New modes of automation and outsourcing of laboratory processes displace a laboratory style of reasoning and reduce the mobility of early-career researchers. As the production of data circulate more freely in Big Biology, the scale of the labour involved becomes comparatively fractional and invisible.

In Chapter 5, we explore the ways in which 'mass inscription' of high-throughput genotyping moves Big Psychiatric genetics towards a statistical style of reasoning, relying on a novel arrangement of expertise to analyse and manage large volumes of genome data. Various kinds of 'boundary work' (Gieryn 1983) between biologists and hybrid disciplines such as 'bioinformatics' expose the tensions and asymmetries of these networks. While the interpretation and management of genome data has become epistemically central to Big Biology, we indicate the ways in which the discipline of bioinformatics is institutionally peripheral to psychiatric genetics (Lewis and Bartlett 2013).

In Chapter 6, we examine the largely invisible 'emotional labour' (Hochschild 1979, 1983) of fieldworkers who collect phenotypic data and blood samples from research participants. Observations of training events and interviews with scientists and especially fieldworkers indicate the ways in which increasing scale amounts to a reduction of the quality of information. Indeed, the recruitment of mainly female psychology graduates constitutes a gendered and increasingly acute division of labour in which fieldworkers must negotiate the affective entanglements of extracting 'data' from research participants.

Chapter 7 explores the ways in which scientists at the Centre account for publics and public engagement. A key argument is that scientists create 'imaginaries' to align biological research with broader cultural values. Imagined futures serve a range of purposes including justifying biological research in psychiatry, installing 'regimes of hope' (Moreira and Palladino 2005), mitigating scepticism and, above all, recruiting publics into their research programmes.

In the final empirical chapter, we consider how the scientific community respond to mounting criticism of their core methodology. After the slow progress and disappointing findings of the first wave of GWAS (2005–2010), arguments about the 'missing heritability' (Manolio *et al.* 2009) of complex diseases engender a unique display of solidarity among scientists during a major conference in 2010. We examine the various circumstances in which scientists lobby to protect their preferred methodology. Upon returning to the field in 2016, we find consortium-based GWAS is bigger than ever. With the Psychiatric Genetics Consortium having trebled in size, recent studies operate at an order of magnitude which are only now beginning to yield biological insights.

In this book, we argue that psychiatric genetics has become a global assemblage that operates along a dynamic continuum of 'cooperative competition' (Hackett 2005) in the context of wider imbalances between competing multinational groups. The intensification of production, the distributed management of resources and the ever-present dynamic of competitive collaboration are forces which act on practitioners. Although the 'labours' of Big Biology have carved out a domain of tractable problems, they have also sharpened the division between quality and quantity, visibility and invisibility, mobility and immobility inside the Centre. Operating in this costly and highly competitive environment, only a minority can enjoy the fruits of mobility and visibility. Where the mobility of genome data is a distinct characteristic of large-scale biological research, by contrast, there are many 'figures' in Big Biology who are unable to 'enhance their own versatility' (Lezaun 2013). Scientists, technicians and fieldworkers must remain *in situ* while other people and other *things* circulate. In the empirical chapters of this book, we will show that although psychiatric genetics has managed to solve the problem of statistical power by embracing a politics of scale, it also produces new hierarchies in which 'fractional' (Beaver 2001) and 'invisible' (Star and Strauss 1999) workers are unable to accrue value and reward in these large networks of biological research.

Notes

1 This is admittedly a crude summary of Crombie's styles. In his own words, the crucial passage reads as follows:

The varieties of scientific method so brought into play may be distinguished as:

a   the simple postulation established in the mathematical sciences,
b   the experimental exploration and measurement of more complex observable relations,
c   the hypothetical construction of analogical models,

d   the ordering of variety by comparison and taxonomy,
e   the statistical analysis of regularities of populations and the calculus of probabilities, and
f   the historical derivation of genetic development.

The first three of these methods concern essentially the science of individual regularities, and the second three the science of the regularities of populations ordered in space and time.

(Crombie 1981: 284)

2   Hacking (1992) proposed that the laboratory style was a novel addition to Crombie's list (a fusion of experimental exploration and hypothetical modelling) but now maintains it is a crystallization of the experimental style (Hacking 2012). We have kept the term 'laboratory style' to highlight the distinctive settings and materials in which scientific reasoning occurs.
3   Although gene discovery has been the most visible and, in some cases, the most controversial method, it is not the only 'method' in psychiatric genetics. Over the last century, the field has developed several research programmes that correspond to different styles of reasoning. For the historically minded scientist, Kuhn's notion of scientific 'paradigms' is often used to demarcate different, and often competing, methodological programmes within a field. Kenneth Kendler (2005), who is a peculiarly reflexive practitioner, is no exception. He describes four 'research paradigms' within psychiatric genetics: (i) basic genetic epidemiology, (ii) advanced genetic epidemiology, (iii) gene discovery, and (iv) molecular genetics. More recently, high-profile techniques of gene discovery, such as Genome-Wide Association Studies (GWAS), have been responsible for identifying new susceptibility genes and thus generating new biological insights, leading to improved methods of calculating polygenic risk (epidemiology) and better understandings of the gene pathways implicated in brain biology (molecular genetics).
4   When Foucault developed his genealogical approach, he used the term *dispositif* (or 'apparatus') to conceive a system of knowledge/power relations. The production of knowledge consists of a heterogeneous ensemble of discourses, institutions, architectural forms, regulatory practices, decisions, laws, administrative measures, scientific statements, propositions, etc. (Foucault 1975). The concept of 'apparatus' offers a much wider definition of conditions of possibility to include a system of discursive and non-discursive relations. For this reason, some STS scholars (Latour 1987, 1988; Keating and Cambrosio 2003) give primacy to 'things' and devices as constitutive of scientific knowledge.

References

Ackerknecht E (1967) *Medicine at the Paris Hospital, 1794–1848*. Baltimore: Johns Hopkins Press.
Arribas-Ayllon M, Bartlett A and Featherstone K (2010) Complexity and accountability: The witches' brew of psychiatric genetics. *Social Studies of Science* 40(4): 499–524.
Bachelard G (1938/2002) *The Formation of the Scientific Mind: A Contribution to a Psychoanalysis of Objective Knowledge*. Manchester: Clinamen Press.
Barry A, Born G and Weszkalnys G (2008) Logics of interdisciplinarity. *Economy and Society* 37(1): 20–49.
Beaver DD (2001) Reflections on scientific collaborations (and its study): Past, present and future – feature report. *Scientometrics* 52(3): 365–377.
Canguilhem G (1991) *The Normal and the Pathological*. New York: Zone Books.
Capshew JH and Rader KA (1992) Big science: Price to the present. *Osiris* 2(7): 3–25.

Collins F, Morgan M and Patrinos A (2003) The Human Genome Project: Lessons from large-scale biology. *Science* 300(5617): 286–290.

Collins HM (2003) LIGO becomes big science. *Historical Studies in the Physical and Biological Sciences* 33(2): 261–297.

Collins HM (2004) *Gravity's Shadow: The Search for Gravitational Waves*. Chicago: University of Chicago Press.

Crombie AC (1981) Philosophical perspectives and shifting interpretations of Galileo. In J Hintikka, D Gruender and E Agazzi (eds). *Theory Change, Ancient Axiomatics and Galileo's Methodology*. Dordrecht: Reidel, pp. 271–286.

Crombie AC (1994) *Styles of Scientific Thinking in the European Tradition* (3 vols.). London: Duckworth.

Davies G, Frow E and Leonelli S (2013) Introduction: Bigger, faster, better? Rhetorics and practices of large-scale research in contemporary biology. *Biosocieties* 8: 386–396.

Dowbiggin IR (1991) *Inheriting Madness: Professionalization and Psychiatric Knowledge in Nineteenth Century France*. Berkeley: University of California Press.

Elwick J (2012) Layered history: Styles of reasoning as stratified conditions of possibility. *Studies in the History and Philosophy of Science* 43: 619–627.

Fleck L (1979) *Genesis and Development of a Scientific Fact*. Translated by TJ Trenn and RK Merton from the German of 1935. Chicago: University of Chicago Press.

Foucault M (1972) *The Archaeology of Knowledge*. London: Tavistock.

Foucault M (1975) *Discipline and Punish*. New York: Vintage Books.

Foucault M (2008) *Psychiatric Power: Lectures at the College De France, 1973–74*. Edited by J Lagrange and translated by G Burchell. Basingstoke: Palgrave Macmillan.

Galison P (1999) Trading zones: Coordinating action and belief. In M Biagioli (ed.). *The Science Studies Reader*. New York: Routledge, pp. 137–160.

Galison P and Hevly B (eds) (1992) *Big Science: The Growth of Large Scale Research*. Stanford: Stanford University Press.

Galison P and Jones CA (1999) Factory, laboratory, studio: Dispersing sites of production. In P Galison and E Thompson (eds). *The Architecture of Science*. Cambridge, MA: MIT Press.

Galton F (1869) *Hereditary Genius: An Inquiry into its Laws and Consequences*. London: Macmillan.

Gieryn TF (1983) Boundary-work and the demarcation of science from non-science: Strains and interests in professional interests of scientists. *American Sociological Review* 48: 781–795.

Gieryn TF (1999) Two faces on science: Building identities for molecular biology and biotechnology. In P. Galison and E. Thompson (eds). *The Architecture of Science*. Cambridge, MA: MIT Press.

Gieryn TF (2002) What buildings do. *Theory and Society* 31: 35–74.

Hackett EJ (2005) Essential tensions: Identity, control and risk in research. *Social Studies of Science* 35(5): 787–826.

Hacking I (1982) Language, truth and reason. In M Hollis and S Lukes (eds). *Rationality and Relativism*. Cambridge, MA: MIT Press, pp. 48–66.

Hacking I (1990) *The Taming of Chance*. Cambridge: Cambridge University Press.

Hacking I (1992) 'Style' for historians and philosophers. *Studies in the History and Philosophy of Science* 23(1): 1–20.

Hacking I (2002) *Historical Ontology*. London: Harvard University Press.

Hacking I (2009) *Scientific Reason*. Taipei: National Taiwan University Press.

Hacking I (2012) 'Language, Truth and Reason' 30 years later. *Studies in the History and Philosophy of Science* 43: 599–609.

Hedgecoe A (2001) Schizophrenia and the narrative of enlightened geneticization. *Social Studies of Science* 31(6): 875–911.

Hilgartner S (1990) The dominant view of popularization: Conceptual problems, political uses. *Social Studies of Science* 20: 519–539.

Hilgartner S (2013) Constituting large-scale biology: Building a regime of governance in the early years of the Human Genome Project. *Biosocieties* 8(4): 397–416.

Hochschild AR (1979) Emotion work, feeling rules and social structure. *American Journal of Sociology* 85: 551–575.

Hochschild AR (1983) *The Managed Heart: Commercialization of Human Feeling*. Berkeley: University of California Press.

Jewson ND (1976) The disappearance of the sick-man from medical cosmology, 1770–1870. *Sociology* 10(2): 225–244.

Keating P and Cambrosio A (2003) *Biomedical Platforms: Realigning the Normal and the Pathological in Late-Twentieth-Century Medicine*. Cambridge, MA: MIT Press.

Kendler KS (2005) Psychiatric genetics: A methodologic critique. *American Journal of Psychiatry* 162(1): 3–11.

Kendler KS (2015) A joint history of the nature of genetic variation and the nature of schizophrenia. *Molecular Psychiatry* 20(1): 77–83.

Knorr-Cetina K (1999) *Epistemic Cultures: How the Sciences Make Knowledge*. Cambridge, MA: Harvard University Press.

Kriege J (1996) *History of CERN, Volume III: The Years of Consolidation 1966–1980*. Amsterdam: North Holland Publishers.

Kuhn TS (1962) *The Structure of Scientific Revolutions*. Chicago: University of Chicago Press.

Latour B (1987) *Science in Action: How to Follow Scientists and Engineers through Society*. Cambridge, MA: Harvard University Press.

Latour B (1988) *The Pasteurization of France*. Cambridge, MA: Harvard University Press.

Latour B (1999) *Pandora's Hope: Essays on the Reality of Science Studies*. London: Harvard University Press.

Lecourt D (1969) *L'Épistémologie historique de Gaston Bachelard*. Paris: Vrin.

Lewis J and Bartlett A (2013) Inscribing a discipline: Tensions in the field of bioinformatics. *New Genetics and Society* 32(3): 243–263.

Lezaun J (2013) Commentary: The escalating politics of 'Big Biology'. *Biosocieties* 8(4): 480–485.

Lopez-Beltrán C (1992) *Human Heredity 1750–1870: The Construction of a Scientific Domain*. PhD Thesis, Kings College London.

Lopez-Beltrán C (2004) In the cradle of heredity: French physicians and *L'Hérédité Naturelle* in the early 19th century. *Journal of the History of Biology* 37: 39–72.

Lopez-Beltrán C (2007) The medical origins of heredity. In S Müller-Wille and HJ Rheinberger (eds). *Heredity Produced: At the Crossroads of Biology, Politics, and Culture, 1500–1870*. Cambridge, MA: MIT Press.

McGuffin P (2017) Obituaries: Irving Gottesman. *British Journal Psychiatry Bulletin* 41(2): 124–125.

Manolio TA, Collins FS, Cox NJ, *et al.* (2009) Finding the missing heritability of complex diseases. *Nature* 461: 747–753.

Moreira T and Palladino P (2005) Between truth and hope: Parkinson's disease, neuro-transplantation and the production of 'self'. *History of the Human Sciences* 18(3): 55–82.

Myers G (1991) Stories and styles in two molecular biology review articles. In C Bazerman and J Paradis (eds). *Textual Dynamics of the Professions: Historical and Contemporary Studies of Writing in Professional Communities*. Madison: University of Wisconsin Press, pp. 45–75.

Myers G (1992) 'In this paper we report …': Speech acts and scientific acts. *Journal of Pragmatics* 17(4): 295–313.

Schizophrenia Working Group of the Psychiatric Genomics Consortium (2014) Biological insights from 108 schizophrenia-associated genetic loci. *Nature* 511: 421–427.

Scott M and Lyman S (1968) Accounts. *American Sociological Review* 31: 46–62.

Shapin S and Schaffer S (1985) *Leviathan and the Air-Pump: Hobbes, Boyle, and the Experimental Life*. Princeton: Princeton University Press.

Star SL and Strauss A (1999) Layers of silence, arenas of voice: The ecology of visible and invisible work. *Computer Supported Cooperative Work* 8: 9–30.

Stephens N and Lewis J (2017) Doing laboratory ethnography: Reflections on method on scientific workplaces. *Qualitative Research* 17(2): 202–216.

Thrift N (2006) Re-inventing invention: New tendencies in capitalist commodification. *Economy and Society* 35(2): 279–306.

Traweek S (1992) Big science and colonialist discourse: Building high-energy physics in Japan. In P Galison and B Hevly (eds). *Big Science: The Growth of Large Scale Research*. Stanford: Stanford University Press, pp. 1–17.

Weinberg AM (1961) Impact of large-scale science on the United States. *Science* 134(3473): 161–164.

1 From 'hereditary madness' to psychiatric genetics

Before the nineteenth century, there was no arrangement for thinking that human *heredity* was a biological concept with explanatory force. Medical discourse was preoccupied with *hereditary* as a description of a family trait or a disease transmitted from one generation to another. To acquire the status of a scientific entity, the concept of 'heredity' required the stabilization of a domain of production, a domain that had special relevance for psychiatry. For heredity to become a self-sufficient cause of mental illness, it required a system of relations that existed in and around the asylum apparatus. Indeed, Foucault (2008) observes that psychiatric power comes to establish itself in a mode of questioning about family history. By asking the mental patient about the illness of his or her family, questioning realizes madness beyond that of pathological anatomy to a horizon of pathological signs belonging to an entire family. Only after this technique was employed in French psychiatric hospitals did notions of 'pathological heredity' and 'degeneration' appear as generalized schemas of transmitted disease.

The task of this chapter is to understand how the concept of heredity later became a coherent tool for psychiatric genetics. We trace the historical transformation of statements describing the cause and transmission of 'hereditary madness' into a scientific explanation of biological laws of heredity. In a purely discursive sense, it follows the emergence of heredity as the reification of a form of madness but this strategy alone is insufficient to understand the transformation of medical-psychiatric discourse. In tracing the conditions of possibility for a science of heredity, the task is to understand the institutional arrangement in which different 'styles of reasoning' (Hacking 1982, 1992) come to be established. A useful framework for structuring our analysis is Ackerknecht's (1967) and Jewson's (1976) periodization of medicine.[1] If medicine of the Middle Ages had centred on *libraries* then the next four centuries would focus on the *bedside*, the *hospital* and the *laboratory* respectively. Our analysis begins with references to hereditary madness in the Renaissance. In the transition between Library Medicine and Bedside Medicine, we find a novel statement of congenital madness that curiously anticipates a modern psychiatric view of heredity.

Early modern discourse on hereditary

Since antiquity, medical knowledge of 'hereditary' had changed little until the sixteenth century. Hereditary referred to the recurrence of family resemblances via metaphors of legal inheritance concerning the distribution of titles and possessions to descendants (Zirkle 1946; Lopez-Beltrán 1992, 1994). For the ancients, inheritance was a useful analogy to explain the transmission of physical traits and moral qualities of character. The first technical use of the analogy in the natural sciences was employed by the physician. The term 'hereditary disease' (*haereditarii morbi*) referred to a class of diseases that occur only in certain families. Statements of this kind can be found in the Hippocratic-Galenic tradition, which recognized that disease, or a disposition to disease, was causally transmitted from parents to offspring. Thus, the French physician, Jean Fernel (1554, cited in Burton 1621/1883: 133) writes:

> such as the temperature of the father is, such is the son's, and look at what disease the father had when he begets him, his son will have after him ... as is as well inheritor of his infirmities as of his land.

The analogy to inheritance implied a rule of 'like begetting like', but what the rule lacked was an inner structure. Analogy could not explain how causal agents acted independently of the particular life forms they were a part of. Our inquiry begins with physicians writing in the sixteenth century who began to push the metaphorical dimensions of hereditary to new limits.

The medical historian, Erwin Ackerknecht (1968), tells us that the Renaissance was a period of 'profound contradictions'. The 'insane' were persecuted as witches or treated for demonic possession at the same time as new medical institutions appeared across Europe offering compassionate treatment. It was amongst this diversity of attitudes that a striking statement appeared that briefly anticipated a modern view of hereditary madness. In a treatise titled *The Diseases Which Deprive Man of His Reason* (1567), the Swiss-German physician known as Paracelsus, outlined a new division of insanity. Regarding those born insane (*Insani*), Paracelsus describes a mode of transmission that breaks from the law of resemblance:

> In the same way we can explain those people who have received insanity from the mother's womb as a heritage, such as a family which is insane or a child who has been born insane: the seed and its function may be defective, or it may be inherited from the part of father or mother. The first reason is that the sperm in itself and in the operation may be lacking in the power of matter which makes and builds the brain ... the circumstance is such that if there is insanity in the brain, the child's mother also has some deficiency in her brain, for the brain of the parents is continued in the brain of the son.... This does not always happen because the sperms become mixed, and either the man or the woman may or may not be insane, and the child may follow the insanity

or take after the one who has greater influence. It may even happen that if both are insane they still would give birth to a healthy child. This is due to the power of nature to which drives out the impediments and adversities.

(1567/1941: 155–156)

The novelty of this statement is not that insanity was congenitally inherited nor that the brain was associated with the defective mind. Rather, it was the awareness of a complex pattern of transmission and a mechanism of inheritance where the defective 'seed and its function' has consequences for brain development. Even Ackerknecht (1968: 24) considers this to be 'a new point of view'.[2] In contrast to humoral pathology where the sick individual determines the cause and nature of disease, it is the disease itself that conditions the patient (Pagel 1982). The fact that congenital madness is inherited from the mother *or* the father, from the mixture of their semen, implies a view of disease and its origins as solid, autonomous entities. Congenital madness was not the work of the devil nor an imbalance of humours but a germ of disintegration passed from one generation to another.

Paracelsus' view of hereditary madness was not typical of early modern discourse on *generation*.[3] He rejected the teachings of scholastic medicine and famously proclaimed that: 'the patients are your textbook, the sickbed is your study'. By rejecting the formal logics of Library Medicine, Paracelsus was advocating a new site of inspection beyond the formal hierarchy of the university apparatus. His style of reasoning was characteristically obscure and personal, governed mainly by analogies that collapsed distinctions and transformed metaphor into reality. Indeed, Vickers (1984: 130) likens his mode of reasoning to a 'calculating machine that can multiply but not divide'. But for all the peculiarity of Renaissance medicine, Paracelsus' view of hereditary madness resonates with the modern reader. How is this possible?

First, Paracelsus' statement occupies an idiosyncratic space between the two systems of possibility: the formal logic of Library Medicine and the 'human totality' (Jewson 1976) of Bedside Medicine. The accuracy of his description of disease transmission arises from acute observation rather than reproduction of scholastic principles. And though many have claimed that his bizarre and confusing analogies were an obstacle to experimentalism (see Vickers 1984 and Pagel 1982), Paracelsus accorded disease *the same* nature as man – each disease is endowed with a 'body' that interacts with other entities. Extrinsic entities – poison, spiritual alignment, a command of God, abnormal imaginations – were thought to interrupt the functioning of the organism. It was this dynamic view of the unity of matter and spirit that allowed Paracelsus to formulate an account of hereditary disease that was more sophisticated than the ancient adage of 'like begetting like'. Indeed, it was Paracelsus' explicitly 'ontological view of disease' (Pagel 1982) that paved the way for scientific approaches that begin to clarify the mechanisms of inheritance in the mid-seventeenth century.[4]

What frustrated efforts to produce a clear description of hereditary in the seventeenth century were the 'speculative excesses' of the previous century

(Lopez-Beltrán 1992). Theories of generation assumed homogeneity of genealogical groups, whereas hereditary diseases posed a troubling exception. The emerging system of Bedside Medicine begins to give prominence to these exceptions. Observed among the day-to-day practice of the physician, variation in familial patterns of disease become themes in need of explanation. Thus, we find various attempts to reconcile the Hippocratic-Galenic tradition (which grants the mixture of male and female semen) with Aristotelian typologies of character and causes. Paracelsus endorsed a material view of hereditary disease and employed a 'dual seed theory' (Boylan 1984) to explain the problem of variation. In 1567, Fernel developed a similar line of reasoning, attributing hereditary diseases to purely material causes of seminal contribution, and hereditary resemblances to immaterial (spiritual) causes linked to the mother's imagination. Other sixteenth century medics, such as Ambroise Paré and André Laurens, combined a dual seminal view of hereditary transmission with immaterial causes that include the influence of virtue and vice. For instance, Paré insisted semen was not a solid but related to the 'ideas' of each body part contained in the blood, which allowed the 'virtue' of disease to be transmitted through the paternal seed and through the maternal blood. As Lopez-Beltrán (1992: 46) observes, it was this 'increasingly immaterial explanation of the "humoralists" that exasperated the following generation'. Nevertheless, we find a range of statements that no longer dismiss hereditary disease as accidental features of generation but begin to offer a useful clarification of irregular transmission.

It was the close observations of sixteenth-century physicians that allowed hereditary disease to introduce *differentiation* into generation theories. The Hippocratic-Galenic tradition had become the prevailing view of 'generation' up to the end of the eighteenth century because it offered a framework with which to account for the instability of hereditary transmission. Galen's dual seminal account of generation and Hippocrates' solid-humoral physiology provided causal flexibility to explain the mechanisms of hereditary influence across generations. However, by the seventeenth century we find increasing scepticism towards the 'excesses' of humoralist and spiritual influences and a general move towards mechanistic accounts of hereditary transmission. A 'sudden outburst' of treatises on hereditary disease followed developing plausible transmission mechanisms based on 'solidistic' causes (often combining humoral and iatrochemical hypotheses).[5] Lopez-Beltrán (1992) cites one particular publication as providing a uniquely clear synthesis of previous themes.

In *Pathologica Haereditaria* (1619), the Irish clergymen, Dermutius de Maera, seeks to limit the claims that all diseases are hereditary – only those in which the defect is located in the solid parts (organs and tissues) are communicated through the semen. Any constitutional disease that does not occur through the semen must be considered an 'accidental influence' exerted by the fluid (nutrients) during the mother's gestation. However, transmission is now widened to include not merely the parents of the offspring but remote ancestors as well. A theme that de Meara explores at length is atavistic transmission which, he argues, must involve the presence of a causal agent passed along the generations from grandparents to grandchildren. This implies that irregular transmission must be the action of 'latent' causes. Irregular transmission is the result of the 'balancing effect' of the healthy semen in one grandparent and the unhealthy semen in another, though the impurity of the seed can produce disease even if the parent did not develop it. Thus, hereditary influence can be sustained or mitigated according to the mixture of healthy and unhealthy constitutions. The clarity of de Maera's account explains differential transmission without recourse to hidden influences such as humours or virtues. This entirely 'solid' account of causation becomes a characteristic of medical thinking in the late eighteenth century (Lopez-Beltrán 1992).

It is important to consider how this pattern of solidist critique of humoralism gained momentum. From a purely discursive point of view, there is a gradual shift in language from the loose, excessively metaphorical descriptions of 'temperaments' to a more precise account of 'constitutions' and solid interactions. It is not sufficient to assume, as Roger (1963) does, that the emergence of solid-to-solid transmission of disease, or its cause, was the result of a growth of Cartesian mechanism. A more practical explanation must be found among the practices of seventeenth- and eighteenth-century physicians. The transition from Library Medicine to Bedside Medicine explains distinct modes of production of medical knowledge (Jewson 1976). Library Medicine was an enclosed system of elite knowledge that privileged theoretical homogeneity of generation. Bedside Medicine was a system of patronage, an apparatus in which patron and physician were closely aligned in the production of medical knowledge. The patient-as-patron therefore was more or less free to offer descriptions of familial disease, thus enabling the physician to deal with the empirical obstacles posed by heterogeneity. Indeed, the growth of solidism parallels the rise of case-collecting among physicians in the seventeenth century (Roger 1963). For instance, dual seminal accounts were favoured by those who used 'genealogical' observations of families, especially among the nobility and royal families, to establish patterns of similitude and difference among the generations. It was the production of theoretical distinctions based on the direct experience and accumulated evidence of treating family disease over several generations that began to give hereditary 'structure and causal meaning' (Lopez-Beltrán 1992: 18). By the first half of the nineteenth century, the concept of *heredity* emerged with all the clarity of explaining a *biological* entity. This process of reification – the transition from metaphorical description to causal explanation – is examined in the next section.

The constitution of heredity

The concept of heredity (*hérédité*) appeared, almost exclusively in the French medical community, in the first two decades of the nineteenth century. Rather than loosely describing patterns of resemblance, irregularity, recurrence or striking peculiarities among families, the concept of heredity now referred to the existence of an *entity*, or at least some criteria for defining it as a force, law or mechanism. After 1830, heredity is in common use permitting physicians to employ a series of distinctions and oppositions. The most important opposition is between 'physiological heredity' and 'pathological heredity'. Physiological heredity is now freed of the moral connotations of vice and virtue, while pathological heredity is subject to further distinctions about the nature and range of transmission. Thus, it is possible to define pathological heredity in terms of whether it is constitutional (innate) or acquired (pre-dispositional), congenital or postnatal, and to focus on the peculiarities of their origin, and the timing of their appearance and recurrence. In other words, the opposition of natural and pathological heredity allowed physicians to separate accidental variation from natural variation (Lopez-Beltrán 1992, 2004, 2007).

The groundwork for developing these distinctions and oppositions had begun at the end of the eighteenth century. Lopez-Beltrán (1992, 2007) traces this work to the essay competitions of the Royal Society of Medicine between 1788 and 1790, the purpose of which was to address the evidence and theoretical support for the existence of hereditary diseases.[6] The competition produced four dissertations of high quality that carefully set out the case for defending the principle of hereditary transmission of disease.[7] The essays had the effect of greatly restricting hereditary diseases to include only the most obvious constitutional and chronic diseases, and establishing consensual criteria for observation and analysis. For instance, it was agreed that the old case-based strategy of selecting 'isolated observations' and 'family tales' were limited, and that rigorous, cumulative methods of genealogical collection were required. Despite their lack of clear physiological description, the essays presented a logical reappraisal of the concepts of latency, homochrony and atavism[8] as the proper basis of causal analysis. By the early nineteenth century, the concept of heredity articulated two kinds of hereditary transmission: the transmission of natural properties and the transmission of diseased properties. Having entered the domain of natural, *biological* variation, heredity is unified under the general term 'physiological heredity'. Pathological heredity is considered a deviation of the same principle – the peculiar transmission of objects predisposing to disease. The normalization of heredity greatly extended its explanatory reach, influencing a new generation of physicians to explore the juxtaposition of normal and pathological heredity (Lopez-Beltrán 1992, 2004, 2007).

By 1820, the French medical community had reached a consensus on heredity. A convincing register of this development can be found among the 60-volume *Dictionarie des Sciénces Médicales*, which 'captured the progressive generalization of the metaphorical notion of hereditary communication into a unified, law-like approach to biological heredity' (Lopez-Beltrán 2004: 47). Between 1812 and 1820, the dictionary had acted as a kind of 'forum' in which key positions were rehearsed and criticized among influential physicians. Given the range of contributions, different medical schools and professional groups begin to converge on heredity as a new domain of intervention. Physicians, naturalists, physiologists and early psychiatrists (known archaically as *aliénistes*) developed alternative accounts of how heredity shaped individual, familial and even national constitutions. It was the alienists who promoted a new division between 'physical' (physiological) and 'moral' (psychological) heredity. The obstacle they faced was developing a style of reasoning where a taxonomy of moral symptoms was dependent on the body's constitution, thus implicating hereditary transmission (Lopez-Beltrán 1992, 2004).

With materialistic approaches gaining favour among physicians in the late eighteenth century, the medical concepts of 'temperament' and 'constitution' began to frame moral qualities on physiological grounds. Pierre Cabanis (1802: 431) argued that all mental phenomena were based on a physical, organic structure; temperamental features are not only transmitted from parent to children but modified by environmental circumstances such as 'education, weather or diet'. This is a crucial consideration for the hygienist programme that now entered theoretical and ideological debates in post-revolutionary France. Prior to 1812, hereditary transmission had appeared mainly in footnotes and short discussions. Alienists had only mentioned 'hereditary influence', but after 1812 it assumes a central explanatory role. For instance, Fodéré (1813) claimed that latency of disease derived by dispositional (diathesis) and 'exciting' causes was a path to developing a generalized view of heredity. Jean Marc wrote in 1812 that hereditary predisposition is 'one the strongest presumptions in favour of the reality of mental disease'. However, it was Etienne Esquirol, Pinel's most talented disciple, who gave heredity the leading role in his 13 articles for the *Dictionaire* (Lopez-Beltrán 1992, 2004).

Before the 1840s, notions of heredity shared a similar status to the concept of *constitution*. Both terms were broad and encompassed incompatible conceptions of the body. Some viewed constitution as an aggregate of organic parts, while others linked it to functional qualities, highlighting the tensions between material/anatomical and functional/physiological explanations. Despite different physiological ontologies struggling to control the domain of heredity, no one in the medical community disputed that constitution was heritable, and often heredity was used to highlight this relationship. Like constitution, heredity became a basic explanatory structure accommodating different hypotheses in the medical community. Physicians wanted to use 'pathological heredity' to inform 'physiological heredity' based on careful observations of patterns of disease communication. Given that signs of pathology were easier to track than normal resemblances, medical authors frequently appealed to more rigorous techniques of theory-testing. As we discuss later in the chapter, empirical approaches lagged behind these developments in theory-building.

The extensive range of articles that appeared in the *Dictionaire* were effective in producing many law-like observations among French medical schools. By 1834, it was possible to state that heredity was the transmission of particular bodily dispositions that tended to reproduce in children the same characteristics (diseases, inclinations or resemblances) as their parents at the same age, or in the presence of the same exciting cause (Lereboullet 1834 cited in Lopez-Beltrán 2004). By now the close association between the term 'disposition' and the idea of 'diathesis'[9] implied a pathological notion of predisposition. For the medical profession, pathological heredity was a lens to inform their understanding of physiological heredity, not the other way around. This is partly because many medical professionals viewed hereditary diseases to be incurable (Waller 2001). Nevertheless, pathological themes linked to biology gained theoretical ground in the second half of the nineteenth century. After the 1840s, the 'moral' and 'psychological' aspects of heredity receive more attention, leading to a whole range of vivid theoretical assumptions. As the concept of heredity became more complex so too did its flexibility in advancing both social and scientific arguments about the pathological 'degeneration' of species, race and national character (Pick 1989).

When the French physician and alienist, Prosper Lucas, produced the remarkable *Traité de l'Hérédité Naturelle* (1847–1850), the reification of heredity was now complete. In two volumes, Lucas assembled a vast array of bibliographic material using a case-by-case method of induction to propose two laws governing hereditary transmission: a 'law of inheritance' (*hérédité*) that represents the memory of life in the natural process of generation, and a 'law of variation' (*innéité*) that generates variation within species.[10] There are many complexities and subtleties in Lucas' system but our concern is the way he addressed the problem of mental or moral inheritance. Using the dichotomies of the physiologists, he divided the constitution (the organization of the organism) into two components: the plastic (or material) and the dynamic. Heredity and inneity acted on both components in a similar fashion – the plastic derived from the material structure of the organism and the dynamic consisted of the emergent properties of the entire set of mental qualities and dispositions. Despite the selection of improbable cases to illustrate his points, and the nominalism of his conceptual apparatus, Lucas' work demonstrates the clearest and most ambitious attempt to impose a synthesis on a valid domain of biological phenomena. Having set the foundations of *biological heredity*, his ideas had a strong influence on medical and psychiatric hereditarianism in France for the next 40 years. Indeed, Lucas' rational and synthetic approach of ordering heredity was compelling enough to persuade Darwin and Galton to propose their own laws of inheritance (Lopez-Beltrán 1992, 2004).

The synthesis of biological laws concerning natural variation and reproduction had strengthened the resolve and imagination of alienists to elaborate their own distinctions of heredity. This project had already started in the early nineteenth century but, as we will see in the next section, French psychiatry sought to consolidate their professional power by claiming control over the domain of heredity.

Hereditarian psychiatry

Earlier, it was noted that hereditarian themes were relatively absent in the writings of alienists until 1812, after which notions of 'physiological heredity', 'predisposition' and 'diathesis' are cited regularly as causes of insanity. The concept of heredity became relevant to psychiatry in post-revolutionary France when Napoleonic reforms gave medical practitioners a more prominent role in public health. The association between public health and heredity was formed after Cabanis (1802) wrote that moral and physical phenomena belonged to the same organic structure, in which case medical treatment and political government had their origins in one and the same principle (see Cartron 2007: 162). Themes of hygiene and heredity allowed medical and moral physicians to fulfil their aspirations of reorganizing civil life (Lopez-Beltrán 2004). Thus, from 1812 onwards, hereditary themes occupy a central explanatory role in the writings of alienists. Among them, Emmanuel Fodere, Antoine Portal and Philippe Pinel played leading roles in medical reforms of post-revolutionary France.

Pinel was a reluctant newcomer to the idea of heredity. In the first edition of his influential treatise, *Traité Médico-philosophique sur l'Aliénation Mental, ou la Manie* (1801), there is only a brief mention of heredity as the 'first cause'[11] of insanity. In the second edition (1809), hereditary predisposition is discussed in a section on statistics. Commenting on the figures of the family background of patients at Bicêtre and La Salpétriére, he cites two causes of madness: predispositional and accidental (latent). On the causes of illness, he concedes: 'It would be difficult not to admit the hereditary transmission of mania when we see everywhere that in certain families some members are affected by the disease over several successive generations' (Pinel 1809: 13). As a moral physician, Pinel was inclined to relegate physiological heredity to the background, allowing moral causes to occupy a central explanatory role, leaving it to the following generation of psychiatrists to promote hereditarian themes. It was Pinel's disciples who used statistics to move heredity from a background cause to being one of the main predisposing causes of insanity. The relationship between statistics and heredity is not incidental. Indeed, hereditarian psychiatry emerged at the time Hospital Medicine converged with the use of medical statistics (see Cartron 2007). The crowded wards of the hospital supplied the raw materials of morbid events and case-histories with which to establish the *signs* of hereditary predisposition among the body of the family.

To understand how statistics became central to hereditarian psychiatry, we must first consider the transformation that occurred at the Parisian hospital schools during the late eighteenth and early nineteenth centuries (Ackerknecht 1967). In the newly emerging field of 'mental medicine', Pinel represented the transition between Bedside Medicine and Hospital Medicine. On the one hand, his speculative nosology constructed pathological entities by grouping together experiential symptoms. On the other, he recognized that insanity was the product of physical causes of which heredity was the 'first cause'. Hospital Medicine was a system of relations that brought the phenomenon of hereditary madness into alignment with the psychiatric profession, allowing access to a greater number of patients through the institutional apparatus of the university hospital and asylum. In fact, the asylum had become the epicentre for precipitating a new type of medicine in the Parisian hospitals producing many talented psychiatrists (Shorter 1997). The arrangement of Hospital Medicine supplied the means of large-scale examination of 'cases' that could be correlated with organic lesions observed on the autopsy table.

At this point, hereditarian themes in psychiatry begin to take hold around the absence of an organic lesion. Foucault (2008) argues that the emergence of heredity in French psychiatry appears to make up for the lack of pathological anatomy.[12] Others have also observed that the failure to find the physical signs or causes of mental illness were drawing the profession into crisis (Ackerknecht 1967; Dowbiggin 1991).[13] Signs of pathology had to be found elsewhere. Foucault notices that from the 1820s onwards, the classic technique of psychiatric questioning 'always includes what we can call the search for medical history' (2008: 270). Asylums now kept careful registers of patient admissions and discharge. The practice of collecting, comparing and counting cases coincides with a method of realizing the existence of hereditary mental illness in the family at precisely the same moment that pathology resisted localization within the individual. Likewise, modern GWAS represent similar attempts of searching for a molecular substratum of illness at the level of the population.

Jewson (1976) remarks that statistical analysis was one of the 'great innovations' of Hospital Medicine. The search for regularities in the population not only enabled clinical observation to be extended and refined, but hospitals established a new base for the collection and accumulation of scientific capital. In psychiatry, where pathological anatomy was lacking, statistical analysis adopted a comparative method of clinical observation by considering variables such as 'climate' and 'social background'. Pinel's student, Etienne Esquirol, was a pioneer of asylum statistics and the first to organize cases into statistical tables. An influential statesman with wide access to hospital registers across France, he was the leading psychiatrist to promote heredity to a physical and even dominant cause of mental insanity. In *Mental Maladies*, he claimed that hereditary predisposition was attributed to 110 out of the 482 cases gathered from the Salpêtrière, and 150 from the 264 wealthy patients at his private clinic (1845: 49). On the basis of his statistical reasoning he concluded: 'Hereditary predisposition is the most common, among the remote causes of insanity, particularly among the rich; and is in the proportion of one sixteenth among the poor. I believe, nevertheless, that the proportion is greater, even among the latter' (1845: 49). In the same passage, he observed the following pattern of transmission:

> Insanity is rather transmissible by mother and fathers. Children who are born before their parents have become insane, are less liable to mental alienation, than those whose births take place afterwards. The same is true of those who are born of parents, who are insane only upon the paternal or maternal side, compared with those, both of whose parents are insane, or who have progenitors on both sides in this condition…. Hereditary mania manifests itself among parents and children, often at the same period of life. It is provoked by the same causes, and assumes the same character.
>
> (1845: 49)

There is nothing remarkable about Esquirol's generalizations of heredity from the statistical data. The same themes of homochrony and latency are present, though what begins to emerge is a peculiar dispositional view of latent causation to account for irregular patterns of transmission. From the 1820s onwards, Esquirol's figures are repeated in many other works, with some psychiatrists claiming that heredity madness had become a 'mathematical truth' (Voisin 1826, cited in Cartron 2007: 167). Jewson (1976) also observes that the increasing use of medical statistics had ushered in an era of therapeutic scepticism. By the 1830s, medical discourse on hereditary madness had become so alarmist and pessimistic that theories of morbid heredity would eventually point towards a prevailing *degeneration*.

Although the spread of the idea of hereditary madness can be attributed to Esquirol's statistical tables, they were not sufficient to engender a theoretical explanation of transmission. Foucault (2008) observes that the examination of family history between 1820 and 1830 was 'anarchical' and not explicitly linked to pathological heredity. Similarly, Lopez-Beltrán (1992, 2004) argues that the first statistical tables of asylum patients did not explain pathological heredity. In fact, the connection between heredity and moral character had been developed earlier, a sophisticated account of which can be found in the reaction of medical authors to the reductionist physiologies made fashionable by Franz Gall and other phrenologists in Edinburgh.

As early as 1817, Fodéré challenged the assumption that hereditary predisposition resided in specific, structural arrangements of the body. Such accounts could not explain how the same arrangement gave rise to different states. Higher mental abilities were too elaborate to be situated in the physical changes of a single organ. Fodéré appealed to a vitalist doctrine to explain hereditary predisposition as an 'emergent' property of the 'principles of life'. Indeed, the dependence of moral and physical qualities in terms of functional, emergent, and dynamic physiology was common in the mid-nineteenth century, especially after the publication of Lucas' *Treatise*. The rise of dynamic accounts of hereditary 'proteism' were based precisely on 'the acceptance of non-localizable, multifaceted, proliferate hereditary basis for degenerate dispositions' (Lopez-Beltrán 2004: 61). As Foucault (2008) puts it, the notion of 'dissimilar heredity' now allowed most forms of insanity to enter the hereditary framework.

An example of this divergent account of heredity is found in Jacques Moreau de Tours' (1859) description of the 'lesion' as a dynamic functional disturbance of the nervous system, which was capable of linking 'oddities and eccentricities' in one generation with hereditary madness in another.[14] Of course, the clearest and most decisive expression of divergent hereditary is found in the writings of Bénédict-Augustine Morel. Having travelled around Europe inspecting different asylums, Morel based his theory of degeneration on observations of working-class communities in isolated rural areas of France where alcoholism, immorality, poor diet, and unhealthy domestic and working conditions suggested a pathological sequence of transmission (Dowbiggin 1991). In 1857, Morel published *Treatise on the Intellectual, Moral, and Physical Degeneracy of the Human Race*, which expanded the definition of heredity to include a flawed condition of the nervous system – a diathesis – capable of producing a variety of neurological and mental disturbances. The degenerative mental and physical traits of these families constituted 'deviations from the normal human type, which are transmissible by heredity and which deteriorate progressively towards extinction' (cited in Ackerknecht 1968: 55).

Morel's concept of *dégénérescence* introduced a new way of thinking about pathological heredity. Heredity was now a technical description for grasping a dynamic *biological* phenomenon. Foucault (2008: 271) describes this reworking of heredity as 'a sort of meta-organic substratum' in which the sick body becomes that of the entire family. Hereditary madness was now polymorphous in manifestation and multifactorial in origin, which greatly extended the explanatory reach of hereditarianism to include forms of intoxication, the social milieu, pathological temperament, moral sickness, inborn or acquired damage, and heredity (Ackerknecht 1968). The dynamic relationship between moral and physical qualities allowed Morel (1857) to posit two new laws of morbid transmission. The 'law of double fertilization' established that degeneracy *emerges* from moral and organic conditions; and the 'law of progressivity' established the *cumulative* effects of transmission through the generations. Together, they described a nefarious chain of pathologies descending into further and more severe deviations (Pick 1989).

Dowbiggin's (1991) sociological reading shows that alienists used the imprecision of hereditary degeneration to propose a new relationship between psychiatry and society. The clinical and moral expertise of psychiatrists could eliminate the moral factors that caused biological deterioration in society. The belief that heredity transmitted a harmful diathesis (causing nerve tissue to respond pathologically to stimuli) was appealing from a medical standpoint. Also, Morel's (1857) proposal for a new method of classification based on aetiological principles rather than psychological symptoms had scientific respectability among medical professionals and the public. The vague relationship between mental and bodily processes allowed hereditarian psychiatrists to claim that asylums had a therapeutic effect. Morel advocated the extension of asylum techniques of behaviour modification and moral instruction to eliminate the social factors that caused insanity. Thus, psychiatry should no longer be confined to the psychological welfare of a single patient but extended to the domain of public health through the 'moralization of the masses'. In this vein, advocates of hereditarianism began to position themselves as experts in 'family hygiene' for the moral reconstruction of French society.

Hereditarianism flourished as asylum conditions deteriorated towards the end of the nineteenth century because it justified the difficulties faced by professional psychiatry (Dowbiggin 1991). Asylums were seen as 'factories of incurability' only because they housed the poorest sectors of a population whose incurability was the result of their hereditary weakness and immoral habits.[15] The decline of hereditarianism was not directly a result of its vague and diffuse reasoning, but intrinsically tied to the fate of the asylums, and with the growing realization that degeneration theory no longer held any use to psychiatrists. The expansion of the welfare state and increasing state investment in education as well as the growing belief that therapy could exist beyond the walls of the asylum, were factors that led to a decline in hereditarian thinking.[16]

Having emerged from inferences drawn from correlative histories of patient records, from social movements in racial and moral hygiene, and the conditions of the working classes, degeneration theory found temporary stability among the shifting fortunes of professional psychiatry. Though later declining in psychiatric circles, we should not underestimate the legacy of its theoretical imagination.[17] As a dynamic account of *biological* heredity, degeneration formed connections with Mendelism and with the early biological psychiatry. Kraepelin (1908) referred to 'hereditary degeneration' as a cause of psychosis, and Ernst Rüdin, the founder of psychiatric genetics, lectured on the topic in 1911 (Weber 1996). Even today, the functional, emergent, and dynamic properties of psychiatric disorders continue to resonate in modern scientific accounts of 'complex', multifactorial aetiology (see Chapter 3).

Science of heredity

By the mid-nineteenth century, the concept of heredity was transformed into a general biological theory that stood at the intersection of several domains including medicine, psychiatry, ethnology, natural history, horticulture and animal breeding. The synthesis it achieved, first in medicine, and later in psychiatry, offered a coherent description of biological laws explaining the hereditary transmission of living organisms. In effect, the transmission of homogeneity of groups, races and species had now been set against a natural background of 'reproduction', while the transmission of irregularities (hereditary variation) became central to the discourse on heredity. The irregular transmission of constitutional traits had now become the rule rather than the exception. Lagging behind these achievements, however, were developments in empirical methods for clarifying and justifying the validity of physiological theories.

Located at the threshold of a science of heredity were two approaches for investigating hereditary transmission. An 'internal' (ontological) approach could infer routes of transmission by imputing the existence of a physiological force or mechanism, but many medical authors had regarded this line of reasoning too speculative given the earlier failures of generation theory (see Lopez-Beltrán 1992). An 'external' (descriptive) approach was considered more reliable inasmuch as one could infer heredity from establishing the facts of transmission among reliable cases. What Lucas had managed to achieve in his general theory of heredity was to invent two opposing forces of nature to account for documented cases of transmission. But as Lopez-Beltrán (1992) observes, Lucas' excessively rationalistic approach was not 'palatable' to British authors who accepted the validity of heredity, yet wanted to develop a style of reasoning based on empirical methods of *probability*. In effect, what had been achieved in the domain of biological heredity from theoretical induction formed the basis of developing a statistical approach, the innovation of which was led by the British polymath, Francis Galton.

The origins of Galton's statistical approach to heredity have been acknowledged in a variety of sources. Many have shown that Galton's ideas about heredity were not spontaneous discoveries, but emerged from concerns regarding the biological deterioration of national fitness (Soloway 1990; Kevles 1985; Waller 2001), and from hereditarian discussions among historians and philosophers in the 1850s and 1860s (Olby 1985; Hilts 1973). Some others have shown that Galton's early ethnological studies contributed to his hereditarian ideas (Hilts 1967; Fancher 1983a). MacKenzie (1981) overlooks this connection to emphasize his eugenic views towards middle-class reform. Alternatively, Lopez-Beltrán (1992) and others (Olby 1985; Hilts 1973; Fancher 1983b) show an indirect link between Lucas' work and the development of Galton's statistical approach in the 1860s.

To appreciate the novelty of Galton's style of reasoning, we should contrast it with the 'pre-scientific' methods of case-collecting used in the seventeenth and eighteenth centuries. Such methods of inferring transmission from a 'striking case of peculiarities' were rhetorically persuasive but vulnerable to scepticism, since authors had many resources to point out exceptions to the rule. By the early eighteenth century, French physicians began to argue that only statistics could provide a sound basis for medicine (Cartron 2007). Rather than being a radical departure from previous methods of case collecting, Lopez-Beltrán (1992, 2006) argues that statistical tables were simply a new way of telling 'transmission stories' by using a more compelling 'probabilistic logic' to organize cases. Following Esquirol's lead in 1810, when French and British alienists had started compiling statistical tables of hereditary illness, external accounts of transmission were still based on 'loose, story-telling, genealogical procedures' (Lopez-Beltrán 1992: 167). Heredity became a sophisticated science when the organization of transmission stories had lost their individuality and started to refer to abstract properties of a population (Hacking 1990). Much like the observational studies of modern GWAS, statistical data of populations became a form of scientific capital. The first step towards a science of heredity required the *systematic* collection of positive and negative cases among stable populations. For alienists, this involved the collection of cases in the asylum, and for Galton, it was the collection of genealogical and biographical data of talented individuals.

When Galton began collecting genealogies of talented individuals he did so independently of whether they were positively or negatively related to the transmission of talent. Esquirol had employed a similar, but less sophisticated, statistical style when he considered that registration of asylum patients would eliminate the bias of seeking hereditary causes: if the percentage of affected relatives was higher, then the inference was justified. However, as critics later observed, asylum statistics gave a distorted picture of 'hereditary burden' because hospital populations were already a biased selection of cases. Without comparison to population tables, it could not be known whether the striking preponderance of cases were representative. Thus, by modern standards, early statistical tables cite an excessively high proportion of affected cases. For instance, Esquirol (1845) estimated that as many as 20 per cent of cases in the Salpêtrière were hereditary; in Britain, George Burrows (1828) concluded that 85 per cent of cases at Wakefield asylum had the hereditary taint, while a decade later Sir William Ellis (1838) calculated 15 per cent of cases had inherited their insanity (see Waller 2001).

Galton was mindful of the criticisms of his methodology, but confident that his procedure of selection showed that talent clustered around kinship, the inheritance of which, he claimed, was much higher than the incidence of chance: 'the overwhelming force of a statistical fact like this render counter-arguments of no substantial avail' (Galton 1865: 160). By invoking the probabilistic principle of coincidence as a rhetorical device, Galton is able to justify the inference of inherited talent with more force than simply stating an occurrence. He was aware that other factors might be at work, the most obvious being social and class factors influencing the distribution of talent. In view of these confounding factors, Galton dedicated the rest of his life to developing the probabilistic argument as an autonomous law.

Galton developed his statistical/probabilistic style of reasoning from earlier ethnological observations of inheritance (Olby 1993). He speculated that inheritance must involve the relationship between *ancestors* and offspring as well as a stochastic process in which heredity is governed by chance. Lucas had also allowed for constancy and variation as 'forces' of heredity, but Galton's empirical attitude was less inclined towards metaphysics. He wanted to transform ethnology into an exact science to provide an adequate description of heredity. The innovation came when he applied Adolph Quetelet's work on 'error theory' to mental characteristics.[18] He was less interested in Quetelet's averages than he was of calculating distributions and deviations from the mean to which he applied the error ('normal') curve to understand the properties of heredity. In doing so, Galton provided the first statistical *explanation* of a phenomenon: regression towards mediocrity over the course of generations.[19] He would later call this 'a simple and far-reaching law of hereditary transmission' (Galton 1886).[20] Like Lucas' account of opposing forces, Galton developed an external account of transmission in which constancy was moderated by variation, a process that pulled back the extremes of character towards the mean of the population. However, the difference between the styles of reasoning of Lucas and Galton highlights the weaknesses of inferring patterns of transmission from peculiar cases. Lucas' inductive approach of developing taxonomies and dichotomies was confusing and unreliable (see Lopez-Beltrán 1992), while Galton's approach utilized the principles of probability to propose a law of an underlying deterministic structure. Galton's invention of regression, and later correlation, disciplined the scope of heredity by suggesting that they were as *real* as the causes of heredity (Hacking 1990).

Galton eventually produced a more sophisticated description of the internal structure of heredity. Building on Spencer and Lewes' earlier claims about the equal contribution of each parent, he developed an account in the 1870s where the whole 'weight' of ancestral contributions were channelled through a process of double inheritance. He supposed that heredity must be governed by some sort of 'stirp' – the sum-total of the hereditary elements ('germs') responsible for the transmission of character from one generation to another. Galton's particulate model inferred a mechanism where both patent and latent elements were selected through a competitive struggle for 'representation' between germs: 'We may thus compare the stirp to a nation and those among its germs that achieve development, to the foremost men of that nation who succeed in becoming its representatives' (1876: 336). He imagined this struggle for representation as a probabilistic process in which the latent elements of previous generations had a declining influence, halving with each generation. This was the idea contained in Galton's 'Ancestral Law of Heredity' proposed in 1897,[21] which allowed the continuity of the 'germ plasm' from more distant ancestors to manifest personal characteristics in the offspring that may not have been present in the parents.

Galton, though, was not the sole inventor of a science of heredity. His contribution forms part of a general stabilization of a domain of production where the scope of biological heredity is eventually disciplined by a statistical style of reasoning. Lucas naturalized heredity as the product of opposing forces of reproduction and variation; Darwin established a discourse where it was possible to discuss inheritance in terms of the selection of small variations in 'species'; and Quetelet made it possible to say that populations had the statistical properties of means and distributions. But it was Galton who transformed heredity into a statistical explanation of phenomena, a mathematical relationship between generations. Indeed, the tools he developed for inductive inference made previous stories of transmission appear 'pre-scientific'. From the collection of both positive and negative cases, Galton provided a coherent methodology with which to mathematize genealogy and demonstrate the blending of inheritance through ancestral influences. He provided a framework that closed off the influence of environmental factors by expressing heredity as entirely the function of ancestry. He gave the study of heredity the nature/nurture and the genotype/phenotype distinction, as well as the idea that twin studies could 'weigh in just scales the effects of nature and nurture' (Galton 1883: 155).

Galton's statistical laws claimed to combine the 'beauty and regularity' of continuous human variation with a utopian ideal of racial improvement. It was these ideas, combined with stable populations and stable diagnostic categories, that paved the way for the first 'family studies' of German psychiatric genetics. By the early twentieth century, hereditary madness, having now acquired the biostatistical properties of laws pertaining to a population, ceased to be a vague domain of resemblance, reversion and variation. In the final section of this chapter, we consider how the application of Mendelian statistics led to further innovations of the statistical style by subjecting genealogical thinking to the laws of Mendelian inheritance.

Mendelian statistics

Prior to the 'rediscovery' of Mendel's laws in 1900, heredity was implicated in the aetiology of a vast range of mental disorders, often engendering fatalistic views ranging from irreversible damage of the 'germ cell' *in utero* to pathogenic diathesis leading to degenerative descent. Despite the increasing acceptance of hereditarian views, there was little understanding of how traits were transmitted. Most theories accepted a form of blending inheritance. Along these lines, Galton's 'Law of Ancestral Heredity' attempted to model particulate inheritance on his statistical theory of 'regression to the mean'; he favoured a theory of discontinuous evolution where incremental changes were neutralized by the mechanism of reversion. In fact, Galton came close to developing a Mendelian particulate theory of inheritance but diverged from this path to focus on continuous rather than discrete traits. With Karl Pearson and WFR Weldon, Galton established the biometric school in 1892 using statistical techniques to study continuous traits at the level of population. In Britain, at least, a science of heredity formed around an explicitly statistical style of reasoning with Pearson's 'correlation coefficient' at the forefront of biometric research.

After Mendel's laws were rediscovered, many biologists flocked to the new theory. The leading Mendelian, at the time, biologist William Bateson, played a crucial role in shaping modern genetics. With his colleagues, Bateson developed an *experimental* or *laboratory* style of reasoning using hybridization and crossbreeding as scientific methods of investigation. Furthermore, his distinct theoretical approach to the problem of variation imputed discrete units of heredity, which he later called 'genes'.[22] The popularity of Mendelism appeared to explain the problem of discontinuous inheritance, which involved no blending of factors. The theory comprised elementary probability theory and the assumption that dominance of one factor could determine the manifestation of a trait. By contrast, the biometricians held an explicitly atheoretical model of heredity based on the degree of measureable similarity of observed characteristics from one generation to another. Indeed, there are strong parallels between this atheoretical model of heredity and the apparently 'hypothesis-free' approach of modern GWAS. For Pearson (1896), heredity was defined as the *correlation* between the characteristics of parents and offspring. Having established a science of heredity before Mendel's work, the biometricians' reaction to 'Mendelian factors' were sceptical and hostile to say the least. The episode known as the biometrician-Mendelian debate has received considerable attention by historians and sociologists of science (Coleman 1970; Froggatt and Nevin 1971; Provine 1971; de Marrais 1974; MacKenzie 1981; MacKenzie and Barnes 1979; Kevles 1981; Olby 1966, 1988).

Mendelism appealed to biologists because its theoretical assumptions justified the validity and continuity of their experimental/laboratory style of reasoning.[23] MacKenzie (1981) explains that those occupying the biometric and Mendelian positions held different theoretical assumptions about the nature of evolutionary change. The biometricians took the orthodox Darwinian view that evolution was a process of gradual, incremental change via the selection of continuous differences. Opposition to this view strengthened in 1894, when Bateson published an empirical study claiming that large discontinuous variations did occur in nature, the source of which should be sought 'in the living thing itself' (Bateson 1894:

78). It seemed that Bateson had come to Mendelism as a result of his views on discontinuous variation in evolution. For Pearson and Weldon, the connection with discontinuous evolution was already a reason to reject Mendelism. Both sides of the controversy can be explained in terms of these divergent views of evolution which arose largely from basic assumptions. For biologists, their assessment of evolutionary theories set the scope for future experimental work and, for this reason, preferred mutation theory to orthodox Darwinism. Mendelism made it possible to do more with their skills than was afforded by Darwinism.[24]

For our purpose, the tensions between biometric and Mendelian approaches are significant in shaping the origins of psychiatric genetics and its future trajectory of research. On the one hand, Mendelism supplied a compelling hypothesis for grounding psychiatric disease in aetiological processes; it provided a new framework for quantifying familial aggregation of schizophrenia to identify the mode of Mendelian inheritance – the so-called 'unit character' transmitted from one generation to another. On the other hand, psychiatric genetics inherited a legacy of assuming a one-to-one relationship between genotype and phenotype, which struggled to explain the disappointing findings of later studies. For the same reasons that Mendelism appealed to Anglophone biologists, it was also commensurate with the goals of German psychiatric medicine. Kendler (2015) explains that Mendelian models were a good fit with the anatomical-clinical disease models for schizophrenia. Rüdin (who we discuss in greater detail in Chapter 2) chose schizophrenia as the object of his family study because it was a coherent category of endogenous psychoses. Rüdin (1911) thought Galton's blended inheritance was insufficient to predict heredity in individuals and outlined a new approach for calculating recessive Mendelian inheritance among psychotic families (Schulze et al. 2004). To understand how Rüdin developed his methods, we need to consider Wilhelm Weinberg's contribution to Mendelian statistics.

The dominant approach among German medical researchers and eugenists was the study of family pedigrees (Gausemeier 2015). Early application of Mendelian ratios searched for exemplary families collected from medical records. However, German eugenicists began to mathematize Mendelism even before Mendel's work gained popularity (Mazumdar 1996). Weinberg was among the first to apply Mendelian calculations to the study of human heredity. He identified very early on that methods of accumulating striking and unusual cases were unsuited to distinguishing patterns of heredity. From a twin study he conducted in 1901, he noticed that if the original proband (the particular subject being studied) was counted with the affected children, the resulting calculations produced an excess of affected offspring, exceeding the expected 25 per cent for homozygous recessive children. Weinberg (1912) proposed two methods of 'correction' for dealing with the excess of recessives: the 'proband' and 'sibling' methods. The first method simply left the probands out of the count, while the second included missing siblings who might have died earlier or had not yet developed the condition. The idea of correcting for the excess of affected children using both methods was a major advance in *ascertainment*,[25] highlighting the need for quantitative techniques to produce realistic calculations. As Gausemeier (2015: 477) puts it, Weinberg's methodological suggestions emphasized the importance of 'constructing generations' rather than 'following lineages'.

Weinberg's breakthrough in Mendelian statistics was a decisive critique of Mendelian approaches using genealogical methods. While medical genealogy read the order of heredity from the visual arrangement of anomalies in a family pedigree, Weinberg's mathematical approach calculated the 'unseen' aspects of recessive inheritance where, for instance, heterozygous carriers produced unaffected offspring (Gausemeier 2015). Weinberg showed that over-representation of heterozygous carriers produced inflated Mendelian ratios. This was considered a major improvement on the American studies carried out at the Eugenics Record Office in Cold Springs, which had compiled an impressive array of family pedigrees extending over several generations. When Rosanoff and Orr (1911) confidently announced that 'insanity' was a recessive Mendelian trait, Weinberg (1913) rebuked these findings as demonstrating a superficial understanding of heredity based on selected pedigrees.

Rüdin's (1916) landmark study of schizophrenia represented a unique synthesis of statistical and laboratory styles of reasoning. Adopting Weinberg's methods of statistical correction marked a break from genealogical empiricism and dealt a serious blow to simplistic applications of Mendelian inheritance (Gausemeier 2015). The principle of recessive inheritance derived from experimental (laboratory) exploration engendered more complex calculations of human heredity. But for all its sophistication, Rüdin's approach never produced the expected ratios for Mendelian recessive inheritance, which at least suggested the possibility of 'polymorphic' heredity. Though future generations of psychiatric geneticists continued to pursue a Mendelian theory of schizophrenia, the integration of biometric and Mendelian approaches closed the divide between two competing theories of inheritance.

In 1918, the statistician, Ronald Fischer, found a way of integrating Mendelism and biometrics when he argued that continuous variation of phenotypic traits was the combined action of many discrete genes acting in an additive manner. There were now two opposing views that divided opinion regarding the inheritance of schizophrenia: a single major (Mendelian-like) locus and a polygenic distribution of liability from many genes of small effect. As we show in Chapter 2, for the next 50 years, psychiatric genetics oscillated between categorical and quantitative models of inheritance: Mendelian models required unambiguous boundaries between affected and unaffected traits, while polygene models relied on subtle, quantitative differences between inherited traits. The breakthrough came in 1967, when Gottesman and Shields (1967) published their polygenic theory of schizophrenia. Using Falconer's (1965) 'liability-threshold model', they argued that schizophrenia was a spectrum containing rare Mendelian manifestations with common polygenic distributions of quantitative traits. The many 'positive' findings of contemporary GWAS support this model. Conditions, like schizophrenia, are believed to be quantitative traits comprising rare variants and common polygenes that aggregate in families (Kendler 2015).

The origins of contemporary GWAS can be traced as far back as the integration of Mendelian and biometrical approaches (Kendler 2015). While Mendelism offered a particulate theory of inheritance, it failed to ground psychiatric conditions in a categorical model. Fischer's resolution of showing that many segregating genes of small effect were distributed quantitatively is now the standard model of polygenic transmission (The International Schizophrenia Consortium 2009). Even the enthusiasm for linkage studies in the 1980s reflects the 'zealousness' of finding 'genes for' schizophrenia, an approach driven by the same categorical reasoning that inspired Rüdin's search for Mendelian ratios (Kendler 2015). In many ways, the failure of linkage studies resembles a similar tension between biometrical and Mendelian inheritance; molecular geneticists claimed they were revealing the underlying biology of psychiatric disease in small, interesting pedigrees, while statisticians were interested in calculating the distribution of quantitative traits in twin studies. Modern GWAS have more in common though with Fischer's (1918) innovative solution suggesting, among other things, that many psychiatric disorders with polygenic liability are continuously distributed in the population; they are quantitative traits with real, molecular properties. On these grounds, at least, scientists believe the old disciplinary boundaries between 'statisticians' and 'biologists' are now obsolete (Kendler 2015). In Chapter 5, we explore this theme further to show that while modern studies presuppose the integration of biological and statistical styles of reasoning, these boundaries are far from obsolete.

Conclusion

The concept of 'human heredity' had become an explanatory scientific term, and later a coherent tool for psychiatric genetics, only after medical knowledge had undergone a series of institutional transformations. Heredity was not the accomplishment of a revolution in medical 'ideas' as such, but of the reorganization of its domain of production. To have an explanatory role in psychopathology, human heredity had to become a material resource – a form of *data* pertaining to a population. In the same way that 'human genomes' have emerged from changes in the mode of data production, the concept of heredity became useful when it formed part of an apparatus of collecting and calculating data about patient populations.

In the transition from Library Medicine to Bedside Medicine, it was the naturalistic observations of *variation* in familial patterns of disease that gave rise to a material view of transmission. Breaking from the assumed homogeneity and resemblance of genealogical groups, the practice of case-collecting among physicians established the problem of variation as a productive domain of inquiry. By the end of the eighteenth century, the arrangement of Hospital Medicine established a stable domain for the 'reification' of hereditary transmission (Lopez-Beltrán 1992, 1994). University hospitals and asylums supplied the means of large-scale examination of cases that could be correlated with organic lesions. It also brought the phenomenon of hereditary madness into alignment with the psychiatric profession, providing access to a greater number of patients.

In France, the popularity of hereditarian psychiatry justified the difficulties faced by the profession which, unlike general medicine, had failed to establish the physical causes of illness (Dowbiggin 1991). The imprecision and causal flexibility of 'dissimilar heredity' (Foucault 2008) compensated for the absence of an organic lesion. In addition to permitting a wider network of correlations between physical and moral traits, the dynamic pathologies of degeneration allowed hereditarian psychiatrists to claim expertise in matters of social, familial and, later, racial hygiene.

At the same time that heredity had entered the domain of biology, there were recurrent disputes regarding the validity of inferring a causal connection from cases. The birth of medical and asylum statistics in both France and Germany were administrative efforts to organize cases into tables; and while they appeared to confirm the alarming extent of hereditary madness in hospitals, they did not explain pathological heredity. A significant breakthrough in the domain of hered-ity occurred when the organization of cases had lost their individuality and started to refer to abstract properties of a population (Hacking 1990). The first steps towards a science of heredity required the systematic collection of positive *and* negative cases among stable populations. Francis Galton led the break-through in statistical reasoning by organizing cases according to *probability*. Galton's probabilistic argument disciplined the scope of heredity by establishing a mathematical relationship between generations. It also established a new mode of production in which scientific information acquired the biostatistical prop-erties of a population. It was the production and accumulation of data as *capital* that became a significant driver of intellectual change.

The biometrician-Mendelian debate highlighted the uneasy alignment of laboratory and statistical styles of reasoning. Both held different theoretical assumptions about evolutionary change and justified different trajectories of experimental research. However, it was Mendelian inheritance that supplied a compelling hypothesis for grounding psychiatric disease in aetiological pro-cesses. Furthermore, the mathematization of Mendelism grounded the *ascertain-ment* of cases in Mendelian ratios as opposed to methods of accumulating 'interesting' cases from hospital populations. In Germany, the breakthrough in Mendelian statistics highlighted the need for quantitative techniques of ascer-tainment based on biological principles rather than genealogical procedures of ordering family pedigree. Weinberg's methodological contribution emphasized the importance of 'constructing generations' (Gausemeier 2015) via statistical reasoning to produce realistic calculations of recessive Mendelian inheritance.

The conditions under which 'hereditary madness' ceased to be a loose, exces-sively metaphorical description of physical and moral traits coincided with a major transformation in the systems of medical reasoning. Psychiatry had embarked on a science of heredity only after the *biologization of hereditary* and the *mathematization of heredity* had established new techniques of scientific examination. But this ensemble of techniques also reveals an 'ambivalent syn-thesis' of laboratory and statistical styles. The short history of psychiatric genet-ics suggests that these styles have been in oscillation ever since Rüdin's landmark study of schizophrenia. As we explore in Chapters 4 and 5, the molecular and bioinformatic styles of contemporary 'molecular psychiatry' are epistemic cultures characterized by these enduring historical tensions.

Notes

1 In applying Ackerknecht's (1967) and Jewson's (1976) periodization of Western medicine, we are not supposing that medical knowledge fell into discrete phases of knowledge production. Rather, the focus is on a series of epistemological transformations in medical practices from which symptoms, signs and pathologies emerged. Library Medicine emphasized the classical learning of physicians, which gave priority to the formal logic of scholastic medicine rather than the specificity of illness. Bedside Medicine began to address the practical management of illness by attending to the classification of patient symptoms. Hospital Medicine supplied the means of large-scale examination of cases, which could be correlated with organic lesions observed on the autopsy table. Lastly, Jewson (1976) adds the medical model called 'Laboratory Medicine', which attended to the physical and chemical processes of cell pathology as the fundamental locus of disease.

2 While Ackerknecht (1968: 27) praises Paracelsus for his unique observation of congenital insanity, he later describes him as being 'an immensely inconsistent confabulator'. Indeed, Paracelsus would later revert to demonical possession as the cause of insanity.

3 In scholastic philosophy, 'generation' referred to the universal modes of creation and corruption in the natural world, a pre-biological account of the processes involved in conception and embryonic development. In the Aristotelian tradition, the generation of the embryo was the product of the action of the male semen on the passive semen of the female, while Galenists thought that the embryo was the mixture of both male and female sperm; the latter implied equality of inherited substance while the former a patrilineal model of inheritance. Such theories of inheritance also held legal implications for the consanguinity of marriage (Sabean 2007).

4 Paracelsus' 'ontological view of disease' (Pagel 1982) anticipated the achievements of William Harvey (1651) postulating that living organisms arose from eggs, Robert Hooke (1665) describing the properties of cells, and Leewenhoek (1677) observing sperm in the semen of man and animals (see Mellon 1996).

5 Some of the more notable and relevant publications of the era include: Mercatus (1594) *De morbis haereditariis liber*, De Meara (1619) *Pathologia Haereditaria*, Burton (1621) *Anatomy of Melancholy*, Lyonnet (1647) *Brevis Dissertatio de Morbis Haereditariis*, Hoffman (1699) *Dissertatio de affectibus haereditarii, illorumque origine*, and Stahl (1706) *Dissertatio inauguralis de haereditaria dispositione ad varios affectus*.

6 In part, the competition was designed to address the earlier sceptical challenges posed by Antoine Louis (1748) who argued that hereditary disease had no real physiological basis.

7 These include the dissertations of Pierre-Joseph Amoreux, Alexis Pujol, Jean-François Pagès and Joseph-Claude Rougement (see Lopez-Beltrán 1992, 2007).

8 *Atavism* referred to the skipping of generations by certain characters, *homochrony* the sudden appearance of the same effects at the same age in different members of the same family, while *latency* described the tendency for disease to remain dormant over several generations.

9 Extending back to antiquity, the idea of diathesis is synonymous with constitutional 'disposition' or 'predisposition' of disease. Lopez-Beltrán (2004: 53) cites Pariset and Villeneuve in 1812 explaining *diathèse* as:

original or acquired: the first set depends on our primitive organization and are the one more ordinarily transmitted to us by our parents; the acquired diathesis are the result of action ... of everything that can act upon our economy.

10 The flexibility of Lucas' model allowed the explanation of cases that defied regularity in terms of variation, and the taming of variation by establishing evidence of regularity. Lopez-Beltrán (2004: 64) provides an elegant summary in terms of the following: 'resemblances are promoted by heredity, dissimilarities by inneity'.

11 It should be mentioned that Pinel was not the first physician to describe hereditary madness in terms of first causes. In *Treatise on Madness* (1758), the English physician, William Battie, also referred to 'original' and 'consequential' causes of madness (see Mellon 1996).

12 On this matter, Foucault writes:

Insofar, as one cannot and does not know how to find any organic substratum of the illness in the patient, one looks for pathological events at the level of the patient's family which are such that, whatever their nature, they will refer to the communication, and consequently existence, of a pathological material substratum. Heredity is a way of giving body to the illness at the very moment that this illness cannot be situated at the level of the individual.

(2008: 271)

13 Ackerknecht (1968) refers to a 'period of disillusionment' among somaticists during the mid-nineteenth century, while Dowbiggin (1991) attributes a 'profound sense of defensiveness and insecurity' among French psychiatrists during this period.

14 Jacques Moreau de Tours (1859) wrote extensively on the effects of heredity on the nervous system, believing it to be a 'lesion of the intellectual organ'. Even though some psychiatrists were sceptical of whether the presence of disturbance resulted from physical inheritance, the new formulation of hereditary predisposition permitted a wider network of correlations between moral and physical traits.

15 According to Morel, asylums were inundated with incurable patients. This contributed to the present state of therapeutic pessimism, because insane people were entering asylums after it was too late to cure them, meaning they were able to reproduce and thereby multiply the numbers of degenerates.

16 Dowbiggin (1991) also cites advances in neurology and the discovery of the mechanism responsible for syphilis, which was previously thought to be hereditary, gave further reason to lose patience with degeneration theory.

17 Though degeneration theory declined in psychiatric circles, its relationship to anthropology and criminology formed a lasting association through the work of Cesare Lombroso (1875). Even today, the term 'degenerate' is strongly associated with a criminal type.

18 Unlike Quetelet's use of error theory to calculate the physical properties of human populations (e.g. average chest size or height), for Galton it made no sense to describe exceptional ability as 'error'. As MacKenzie (1981) explains, error theory hindered the analysis of human variability as the source of racial improvement. Galton's departure from error theory to focus on 'race variability' was political rather than theoretical.

19 In *Hereditary Genius* (1869: vi), Galton sketched out an early version of regression as a statistical theory of heredity in the following terms:

The theory of hereditary genius ... has been advocated by a few writers in past as well as in modern times. But I may claim to be the first to treat the subject in a statistical manner, to arrive at numerical results, and to introduce the 'law of deviation from an average' into discussions on heredity.

20 In Galton's later analyses of physical stature, he articulated his conclusion on regression with clear, mathematical precision: 'The number of individuals who are nearly

mediocre is so preponderant, that an exceptional man is more frequently found to be the exceptional son of mediocre parents than the average son of very exceptional parents' (1889: 99).

21 In 1897, Galton proposed a law of 'filial regression' that would bring him full circle with the assumptions he made 30 years earlier regarding hereditary talent and character. He proposed that parents contribute one-half of the total heritage of the off-spring, the grandparents one-quarter, the great grandparents one-eighth, and so on. In this sense, he was arguing for the possibility of remote ancestors manifesting traits in the offspring, a form of latency that could explain how children could resemble their grandparents.

22 The concept of 'genes' is somewhat misleading by today's standards because we are accustomed to thinking of them as physical entities, but for the early Mendelians these factors were purely theoretical.

23 Even before the controversy with Mendelism, many biologists were hostile to statistics and found the explicitly quantitative study of life distasteful (Kevles 1985).

24 MacKenzie (1981) explains how Mendelism gained widespread acceptance among the new generation of professional biologists after the development of Mendelian chromosome theory in 1910–1915. The new generation had been trained in an experimental and mechanistic style and the establishment of Mendelian chromosome theory afforded the opportunity to use these skills on fast-breeding *Dropsophia*. These techniques become more attractive because they made the problem of heredity experimentally tractable. Mendelism offered a means of extending the scope of experimental biology: 'it was a theory that enhanced the value of the competences of experimental biologists' (1981: 128).

25 Ascertainment is a technical term in statistical studies to describe the method of collecting data. While it may refer to a neutral description of data collection, historically, the term highlights a systematic distortion (or 'bias') in measuring the true frequency of a phenomenon. A classic distortion in early genetics studies is the reporting of higher frequencies of a Mendelian condition due to the way data were collected. For example, a physician conducting a study based on their own practice is likely to see a preponderance of affected cases rather than unaffected cases, thus distorting the true frequency of disease.

References

Ackerknecht E (1967) *Medicine at the Paris Hospital, 1794–1848*. Baltimore: Johns Hopkins Press.

Ackerknecht E (1968) *A Short History of Psychiatry*. Translated by S Wolff. New York: Hafner Publishing Company.

Bateson W (1894) *Materials for the Study of Variation*. London: Macmillan.

Boylan M (1984) The Galenic and Hippocratic challenges to Aristotle's conception theory. *Journal of the History of Biology* 17(Spring): 83–112.

Burton R (1621/1883) *The Anatomy of Melancholy*. Philadelphia: E. Claxton & Company.

Cabanis PJG (1802) Rapports du physique et du moral de l'homme. In C Lehec and J Cazeneuve (eds) (1956). *Oeuvres Philosophiques de Cabanis* (2 vols.). Paris: Presses Universitaires de France.

Cartron L (2007) Degeneration and 'alienism' in early nineteenth-century France. In S Müller-Wille and HJ Rheinberger (eds). *Heredity Produced: At the Crossroads of Biology, Politics, and Culture, 1500–1870*. Cambridge, MA: MIT Press.

Coleman W (1970) Bateson and chromosomes: Conservative thought in science. *Centaurus* 15: 28–314.

De Marrais R (1974) The double-edged effect of Sir Francis Galton: A search for the motives in the biometrician-Mendelian debate. *Journal of the History of Biology* 7(1): 141–174.

Dowbiggin IR (1991) *Inheriting Madness: Professionalization and Psychiatric Knowledge in Nineteenth Century France*. Berkeley: University of California Press.

Esquirol E (1845) *Mental Maladies: Treatise on Insanity*. Translated by EK Hunt. Philadelphia: Lea and Blanchard.

Falconer DS (1965) The inheritance of liability to certain diseases, estimated from the incidence among relatives. *Annuals of Human Genetics* 29: 51–76.

Fancher RE (1983a) Francis Galton's African ethnography and its role in the development of his psychology. *British Journal for the History of Science* 16(1): 67–79.

Fancher RE (1983b) Alphonse de Candolle, Francis Galton and the early history of the nature-nurture controversy. *Journal of the History of the Behavioral Sciences* 19(4): 341–352.

Fisher RA (1918) On the correlation between relatives on the supposition of Mendelian inheritance. *Transactions of the Royal Society of Edinburgh* 52(2): 399–433.

Fodéré FE (1813) *Traité de médecine légale et d'hygiène publique, tome V, 3e partie. Police médicale et hygiène publique*. Paris: Mame.

Foucault M (2008) *Psychiatric Power: Lectures at the College De France, 1973–74*. Edited by J Lagrange and translated by G Burchell. Basingstoke: Palgrave Macmillan.

Froggatt P and Nevin NC (1971) Galton's law of ancestral heredity: Its influence on the early development of human genetics. *History of Science* 10: 1–26.

Galton F (1865) Hereditary character and talent. *Macmillan's Magazine* 12: 157–166.

Galton F (1869) *Hereditary Genius: An Inquiry into its Laws and Consequences*. London: Macmillan.

Galton F (1876) A theory of heredity. *Journal of the Anthropological Institute* 5: 329–348.

Galton F (1883) *Inquiries into Human Faculty and its Development*. London: Macmillan.

Galton F (1886) Anthropological miscellanea: Regression towards mediocrity in hereditary stature. *Journal of the Anthropological Institute* 15: 246–263.

Galton F (1889) *Natural Inheritance*. London: Macmillan.

Galton F (1897) The average contribution of each several ancestor to the total heritage of the offspring. *Proceedings of the Royal Society of London* 61: 401–413.

Gausemeier B (2015) Pedigrees of madness: The study of heredity in nineteenth and early twentieth psychiatry. *History and Philosophy of the Life Sciences* 36(4): 467–483.

Gottesman II and Shields J (1967) A polygenic theory of schizophrenia. *Proceedings of the National Academy of Sciences* 58(1): 199–205.

Hacking I (1982) Language, truth and reason. In M Hollis and S Lukes (eds). *Rationality and Relativism*. Cambridge, MA: MIT Press, pp. 48–66.

Hacking I (1990) *The Taming of Chance*. Cambridge: Cambridge University Press.

Hacking I (1992) 'Style' for historians and philosophers. *Studies in the History and Philosophy of Science* 23(1): 1–20.

Hilts VL (1967) *Statist and Statistician: Three Studies in the History of 19th Century English Statistical Thought*. PhD, Harvard. Published in a facsimile by Arno Press, 1981, New York.

Hilts VL (1973) Statistics and social science. In RN Giere and RS Westfall (eds). *Foundations of Scientific Method: The 19th Century*. Bloomington: Indiana University Press, pp. 206–233.

The International Schizophrenia Consortium (2009) Support for the involvement of large copy number variants in the pathogenesis of schizophrenia. *Human Molecular Genetics* 18(8): 1497–1503.

Jewson ND (1976) The disappearance of the sick-man from medical cosmology, 1770–1870. *Sociology* 10(2): 225–244.

Kendler KS (2015) A joint history of the nature of genetic variation and the nature of schizophrenia. *Molecular Psychiatry* 20(1): 77–83.

Kevles DJ (1981) Genetics in the United States and Great Britain 1890–1930: A review with speculation. In C Webster (ed.). *Biology, Medicine and Society 1840–1940*. Cambridge: Cambridge University Press, pp. 193–215.

Kevles DJ (1985) *In the Name of Eugenics: Genetics and the Uses of Human Heredity*. Berkeley: University of California Press.

Kraepelin E (1908) Zur Entartungsfrage. *Zentralblatt für Nervenheilkunde und Psychiatrie* 31: 745–51.

Lombroso C (1875) *L'uomo deliquente* [*The Delinquent Man*]. Milan: Hoepli.

Lopez-Beltrán C (1992) *Human Heredity 1750–1870: The Construction of a Scientific Domain*. PhD Thesis, Kings College London.

Lopez-Beltrán C (1994) Forging heredity: From metaphor to cause, a reification story. *Studies of the History and Philosophy of Science* 25(2): 211–235.

Lopez-Beltrán C (2004) In the cradle of heredity: French physicians and *L'Hérédité Naturelle* in the early 19th century. *Journal of the History of Biology* 37: 39–72.

Lopez-Beltrán C (2006) Storytelling, statistics and hereditary thought: The narrative support for early statistics. *Studies in History and Philosophy of Biological and Biomedical Sciences* 37: 41–58.

Lopez-Beltrán C (2007) The medical origins of heredity. In S Müller-Wille and HJ Rheinberger (eds). *Heredity Produced: At the Crossroads of Biology, Politics, and Culture, 1500–1870*. Cambridge, MA: MIT Press, pp. 105–132.

MacKenzie D and Barnes B (1979) Scientific judgment: The biometry-Mendelism controversy. In B Barnes and S Shapin (eds). *Natural Order: Historical Studies of Scientific Culture*. London: Sage, pp.191–210.

MacKenzie DA (1981) *Statistics in Britain: The Social Construction of Scientific Knowledge*. Edinburgh: Edinburgh University Press.

Mazumdar PMH (1996) Two models for human genetics: Blood grouping and psychiatry in Germany between world wars. *Bulletin of the History of Medicine* 70: 609–657.

Mellon CD (1996) *Hereditary Madness: The Evolution of Psychiatric Genetic Thought*. New Mexico: Genetics Heritage Press.

Moreau de Tours JJ (1859) *Psychologie Morbide*. Paris: V. Masson.

Morel BA (1857) *Traité des degénérescences physiques, intellectuelles et morales de l'espèce humaine*. Paris: JB Bailliére.

Olby R (1966) *Origins of Mendelism*. London: Constable.

Olby R (1985) *Origins of Mendelism*, second (enlarged) edition. Chicago: University of Chicago Press.

Olby R (1988) The dimensions of scientific controversy: The biometric-Mendelian controversy. *British Journal for the History of Science* 22: 299–320.

Olby R (1993) Constitutional and hereditary disorders. In WF Bynum and R Porter (eds). *Companion Encyclopedia of the History of Medicine*. Oxfordshire: Routledge, pp. 412–437.

Pagel W (1982) *Paracelsus: An Introduction to Philosophical Medicine in the Era of the Renaissance 2nd Edition*. Basel: Karger.

Paracelsus (1567) The diseases that deprive man of his reason. Translated by George Zilboorg. In HE Sigerist (ed.) (1941). *Four Treatises of Theophrastus von Hohenheim Called Paracelsus*. Baltimore: The Johns Hopkins Press, pp. 127–212.

Pearson K (1896) Mathematical contributions to the theory of evolution, III: Regression, heredity and panmixia. *Philosophical Transactions of the Royal Society of London* 187: 253–318.

Pick D (1989) *Faces of Degeneration: A European Disorder, c.1848–1918*. New York: Cambridge University Press.

Pinel P (1809) *Traité médico philosophique de l'aliénation mentale*, second edition. Paris: Brosson.

Provine W (1971) *The Origins of Theoretical Population Genetics*. Chicago: Chicago University Press.

Roger J (1963) *Les Sciences de la Vie dans la Pensée Française*. Paris: Armand Colin.

Rosanoff AJ and Orr FI (1911) A study of insanity in the light of the Mendelian theory. *American Journal of Psychiatry* 68(2): 221–261.

Rüdin E (1911) Einige Wege und Ziele der Familienforschung mit Rücksicht auf die Psychiatrie. *Zeitschrift für die gesamte Neurologie und Psychiatrie* 7: 487–585.

Rüdin E (1916) *Studien über Vererbung und Entstehung geistiger Störungen, Bd. 1: Zur Vererbung und Neuentstehung der Dementia Praecox*. Berlin: Springer.

Sabean DW (2007) From clan to kindred: Kinship and the circulation of property in pre-modern and modern Europe. In S Müller-Wille and HJ Rheinberger (eds). *Heredity Produced: At the Crossroads of Biology, Politics, and Culture, 1500–1870*. Cambridge, MA: MIT Press, pp. 37–59.

Schulze TG, Fangerau H and Propping P (2004) From degeneration to genetic suscepti-bility, from eugenics to genethics, from Bezugsziffer to LOD score: The history of psy-chiatric genetics. *International Review of Psychiatry* 16(4): 246–259.

Shorter E (1997) *A History of Psychiatry: From the Era of the Asylum to the Age of Prozac*. New York: Wiley.

Soloway RA (1990) *Demography and Degeneration: Eugenics and the Declining Birth-rate in Twentieth-Century Britain*. Chapel Hill: University of North Carolina Press.

Vickers B (1984) Analogy versus identity: The rejection of occult symbolism, 1580–1680. In B Vickers (ed.). *Occult and Scientific Mentalities in the Renaissance*. Cambridge: Cambridge University Press, pp. 95–163.

Waller JC (2001) Ideas of heredity, reproduction and eugenics in Britain, 1800–1875. *Studies in History and Philosophy of Biology and Biomedical Sciences* 32(3): 457–489.

Weber MM (1996) Ernst Rüdin, 1874–1952: A German psychiatrist and geneticist. *American Journal of Medical Genetics* 67: 323–331.

Weinberg W (1912) Weitere Beiträge zur Theorie der Vererbung. *Archiv für Rassen- und Gesellschaftsbiologie* 9: 165–174.

Weinberg W (1913) Über neuere psychiatrische Vererbungsstatistik. *Archiv für Rassen- und Gesellschaftsbiologie* 10: 303–312.

Zirkle C (1946) The early history of the idea of the inheritance of acquired characters and of pangenesis. *Transactions of the American Philosophical Society* 38: 91–151.

2 The birth of psychiatric genetics

Psychiatric genetics emerged from a small, but diverse, network that took shape in Germany at the beginning of the twentieth century. Experimental biology, Mendelian statistics and psychiatric classification were styles of reasoning that crystallized in the milieu of the 'research institute'. Together, they produced a method of calculating Mendelian inheritance of schizophrenia that crossed the threshold of a mature science of heredity. The birth of psychiatric genetics also intersects with eugenic themes of racial hygiene and Nazi health policy. Many of its classical methods – family and twin studies, for example – emerged from a biopolitical vision of detecting and preventing severe psychoses in the German population. For these, and many other reasons, controversy occupies a central role in the history of psychiatric genetics. We show how twin studies, in particular, evolved from criticisms that led to subsequent modifications and improvements in their design and execution. We also examine the efforts of researchers to stabilize a statistical style of reasoning by constructing a narrative of uniformity and progress. Finally, we consider the durability of a discipline that entered a period of 'enlightenment' in the 1980s.

A new statement on method

We begin by tracing a novel statement that marks the birth of psychiatric genetics: the segregation pattern of schizophrenia in siblings *does not* conform to a simple Mendelian ratio. We shall treat this statement not as a 'truth' with coherent, universal properties, but as a 'candidate for truth' (Hacking 1992) that emerges from a small network of production. Our first task is to re-examine this statement as a solution to methodological problems of investigating Mendelian inheritance among clinical populations. We then demonstrate the statement's novelty, contrasting it to earlier Mendelian studies in neuropsychiatry, to show the exceptional difficulty of testing a relatively simple Mendelian hypothesis. By tracing a methodological break from previous studies, we can appreciate the birth of psychiatric genetics as a new kind of science of heredity.

Between 1907 and 1911, Ernst Rüdin began collecting cases in what would be the first large-scale family study on *dementia praecox* (later relabelled 'schizophrenia'). Rüdin excluded a dominant gene theory on the grounds that many of the cases he collected had unaffected parents, thus the aim of the study was to test whether dementia praecox behaved as a Mendelian recessive trait. The study was not only the largest of its kind, including 755 probands and their 2,732 siblings, but the first to use standardized diagnostic procedures and systematic ascertainment of probands based on the certainty of diagnosis rather than family history (Rüdin 1911, 1916).

The publication of Rüdin's monograph in 1916 contained a methodological statement outlining new standards of objectivity for a science of heredity, an approach he called 'empirical heredity prognosis'. Using the system of classification developed by Emil Kraepelin, he applied diagnostic criteria based on prognosis, rather than aetiology, to select a category of progressively deteriorating, non-affective psychosis. Dementia praecox formed the basis of his family study because it was believed to be a stable pattern of deterioration caused by endogenous factors. Diagnoses were made on the basis of cross-sectional and longitudinal data of which only cases of diagnostic certainty were included. The same criteria for diagnosis were applied to relatives as well as the probands. Certainty of diagnosis for the relatives relied on direct observation, hospital records or 'precise description' by third parties. Rüdin adopted a narrow view of dementia praecox, excluding cases of brief or atypical psychosis, delusional disorder or spectrum personality disorder (Kendler and Zerbin-Rüdin 1996).

Collection of longitudinal data of probands and relatives involved recontacting families to establish the course and outcome of the condition. In the first instance, Rüdin used first-hand information, such as interviews or letters, and when this was not available other sources of information were collected such as medical records, parish registries, official records of estates, case histories from clinics, family pedigrees, and records from police, prisons and the military (Kendler and Zerbin-Rüdin 1996). All the proband-family information was compiled into a file, including a detailed pedigree, from which a standard card was completed for every proband. Using Kraepelin's method of 'counting cards' (*Zahlkarte*), Rüdin employed a system of 'standardized, chronological, and structured documentation of the course of a mental illness for large groups of patients' (Weber 1996: 326).

Having collected the family data, Rüdin used new statistical techniques to overcome two problems: correcting for variable age of onset and multiple ascertainment bias. Some relatives of the proband were still at risk of developing the condition, and several probands were recruited from the same family. Rüdin sought the help of Wilhelm Weinberg – the leading statistical geneticist in Germany at the time – to develop various 'correction' techniques to estimate morbid risk (see Chapter 1 for a discussion of these techniques). Weinberg's Sibling and Proband method was used to address the issue of ascertainment bias and the Abridged Weinberg method for age correction (Weinberg 1903, 1908, 1913).

The results of Rüdin's study were perhaps less remarkable than the method itself since the pattern of morbidity found among siblings fell well-below the ratios expected for a recessive trait. In conclusion, he ruled out a simple monogenic hypothesis and speculated whether genetic and environmental factors played an aetiological role in dementia praecox. He also proposed a possible two-locus recessive model as a closer fit with the results. In the final assessment, Rüdin found a relatively low morbid risk of 4.5 per cent for siblings, a decreased risk for parents compared to offspring and, more strikingly, a non-Mendelian pattern of segregation among the siblings. Despite the modesty of these findings, it was the apparent integrity of Rüdin's approach that established his international reputation as a psychiatric geneticist.

Rüdin's family study is considered the first modern scientific study in psychiatric genetics. Even by modern evaluations, the study is praised for its rigorous standards of objectivity. Practitioners describe the methodology as 'scientifically sound and durable' (Gottesman and Shields 1982), 'disciplined' and 'robust' (Mellon 1996), the findings of which are said to be 'virtually uncontested by modern studies' (Schulze *et al.* 2004: 251). Kendler and Zerbin-Rüdin (1996: 338–339) describe his systematic ascertainment as 'very unusual' given that previous studies presented strong family loading, concordant twin pairs, or 'interesting families'. The modesty of Rüdin's findings established an 'incidental' object at the birth of psychiatric genetics – a *complex* disorder in which 'internal' and 'external milieu' seemed to play an aetiological role (Rüdin 1916). To appreciate the novelty of Rüdin's statement fully, we need to differentiate it from other statements that applied Mendelian ideas to mental illness.

Mendelism had an immediate impact on neuropsychiatry, partly because it was complementary to biomedical disease models (Kendler 2015), but also because it offered a relatively simple theoretical hypothesis. For instance, Charles Davenport (1911) enthusiastically applied Mendelian inheritance to investigate a panoply of mental and physiological disorders. By today's standards, his attempts to lump together characteristics as broadly conceived as alcoholism, feeblemindedness, pauperism and criminality into the category of 'neuropathic conditions' was grossly oversimplified (Kevles 1985). The American psychologist, HH Goddard, also drew on Mendelian laws to explain the transmission of feeblemindedness. Measuring the mental age of 327 children, he concluded that 'feeblemindedness is in all probability transmitted in accordance with Mendelian Law of heredity' (1914: 589–590). Around the same time, in New York, Rosanoff and Orr (1911) obtained data from hospital records and family interviews to publish the first family pedigree of insanity. They pooled a wide variety of functional neuropathy, including epilepsy and feeblemindedness, into one clinical category. These 'primitive techniques' (Gottesman and Shields 1982) of ascertainment and diagnosis simply confirmed what the study had set out to prove: 'It would seem, then, that the fact of the hereditary transmission of the neuropathic constitution as a recessive trait, in accordance with the Mendelian theory, may be regarded as definitely established' (Rosanoff and Orr 1911; 228).

By the first decade of the twentieth century, applications of Mendelism in neuropsychiatry had not yet crossed the 'threshold of scientificity' (Foucault 1972). That is to say, they had not yet acquired the epistemological threshold of distinguishing positive knowledge of disease from the wider moral universe of meanings attributed to 'defective' individuals. The bias of selecting probands from hospital populations was prevalent among nineteenth-century studies of hereditary predisposition, where selection was based on 'interesting' family pedigrees, and broad diagnostic classifications. The arbitrary and haphazard criteria of many early family studies conflated clinical homogeneity with aetiological homogeneity (Mellon 1996). Neuropsychiatry 'influenced as it was by anatomy and physiology, eagerly adopted and aggressively applied' (Gottesman and Shields 1982: 38) the simple principles of Mendelism at the expense of nosology. The break with neuropsychiatry comes from a clinically informed psychiatry that begins to orient its gaze to the course and outcome of disease. In the next section, we examine how a new style of testing the truth and falsity of Mendelian inheritance emerges from a small, but diverse, network of biological psychiatry.

Tracing a network

What conditions were necessary for Rüdin to produce his novel method of investigating inheritance of schizophrenia? To answer this question, we look beyond the efforts of a solitary figure and trace the formation of a network of patients, scientists, and techniques that grounded Mendelian inquiry in stable procedures of clinical observation. First, we go back and consider the institutional context of German psychiatry to understand the development of a new clinical approach.

A new nosology

By the end of the nineteenth century, the decline of hereditarian views reinstated a sense of therapeutic pessimism among European and American hospitals.[1] In Germany, the situation was different; German asylums were well-funded, state-supported and tightly linked to universities and research institutes. Teaching and research were linked via two mechanisms: the doctoral dissertation and the habilitation (the latter demonstrating a serious contribution to the field as a post-doctoral researcher). Also, the physical proximity between psychiatry departments and medical departments, made the presentation of patients more accessible for students. It was this distinctly German apparatus of Hospital Medicine and Laboratory Medicine that led to the 'first wave' (Shorter 1997) of biological psychiatry.

At the time, there were two experimental styles of reasoning within biological psychiatry: pathological-anatomical localization and neurology. Both approaches embraced the 'spirit of localization', adopting a style of physical examination in which the patient's verbal statements were replaced with the interpretation of bodily responses (Foucault 2008). In neurology, a hierarchy of voluntary and involuntary, and automatic and spontaneous effects, permitted the isolation of the patient's will or intention. In the pathological-anatomical approach, the organization of symptoms were correlated with the subtle detection of lesions in the brain tissue in a criss-cross fashion, a constant checking by way of positive and negative inferences. Common to both approaches was the capture of symptoms-as-signs within a framework of regularity. The stability of the sign made it easier to deduce causes or generate inferences of function. In other words, the dimension of *time* in psychiatry was applied insofar as it permitted the continuity of the sign to appear as a candidate for diagnosis.

In 1896, Emil Kraepelin proposed 'a new way of looking at mental illness'. Diagnosis was assigned to the course and outcome of illness rather than the moment of its clinical presentation. In 1890, Kraepelin immediately began a research project of tracking a patient cohort. He had his residents complete index cards for all patients (to avoid the bias of including only 'interesting' cases) by noting clinical features during the period of diagnosis and prognosis. Clinical data were analysed statistically, which suggested that a large proportion of patients ended up in a state of dementia 'in spite of individual differences' (Kraepelin 1983, cited in Berrios and Hauser 1988). From the presentation of dementias, he identified a subcategory of premature dementia which he called *dementia praecox* (discussed earlier). Having reached this conclusion, he sought to identify early indicators for the degenerative process.[2] Later he refined the research process so that index cards contained patient information from the follow-up interviews. Aggregating all the information in a single source allowed Kraepelin to search for correlations between early presentation and later changes over the illness course. It was during this period of sorting through the cards that he reached a startling conclusion. In 1896, he wrote: 'I have abandoned any effort to classify [psychosis] on the basis of the clinical presentation' (Kraepelin 1896: v). This marked a decisive shift from deducing the causes of psychiatric illness to classifying illness in such a way as to permit the prediction of the outcome.[3] Kraepelin introduced the idea that prognosis, not cause, formed the basis of reliable diagnosis. The combination of clinical observation, patient interviews, note-taking and the aggregation of patient data allowed patient experience to appear within the longitudinal study of illness. The body of pathological anatomy and neurology played no part in revealing the secrets of the disease process.

When Kraepelin published the sixth edition of the *Textbook* in 1899, his classification of illness had reached its fullest expression. He divided psychiatric illness into 13 major groups; but what transformed Western psychiatry was the isolation of two particular groups that became known as the 'Kraepelinian dichotomy' (Brockington and Leff 1979). Psychotic illness was split into affective and non-affective components, which he labelled 'manic-depressive psychosis' and 'dementia praecox'.[4] The fact that this distinction still remains in the *Diagnostic and Statistical Manual of Mental Disorders* is a testimony of its durability and significance. That said, contemporary genetic research disputes this taxonomy. Recent genome studies indicate that schizophrenia and bipolar disorder are quantitative traits that share common polygenes, which challenge this dichotomy (Craddock and Owen 2005, 2010). Even so, at the time, Kraepelin introduced a new clinical style of reasoning within psychiatry by identifying common patterns of symptoms over a period of time rather than by simple similarity of major symptoms. It was this breakthrough that stabilized psychiatric nosology and set the foundation for subsequent studies of heredity. Another development that stabilized a science of heredity was the biologization of family history, i.e. genealogy.

The genealogical turn

In Germany, degeneration theory was greeted with a mixed reaction from the medical profession. Some psychiatrists dismissed it as an absurd hypothesis since any oddity or eccentricity could be interpreted as a sign of progressive pathological heredity (Jung 1866). In the second half of the nineteenth century, statistical surveys of asylum patients using standard criteria failed to settle the matter of pathological heredity. The high incidence of 'unassured' cases combined with poor access to patient medical records produced an incomplete clinical picture (Hagen 1876). In the last two decades of the nineteenth century, psychiatrists had lost faith in statistical approaches and turned their attention to the genealogical study of individual families (see Gausemeier 2015).

In psychiatry, pedigrees had been used as a visual tool to show progressive degeneration in the family tree (Krafft-Ebing 1869; Damerow 1865). By 1900, genealogical practices were promoted in the German medical community by those opposed to degeneration theory. The German psychiatrist Robert Sommer (1901) criticized previous studies that only selected families to show a striking accumulation of cases. The same selection bias operated in asylum statistics since capturing cases of patients with diseased relatives could only give a distorted picture of 'hereditary burden' (Grassmann 1896). An influential text among German medical practitioners was Ottokar Lorenz's (1898) *Handbook of Scientific Genealogy*. Lorenz argued for the reorientation of genealogy in light of recent chromosomal theories of heredity in the 1880s and 1890s. Citing Weismann's germ-plasm theory, biological principles ruled out the heredity of acquired characteristics and established the equivalence of the sexes. Previously, genealogists had only considered the male lineage important. The 'correct' procedure was to construct an ancestral chart (*Ahnentafel*) to show the complete ascending ancestry of male and female 'germ-plasm' for a single individual. Lorenzo transformed genealogy from the collection of facts about family history into a technique for ordering ancestry according to biological principles of heredity. The *Handbook*'s appeal lay in the key message that genealogy was central to linking the humanities and the biological sciences (Gausemeier 2008).

The biologization of heredity established new networks among amateur genealogists, medical practitioners, psychiatrists, social scientists, public health officials, lawyers and activists in the eugenics movement. Sommer actively promoted genealogy as a hybrid science and campaigned for the central collection of clinical and asylum data, and the standardization of methods (Sommer 1912). New initiatives formed around the genealogical collection of individual and family histories for the purpose of racial hygiene and the establishment of national genealogical registers, only some of which were partially realized (Gausemeier 2015). Genealogy became the preferred technique for assembling databases of the 'inferior', which Rüdin used to full effect in his family study of schizophrenia.

The Munich School

Kraepelin ended the first wave of biological psychiatry only to re-establish it in the form of experimental science. The second wave of biological psychiatry incorporated the features of Hospital Medicine and Laboratory Medicine by assembling a diverse network of investigators. When Kraepelin established a university psychiatric clinic in 1904, he surrounded himself with many talented laboratory researchers, such as Nissel, Alzheimer, Plaut, Isserlin and Rüdin himself. Although he remained agnostic about aetiology, Kraepelin's ambition was to create an intellectual milieu of methodological diversity to advance the field of clinical psychiatry (Hippius *et al.* 2008).

After completing his habilitation, Rüdin arrived at Munich in 1909 to take up a research post with his teacher and mentor. Kraepelin's psychiatric clinic accommodated over 100 beds and an out-patient clinic over which Rüdin was now responsible. The new position provided a base for the collection of cases for his family study. He also utilized Kraepelin's standardized approach for the systematic documentation of cases; indeed, many of the diagnoses were believed to have been reviewed by Kraepelin himself (Kendler and Zerbin-Rüdin 1996). By 1911, Rüdin sketched a theoretical vision of a research programme based on the systematic compilation and statistical evaluation of data relating to psychopathology, physical medicine, genealogy, demographics and physical anthropology for large-scale studies (Rüdin 1911). At a time when German psychiatrists were appealing to heredity to understand and prevent psychiatric disorders, Rüdin was the first to assemble a mathematical and empirical science of heredity (Ritter and Roelcke 2005; Gausemeier 2015).

A year after Rüdin published his landmark family study, Kraepelin established the German Institute for Psychiatry. The 'Munich School' became an international model for the organization of psychiatric research with laboratories for experimental psychology, neuropathology, chemistry and later serology, genealogical research and a large archive of case histories. Although the Institute was financially precarious (Engstrom *et al.* 2016), it provided the conditions for combining systematic clinical observation with hereditary science. Indeed, Kraepelin's predilection for neutral scientific inquiry and methodological diversity was not the sole reason for supporting genetic research. He believed dementia praecox was primarily a hereditary disease attributed to 70 per cent of cases (Kraepelin 1899/1902). With the rediscovery of Mendelian heredity, Kraepelin maintained that the future of psychiatry may well reside in 'the discovery of laws that govern the transmission of diverse traits associated with insanity and wherever possible to illuminate the conditions under which there first appears the germ of a disease that can be transmitted from parent to offspring'

(Kraepelin 1962: 134). Enthusiasm to explore psychosis as a Mendelian trait permeated the Munich School, and provided the ideal conditions for Rüdin's research.

We have now reached a position to reconsider the birth story of psychiatric genetics. Rüdin's large-scale family study formed part of a network of production that established the conditions of possibility for psychiatric genetics. Having introduced a new clinical style of reasoning that subjected psychiatric nosology to statistical observation and experimental testing, Kraepelin acquired the mandate to establish a network of expertise in Munich. The significance of this network is in the way it combined Hospital Medicine and Laboratory Medicine to form an ensemble of researchers and methodological techniques around patient populations. It also co-opted the statistical expertise of Weinberg to address the problem of ascertainment bias and variable onset of risk. Kraepelin was not only an influential nosologist but a capable 'research manager' and a charismatic leader who envisioned psychiatry's role of restoring the health of German society (Engstrom *et al.* 2016). After securing the resources to establish the first research institute for psychiatry, the Munich School formed part of an international network of highly porous relations extending across Europe and North America (Ritter and Roelcke 2005). By the time Rüdin became the director of the Genealogic-Demographic Department in 1917, the Institute had become the leading centre for psychiatric genetics research. Many of those who visited Rüdin's department became major figures of the next generation in psychiatric genetics, including Essen-Möller, Juda, Kallmann, Luxenburger, Schulz, Slater, Strömgeren and Sjögren (Zerbin-Rüdin and Kendler 1996). Though Rüdin deserves credit for shaping a new field of scientific inquiry, it was Kraepelin the research manager who pulled together the resources and expertise for a science of heredity to take hold. As we will see in later chapters, the parallels between Kraepelin and the director of 'the Centre' at our ethnographic site are striking.

Rüdin's legacy

Social scientists have observed the ways in which 'discourse' (Gilbert and Mulkay 1984), 'narratives' (Myers 1991) and 'birth dramas' (Knorr-Cetina 1999) work to orient the field of science. Typically, they reconstruct the past to neutralize controversies and bolster objectivity. Along these lines, contemporary researchers often give a heroic account of Rüdin's methodological achievement. While some acknowledge Rüdin's 'Nazi involvement' (Mellon 1996) and the 'possible misuse and abuse of findings' (Zerbin-Rüdin and Kendler 1996: 336), it is rare for practitioners to directly confront the eugenic origins of their discipline. Stronger accounts can be found among those writing outside the discipline (see Kevles 1985; Proctor 1988; Weber 1991, 1993; Ritter and Roelcke 2005; Joseph 2013). However, the image of Rüdin as an advocate of 'racial hygiene', or the Munich Institute as a 'think tank' for Nazi health policy, is not part of the official birth story of psychiatric genetics. In this section, we want to briefly consider how modern researchers manage this troubling legacy.

In 1996, a special issue of the *American Journal of Medical Genetics* marked an unusual moment of reflection regarding the legacy of German psychiatric genetics. With contributions from key scientists (Kendler and Gottesman), Rüdin's daughter (Zerbin-Rüdin) and a medical historian (Weber), the collection combined a retrospective of Rüdin's methodological contribution with a stark account of his involvement in Nazi health policy (see Weber 1996). In the introduction of the special issue, Gottesman and Bertelsen (1996) proceed to mitigate Rüdin's involvement with the Nazi regime by stating that: his work was 'abused' by the Nazi regime, eugenics was rife in other countries, he was 'caught up' in a system of abuse, and that colleagues had thought kindly of him. This is at odds with Weber's (1996) meticulous historical account (summarized below) that indicates, among other things, that Rüdin was *actively* involved in the development of Nazi health policy.

The unofficial story of Rüdin's legacy proceeds as follows. Influenced by his brother-in-law, the physician and social Darwinist, Alfred Ploetz, Rüdin became an advocate of the racial hygiene movement. Ploetz founded the *Archives of Racial and Social Biology* on which Rüdin worked as a reviewer and later a full-time editor. After studying medicine and deciding to purse an academic career in psychiatry, Rüdin became a loyal follower of Kraepelin's work on psychoses. Kraepelin himself was not a proponent of racial hygiene, but was active in German Nationalist circles and openly supported ideas associated with social Darwinism (Weber 1996). Having succeeded Aloysius Alzheimer as senior physician at the Munich Hospital in 1909, Rüdin continued to support racial hygiene along utopian lines, and gave frequent expert advice on eugenic abortion and involuntary sterilization. Many cite (Proctor 1988; Engstrom *et al.* 2016) the acute economic and political crises of the Weimar Republic as reasons why eugenic models were popular in Germany. The medical community often justified euthanasia in economic terms of relieving the 'financial burdens' of caring for 'defectives and sick persons of all types' (Rüdin 1911 cited in Ritter and Roelcke 2005: 268). Even today, this terminology can be heard when rates of mental illness are discussed in terms of a 'burden' on a society (see Chapter 7).

When the National Socialists seized power in 1933, Rüdin viewed this as an opportunity to intensify research on racial hygiene. Weber (1996) cites numerous documents indicating that Rüdin suffered no crisis of conscience with regard to cooperating with the Nazi regime. Though he was not responsible for drafting the text of the sterilization law of 1933, he provided expert commentary, and continued to play a central role in propagating the racial hygiene doctrine in the 'Third Reich'. He also received ample funding from the National Socialist government to continue research activities. In his letter of thanks to Hitler, he stated that he would continue to structure his research so that 'results will contribute to providing an even firmer basis for the further expansion and realization of your racial hygiene program in the German *Volk*' (Rüdin 1936, cited in Weber 1996: 328). By 1940, Weber describes Rüdin as 'entangled in the oligarchic power structure of national socialism' (1996: 329) and becoming involved in long disputes with the SS *Ahnenerbe* who prevented further research. Though Rüdin was not directly involved in preparations for the execution of any murders in the 'T4 action' (the euthanasia of 80,000 mentally handicapped and 'inferior' individuals) nor did he protest these actions despite requests from his colleagues. In the final assessment, Weber (1996) claims that Rüdin was directly responsible for the enforcement of sterilization, damaging the reputation of the Institute, and burying the academic field of psychiatric genetics under the suspicion of Nazi eugenics.

The 1996 special issue of the *American Journal of Medical Genetics* provoked several angry responses from scientists who objected to Kendler's and Zerber-Rüdin's (Rüdin's daughter) apparent sidestepping of Rüdin's eugenic legacy (Gershon 1997; Gejman 1997; Lerer and Segman 1997). Taking the stronger view, Lerer and Segman argued that 'Nazi-tainted science' should not be cited in scientific literature, while Gershon and Gejman insisted that any historical review of Rüdin's work should include the full extent of his involvement in Nazi euthanasia and compulsory sterilization. Common to these views is the assumption that eugenic ideology and scientific practice are not separate spheres of activity. Given that Rüdin's support for racial hygiene preceded his scientific work, one can only assume that eugenics was a motivation for his research. Even Gottesman and Bertelsen (1996: 319) concede that Rüdin's genetic research was developed so that 'mental illness could be predicted and prevented'.

Kendler's (1997) reply is curious. As one of the leading twin researchers in the field, he clearly seeks to preserve a legitimate birth story of psychiatric genetics. He argues that Rüdin's original family study of schizophrenia was conducted ethically; it was published 17 years before the Nazis came to power; eugenics was common during this period (Rüdin was not the only intellectual contributor of Nazi policy); and that censorship of scientific literature on the basis that it was abused by others would exclude huge swathes of legitimate science. As such, there is no secure ground for establishing criteria for exclusion. In order to preserve Rüdin's place in history, Kendler assumes that separating science and politics is achievable, even though others claim that Rüdin held precisely the opposite view (see Ritter and Roelcke 2005: 265).

What purpose does this reflection serve? The 1996 special issue on German psychiatric genetics coincides with a period of 'enlightenment' in psychiatric genetics. By the mid-1990s, we see an array of strategies attempting to reconstruct the discipline as cautious, reflexive and responsible (Hedgecoe 2001). The reconstruction of origins, albeit from different perspectives, seeks to control a narrative of scientific progress by suspending the elements of 'good' science as the basis of continuity, and by signalling its moral distance from 'bad' ideology. The tension between science and politics is never fully reconciled because a science of heredity was already embedded in networks of German Nationalism and wider strategies of biopolitical reform. It seems plausible that methods of detecting and preventing the lives of the mentally unfit formed part of the wider conditions of possibility of psychiatric genetics. Efforts to minimize or contain this history deny that these political goals are *constitutive* of scientific inquiry. However, rather than evolving independently of these abuses, we show that psychiatric genetics is a peculiar case in which disciplinary responses to historical abuses have actively shaped its key methodologies.

Twin studies

One of the most respected and yet controversial methods in psychiatric genetics is the twin study. Following Galton's (1876) earlier observations, the first systematic twin study was performed at the Munich Institute in the late 1920s. By the 1970s, twin research provided some of the strongest evidence for implicating genetic factors in the aetiology of schizophrenia. Important to note is that the origins of twin studies are also the product of German eugenic thinking. Our task is not to dwell on these eugenic themes, but to understand the co-evolution of scientific reasoning and controversy as a 'self-authenticating' (Hacking 1992) process. In what follows, we focus on how the *clinical* and *statistical* styles of reasoning in twin research have evolved in relation to scientific criticism.

Twins studies adopt the relatively simple, comparative design of investigating the prevalence of a trait or condition across zygosity of twin pairs. It is assumed that monozygotic (MZ) twins are genetically identical and that dizygotic (DZ) twins share, on average, half their genes. It is also assumed that any dissimilarity between MZ twins must be attributed to environmental factors. The extent to which MZ and DZ twin pairs resemble each other is calculated by the rate of 'concordance' (the presence of the same trait in the twin pair).[5] What belies the simplicity of the twin design are formidable hurdles of sampling twin populations, determining zygosity, establishing diagnosis and calculating concordance. The task then is to understand how an impression of universal validity is maintained by scientists given the inconsistent methods and standards applied across these studies.

The first twin study in psychiatric genetic was conducted by Hans Luxenburger in 1928.[6] He obtained index cases from the Munich Psychiatric Clinic and from the resident population of Bavarian mental hospitals, and reviewed 16,000 medical records from which 19 MZ and 13 DZ same-sex pairs were identified (Gottesman and Shields 1982). His main findings are an interesting departure from Mendelian theory: the frequency of twins among schizophrenic patients was not different from that of the general population, and the concordance of MZ pairs was 58 per cent compared to 0 per cent for DZ pairs (Schulze *et al.* 2004). Similar to Rüdin's findings, the first twin study of schizophrenia suggested a combined aetiology of environmental and hereditary factors. Subsequent studies have shown considerable variation in methods of sampling, diagnosis and calculation, with concordance of MZ twins ranging from 0 per cent to 86 per cent.

A common technique of narrating the canon of twin research is to display tables listing the studies by year and their results by concordance. Tables are used by practitioners to show the continuity of concordance across studies, inviting the reader to compare these studies as uniform items of information. However, the many versions of tables that appear in the literature are anything but uniform. Studies are sometimes omitted for reasons unstated, or excluded on the basis of modern standards; their findings are recalculated to show higher rates of concordance, or partitioned to give an impression of scientific progress. For instance, Gottesman and Shields (1982) distinguish between 'older' and 'newer' studies to justify higher rates of concordance (we will return to this issue later). Sullivan *et al.* (2003) distinguish between methodologically 'inferior vs superior' studies in terms of whether they adopt the gold standard criteria of systematic recruitment and diagnosis, and blinding diagnostic status and zygosity. Critics also reproduce these tables to show exaggerated concordance rates of earlier studies that used non-blind diagnosis and resident hospital samples (Boyle 1990; Joseph 2003). Indeed, tables are *reality techniques* used by different interest groups to affirm or cast doubt on the aetiology of schizophrenia. To give an example, we reproduce a similar kind of table to present the main twin studies cited in the literature (see Table 2.1).

The distinction between earlier and newer twin studies coincides with criticisms that begin to surface in the 1950s and 1960s. In his substantial review of the 'primary biases in Twin Studies', Price (1950) claimed that MZ twins do not necessarily share the same environmental or prenatal factors (e.g. a proportion of MZ twins are dichorial). The geneticists Neel and Schull (1954) also raised concerns that concordant twins were more likely to come to the attention of researchers than discordant twins. Jackson (1960) focused on the unreliability of diagnosis where subjects stood a better chance of being diagnosed with schizophrenia the longer they were hospitalized. He also disputed the assumption that

Table 2.1 Pairwise concordance rates in schizophrenia twin studies

Author	Year	Country	MZ	%	DZ (SS)	%
'Early studies'						
Luxenberger	1928	Germany	19	58	13	0
Rosnaoff *et al.*	1934	USA	41	61	53	13
Essen-Möller	1941	Sweden	11	27	15	15
Kallmann	1946	USA	174	69	296	11
Slater	1953	UK	37	65	58	14
Inouye	1961	Japan	58	59	20	15
'Newer studies'						
Tienari	1963	Finland	17	0	20	5
Gottesman and Shields	1966	UK	22	40	33	9
Kringlen	1967	Norway	55	25	90	4
Fischer *et al.*	1969	Denmark	21	24	41	10
Pollin *et al.*	1969	USA	95	14	125	4–8
Koskenvuo *et al.*	1984	Finland	73	11	225	2
Onstad *et al.*	1991	Norway	24	33	28	4
Franzek and Beckman	1998	Germany	9	67	12	17

Source: adapted from Joseph (2003: 142).

identical and fraternal twins grow up in similar environments, proposing that identical twins have a unique psychological bond ('ego fusion') contributing to their higher concordance. Similarly, Rosenthal (1962a, 1962b) published a series of papers highlighting the problems of ascertainment among hospitalized samples, resulting in an excess of concordant pairs.

These criticisms coincide with a growing awareness among scientists of sampling and diagnostic bias. For instance, in their historical review of twin studies, Gottesman and Shields (1982) contrast Rosanoff and colleagues' (1934) 'crude' use of diagnostic standards with Essen-Möller's (1941) systematic methods of sampling via national registers. Kringlen (1967) also writes approvingly of Essen-Möller's techniques of determining zygosity, supplementing personal investigation (similarity method) with information derived from blood group (serology) and fingerprinting; whereas other studies (e.g. Luxenburger, Rosanoff and Kallmann) relied exclusively on the similarity method. The fact that ascertainment appears to be taken more seriously by the 1950s is illustrated in Slater's 1953 study. Building on Essen-Möller's methods, Slater developed a systematic approach of ascertaining twins at the Maudsley and Bethlem Royal Hospital matching national registers with hospital case registers. Zygosity was determined by the similarity method alongside anthropometric data and fingerprint analysis. He also presented case materials 'giving the reader the possibility of forming his [*sic*] own opinion as regards diagnosis' (Kringlen 1967: 84).

One study that has received a great deal of criticism is Kallmann's twin study (Kallmann 1946). Aside from being the largest twin study on schizophrenia, it also reports the highest rate of concordance. Kallmann collected 794 schizophrenic twin index cases from the resident population of state hospitals in New York from 1937 to 1945, comprising 174 MZ pairs and 517 DZ pairs. There were several stages in which concordance was calculated. Initially, 50 per cent of 174 MZ pairs and 6 per cent of 517 DZ pairs were concordant for a hospital diagnosis of schizophrenia. After 'diagnostic revision', 59 per cent of MZ pairs and 9 per cent of DZ pairs were concordant for 'definite schizophrenia'. When cases of doubtful schizophrenia were included, the rate increased to 69 per cent and 10 per cent, and after applying the Abridged Weinberg method of age-correction, the concordance figures rose to 86 per cent and 15 per cent. Kallmann's conclusion that schizophrenia was *predominantly* a genetic condition became the focus of intense criticism in the 1960s (see Jackson 1960 and Rosenthal 1962a). In defending Kallmann from accusations that he applied his diagnostic standards too 'loosely' or that knowledge of zygosity may have led to 'contaminated' diagnosis, even Shields *et al.* (1967) concede that 86 per cent concordance was an artefact of oversampling chronic hospital cases.

Critics of twin studies tend to underestimate the reflexivity of twin researchers regarding their own methods. They often impute the deficiencies of older studies to all twin studies, therefore denying *any* improvement in the technique. Indeed, Joseph (2003) argues the whole premise of the twin study design is flawed. Moderate critics such as Rosenthal (1962a, 1962b) and Neale and Oltmanns (1980) are critical of earlier twin studies, but appeal to improved techniques of sampling since the 1960s. The fact that practitioners are highly responsive to criticisms is evident in Gottesman and Shield's 1966 study.[7] The elaborate description of their methods is a coherent synthesis of previous criticisms: determining zygosity via similarity, blood type and fingerprinting, sampling via systematic ascertainment of hospital registers, employing the use of hospital notes, case histories, semi-structured interviews and personality tests, as well as the submission of data to independent judges for diagnostic assessment. In fact, they explicitly orient their methodology to address past criticisms: 'We thus have a study which meets many of the criticisms of earlier twin research on schizophrenia' (Gottesman and Shields 1966: 811).

Even if we can establish that criticisms in the 1960s played a decisive role in improving the methodology of twin studies, critics have numerous resources with which to mobilize their objections. For instance, Boyle (1990) raises two objections relating to modern twin studies. First, the use of broad criteria to infer a 'schizophrenia spectrum' (Gottesman and Shields 1972) inflates concordance rates and accentuates differences between MZ and DZ twins.[8] Second, practitioners prefer an ambiguous method of calculation that produces systematically higher concordance rates (the *probandwise* method rather than the *pairwise* method).[9] Gottesman and Shields (1982) also view concordance as the basis for distinguishing older and newer twin studies. Their demarcation serves to contain the deficiencies of older studies from contaminating the improvements of newer studies. Concordance is calculated in terms of pairwise rates for the early studies and probandwise rates for the older studies. The reason they give for this is because the newer studies are considered more representative of the population 'at least in those operating with accurate twin and psychiatric registers', and because the information available in the older studies 'does not permit other calculations' (1982: 112). Geneticists also argue that this method is more accurate in supplying risk information to individuals (McGue 1992), while critics argue that the practice of 'counting subjects twice' is a convenient way of inflating concordance rates.[10]

The fact that critics object to how scientists review their own literature draws attention to the malleability of research findings. The twin study literature is not an immutable archive but a pliable resource for shaping a stable narrative. In other words, scientists *can* and *do* engage in various kinds of 'curatorial work' to justify discrepancies and reinterpret findings in order to insulate the canon of research from ongoing criticism. Our point is not to impute a disingenuous motive to scientists' curatorial practices, but to show how consistency of scientific research is constructed in the literature. Gottesman and Shields (1982) employ a variety of strategies to achieve this: they divide the literature to foreground methodological progress of twin studies (segmentation), they re-describe deviant studies to foreground the fragility of discordant findings (contextualization), they collapse methodological differences to imply uniformity (conflation) and recalculate the findings of recent studies to report preferred rates of concordance (reinterpretation). By adopting these strategies, Gottesman and Shields reach the following conclusion:

Allowing as we have for the small sizes in some of the twin studies and for certain key dimensions, many of the alleged discrepancies among all the twin studies are attenuated. We feel quite comfortable in concluding that the twin studies of schizophrenia as a whole represent variations on the same theme and are, in effect, sound replications of the same experiment. No doubt critics will feel less comfortable with such a conclusion.

(1982: 115)

To assert that twin studies are the 'same experiment' replicated across different countries at different periods is a striking statement of uniformity. Not all twin researchers agree with this statement (Kringlen 1976). As we have seen, critics routinely foreground the methodological inconsistencies of sampling, diagnosis and interpretation to show that twin studies are prone to human bias and error. Gottesman and Shields' reconstruction of the literature illustrates the ways in which consistency can be achieved by dividing, re-describing, conflating and reinterpreting twin studies to present 'variations of the same theme'.

Dialectics of twin and adoption studies

Prior to the 1960s, twin studies were a relatively isolated research programme overshadowed by popular 'environmentalist' theories. Intense criticism in the 1960s, combined with Tienari's reporting of 0 per cent concordance in 1963, might have relegated twin studies to obscurity. But psychiatric genetics was remarkably resilient during this period. Writing about the preliminary results of their 1966 twin study, Gottesman and Shields (1966) clearly stated their purpose was to 'find out what effects would be on the results when care was taken to avoid, or to make provision for, the alleged sources of error and bias in the earlier "classical" studies conducted before 1953' (1972: xvi). Twins researchers were not merely responding to criticism but actively reshaping their methodologies in relation to criticism. By the late 1960s, a new approach had been developed to specifically address the shortcomings of previous studies, an approach that would dramatically turn the tide of opinion in favour of a genetic aetiology of schizophrenia.

In 1966 and 1968, two 'adoption studies' were published that appeared to disentangle the effects of genetic and environmental contribution to schizophrenia. Neale and Oltmanns (1980: 142) described the approach as 'ingenious' claiming that they 'provided almost irrefutable confirmation of the importance of genetic factors'. Leonard Heston identified 47 adopted offspring of institutionalized women diagnosed with schizophrenia. The offspring were adopted a few days after birth between 1915 and 1945. Using an experimental-control design, he compared the index group with 50 unaffected adoptees who were matched in terms of gender, type of placement and length of time in care. Records for each adoptee were compiled from psychiatric hospital records, personal interviews and psychological tests. Three psychiatrists (including Heston) evaluated the records 'blindly and independently'. The results showed that five experimental and 0 control subjects received a diagnosis of schizophrenia with a significant probability of 0.024. Heston concluded: 'this study supports a genetic aetiology of schizophrenia' (1966: 823).

In 1967, the preliminary findings of the American–Danish adoption studies were presented to a conference of biological and psychosocial scientists. Gottesman (1991: 83) tells us that 'the entire field of schizophreniology was converted, at least in public pronouncements, to some kind of interactionist stance for advancing against a common enemy – ignorance about the true cause of schizophrenia'. Others would write that the findings were a 'steamroller', which 'obviously abolished a number of more or less fragile observations and assumptions. It changed the scene in psychiatric genetics' (Strömgren 1993: 11). However, other twin researchers were less impressed with the way in which these studies were 'propergandized' (Kringlen 1976). Nevertheless, when the American-Danish study was published in preliminary form in 1968 and 1975, the reaction temporarily stunned the critics.

Leading the study were Kety, Rosenthal, Wender and their Danish associates. The sampling was complicated, to say the least. The first phase, published in 1968, was based entirely on institutional records, while the next phase, published in 1975, was based, in part, on interviews conducted with biological and adoptive relatives of index and control adoptees. Accessing various registers and official records in Greater Copenhagen, the investigators compiled a group of 507 adoptees who had been admitted to a psychiatric unit. The records were screened and assessed from which an index group of 34 adoptees received a diagnosis of chronic, acute or borderline schizophrenia. A control group was also selected consisting of 33 adoptees with no psychiatric history. Index and control adoptees were matched in terms of age, sex, age at adoption and socioeconomic status of the adoptive family. Researchers then attempted to locate biological and adoptive relatives, from which a total of 463 were identified. Again, searches were made for psychiatric history among the relatives; where no such records were found, blind consensus diagnoses were made by the researchers. At no point though had contact been made with any of the adoptees or their relatives. In 1968, the group reported a higher prevalence of 'spectrum' disorders among index biological relatives compared to the control biological relatives. From 150 biological relatives, 8.7 per cent had a diagnosis of schizophrenia compared to 1.9 per cent with the same diagnoses among the biological relatives of the controls. The researchers concluded that: 'genetic factors are important in the transmission of schizophrenia' (Kety *et al.* 1968: 361).

Space does not allow a full discussion of the adoption studies literature nor how critics proceeded to unravel their apparent flaws. Suffice it to say, the controversy of adoption studies contains variations of the same theme. On the one side, studies have continued to change, using increasingly sophisticated techniques of sampling and diagnosis to mitigate bias and error. Unlike twin studies, adoption studies used the superior case-control design and, drawing on the methods developed by Slater, and later refined by Gottesman and Shields, employed an arsenal of psychological testing, personal interviews, blind diagnoses, independent judges, inter-rata reliability and standardized diagnostic procedures (e.g. DSM II). On the other side, critics drew attention to issues of contaminated diagnosis (which was not always assigned blindly or independently) and insufficient case histories. The use of broad definitions of schizophrenia were also a frequently cited concern. While researchers justified the inclusion of borderline cases as genetically related, critics argued that broad definitions artificially inflated the statistical difference between index groups and control groups. Perhaps one of the most high-profile attacks on the adoption method was mounted by Rose *et al.* (1984) in their book, *Not in Our Genes*. They revealed that researchers had prepared so-called 'pseudo-interviews' by filling interview forms for dead relatives on the basis of what they 'guessed the relative would have answered' (1984: 225).

An interesting feature of the dialectics of twin and adoption studies and their critics is that researchers are persistent in their efforts to improve their techniques while continuing to absorb or neutralize criticism. Radical critics, by contrast, come and go, though some have been unusually persistent, for example, Kamin, Rose and Joseph. By the 1970s, the legacy of Jackson's influential critique of twin studies had been worn smooth and eventually relegated to a 'vocal critic of genetic interpretations' (Gottesman and Shields 1982: 73). However, it is interesting to consider the rivalry between twin and adoption researchers during this period and the kinds of arguments they drew upon.

While twin researchers were happy to bask in the popularity of genetic studies of schizophrenia, Kety *et al.* (1968) viewed their own approach as a significant improvement on previous methods. Family studies and twin studies were 'inconclusive', they would write, and 'fail to remove the influence of certain environmental factors' (1968: 345). In a similar vein, Rosenthal argued:

> In both family studies and twin studies, it has not been possible to obtain leverage on the possible role of environmental variables in producing behavioural disorder under scrutiny. Environmental factors have always been conceived in the crudest terms in these 'genetic' studies, and no effort has ever been seriously made to control for them. Genes and environment have always been confounded in the same families.
>
> (1972: 64)

Although it is common to put twin and adoption studies in the same camp of endorsing a genetic aetiology, the dialectics of twin and adoption studies increasingly moderate a genetic hypothesis.

Previous studies explained non-Mendelian distributions in terms of statistical distributions shored up but not necessarily explained by an additive, polygenic model. By the late 1960s and early 1970s, it was now possible to claim that early studies made no attempt to investigate the environment to explain the significant variation across these studies. Even the Norwegian twin researcher, Einar Kringlen, who admits being 'very much impressed with the elegant experimental design' of adoption studies (1976: 429), accuses Gottesman and Shields of adopting a 'weak' understanding of the environment: 'every time an alternative environmental explanation of data crops up, giving room for a tiny little environmental factor, the authors fall upon this poor factor and kill it' (1976: 431).

What begins to emerge in the 1970s is a more robust version of the environment as a 'variable' with explanatory force rather than an unexplained residue of statistical analysis. These arguments would have a significant impact on the genetic hypothesis initiating a surge of 'theoretical imagination' in the 1980s where previous discordant elements were now preserved and modified within a new theoretical framework. In the next section, we consider the ways in which schizophrenia serves as a model for stabilizing the field of psychiatric genetics.

Theoretical imagination of schizophrenia

Since the birth of psychiatric genetics, schizophrenia has been the stock model of the field, an exemplar for integrating clinical, statistical and laboratory styles of reasoning. By the 1980s, the consensus position among twin and adoption researchers was a polygenic theory of schizophrenia. Some still adhered to a modified Mendelian model involving a dominant gene of 'incomplete penetrance'. Indeed, both models appeared to explain the data equally well. However, the polygenic model allowed environmental factors to play an active, albeit unspecific, role in explaining the considerable variation of the clinical picture. Hedgecoe (2001) argues that genetic theories of the 1980s and 1990s illustrate a phenomenon of 'enlightened geneticization' where researchers construct a narrative that increasingly acknowledges environmental factors while continuing to prioritize a genetic aetiology of schizophrenia. In this section, we examine how clinical and aetiological *heterogeneity* are theoretically integrated in the 1980s to create new pathways for research.

When psychiatric genetics appeared at the beginning of the twentieth century, the assumption that 'schizophrenia' was a genetic disorder was taken for granted. Indeed, the task of devising suitable research methods was not intended to prove the existence of genetic contribution but to test whether major psychoses were transmitted in a Mendelian fashion. In this sense, Mendelian theory was constitutive of the methods devised in the early years at Munich. The fact that Rüdin and Luxenburger found no evidence of simple Mendelian transmission did not deter the diaspora of Munich-trained researchers from continuing to test a Mendelian hypothesis. Kallmann (1946: 309) speculated that predisposition to schizophrenia was 'probably recessive and autosomal'. Slater (1958) insisted on a partially dominant (incompletely penetrant) gene as the simplest explanation for observed rates of schizophrenia in families. But by the 1960s, all attempts to show that schizophrenia was a simple Mendelian disease had failed (Kringlen 1967). The model that became widely favoured among researchers was polygenic inheritance.

Polygenic inheritance was an old idea (Nilsson-Ehle 1909) that gained ascendency by synthesizing several competing perspectives. Though it lacked the elegance of simple Mendelian inheritance, it allowed researchers to unify schizophrenia around a *continuum* ranging from clinical normalcy to schizoid behaviour and deteriorated dementia. This explained why the concept of the 'schizophrenia spectrum' became popular among twin researchers in the 1960s. It also explained the considerable clinical variation found among families and frequencies of illness in the population. The prevalence rates of schizophrenia ruled out a simple monogenic model because most single-gene disorders tended to be rare; it was more common than the population risk of 1 per cent, which indicated that the condition was *familial*. But the familiality of schizophrenia was obscured by the fact that a vast majority of affected individuals had 'negative family histories' (Gottesman 1991: 103).

The heterogeneity of schizophrenia was a major theme throughout the 1960s and 1970s as researchers set about intensively modelling the family incidence of risk. A striking observation of the literature is the contradictory models derived from different datasets or from different combinations of family studies. Isolated pedigrees in Sweden (Böök 1953) or Iceland (Karlsson 1968) were considered alongside meta-analyses of twin studies (Rosenthal 1970; Kidd and Cavalli-Sforza 1973), or re-analyses of large studies (Elston and Campbell 1970; Elston *et al.* 1978). Some claimed that monogenic theories (comprising single locus, two-locus or even four-locus models) fit the observed family data, while others suggested polygenic models were more appropriate.[11] By the 1980s, the oscillation between modified Mendelian and non-Mendelian aetiology settled upon the latter, with a single locus model being virtually ruled out (Rourke *et al.* 1982). The picture that emerged prior to the gene-finding era of linkage studies was a consolidation of *genetic heterogeneity*. Heterogeneity reconfigured the architecture of schizophrenia to allow major loci to form part of a 'polygenic background' comprising multiple genes, incomplete penetrance and non-genetic factors. Thus, there was no gestalt switch to a new 'paradigm' in quantitative (and later 'molecular') genetics but an incremental move towards subordinating Mendelism to a multidimensional model of aetiology.

The move towards a polygenic model was a significant theoretical milestone in psychiatric genetics that achieved a number of practical purposes. Schizophrenia was unified as a multi-genic continuum rather than a disparate collection of genetic and/or non-genetic conditions. It also sustained a position of productive 'uncertainty' within the field (Gottesman 1979) that freed research from having to establish a one-to-one correspondence between genotype and phenotype. Instead, the presumed interaction of genes was necessary to produce a 'threshold liability' (Falconer 1965). Liability was explained by the 'diathesis-stress model', first proposed by Meehl in 1962, which resurrected the nineteenth-century concept of 'diathesis' to propose a genetic theory of constitutional predisposition. In its modern instantiation, diathesis explained how a small number of genes with large effect could lead to specific defects in the central nervous system, such as 'synaptic slippage' (Meehl 1966) or 'neural integration' (Rosenthal 1970). Modern genetic theory enrolled the notion of diathesis to describe a pathological response to environmental stressors.

The diathesis-stress model also provided common theoretical ground for twin and adoption researchers. It enabled twin researchers to continue to infer the existence of several major genes that varied in a 'dynamic system' of nonspecific environmental factors (Gottesman and Shields 1982). For adoption researchers, it showed that genetic factors were 'relatively weak unspecific polygenic dispositions' (Kringlen 1967: 159) influenced by specific environmental influences such as differences in rearing and protective effects. The flexibility of polygenic theory allowed a 'looseness of fit' (Hacking 1992) between rival approaches on both sides of the gene–environment continuum so that 'twin and adoption' studies could be integrated as a unified programme of research. Genetic predisposition could be interpreted so that environmental *or* genetic factors were aetiologically predominant depending on whether one viewed the origins of schizophrenia residing within the individual or within society (Lewontin 1991).

The problem that confronted psychiatric genetics in the 1980s was how to deal with the *uncertainty* of clinical and genetic heterogeneity. In an extreme sense, heterogeneity threatened to dissolve the schizophrenia concept into a cluster of monogenic and environmental disorders. The increasing modification and adaption of genetic models was an effort to develop tractable solutions to this problem. Gottesman and Shields (1982) argued that monogenic theories cannot continue to motivate a search for inherited traits because the path was too difficult to follow; researchers were unlikely to find a 'gene for' schizophrenia because monogenic theories were unable to account for heterogeneity in transmission, nor could they account for schizophrenia being more common than other 'mendelizing' disorders such as cystic fibrosis. By contrast, the flexibility of the polygenic model offered psychiatric genetics an open future. It provided an adequate explanation of the data, by allowing major genes to play some role within a framework of 'common polygenes' unified around a spectrum of schizophrenia, and it permitted an investigation of 'partial risk factors' regarding diathesis and environmental stressors. Rather than an intractable problem, heterogeneity became a resource for driving future research.

By the 1980s, psychiatric genetics reached the following theoretical limits: schizophrenia was a common condition with multiple common small effect genes interacting with environmental exposures to exceed a biological threshold. This was the hypothesis that best fit the twin and adoption data, confirming that schizophrenia was familial even though most patients had no close affected relative. Even today, the 'common disease-common variant' model is the principal hypothesis informing modern genomic research. Although no single major effect gene has been detected we cannot say, following Kuhn (1962), that the 'Mendelian paradigm' collapsed under the weight of its own contradictions. A monogenic theory had borrowed so heavily from other genetic models that it could not be completely refuted. Indeed, the three major models cited by Gottesman and Shields (1982) – (1) distinct heterogeneity, (2) monogenic theory and (3) multifactorial polygenic theory – overlapped to the extent that the 'differences among proponents of different models are simply semantic or simply associated with intuitive preferences' (1982: 219). Polygenic models gained ascendency because it transformed genetic heterogeneity into a potentially tractable problem.

The idea that heterogeneity was now a source of imagination can be seen in the way Gottesman and Shields (1982) enrolled a bewildering range of concepts to open up new pathways of investigation. They introduced the 'endophenotype' concept to measure underlying liability (measurable components unseen by visual methods of diagnosis) that would later have an enormous impact on the field (see Gottesman and Gould 2003). They invoked Waddington's (1966) concept of the 'epigenetic landscape' to explain circuits of gene regulation and their implications for ontogenesis. The 'heuristic implications' of the polygenic system facilitated a vision of multidisciplinary research focusing on:

> partitionable facets of the syndrome such as neurotransmitter receptor morphology, number, and subtype, paranoid features, genetic polymorphisms of proteins in brain and blood, variations in brain scans, and neurophysiology, on the chance that ordinary twin, adoption, and family studies will reveal one or more of the high-value genes segregating in a clear Mendelian pattern.
>
> (Gottesman and Shields 1982: 226)

Rather than killing off the monogenic model, it was now absorbed and modified as a component of the polygenic system. The multifactorial polygenic model provided the most creative path for imagining the future of psychiatric genetics as a genuinely multidisciplinary response to increasing heterogeneity. Propped up by the apparent stability of family studies, heterogeneity had become, by the 1980s, a pliable and productive resource for promising new directions of research.

* * *

For most of its short history, psychiatric genetics has adopted an *epidemiological* approach of clinical and statistical reasoning to generate inferences about the proportion of genetic liability in psychiatric disorders. It was the durability of these styles of reasoning that gradually evolved in relation to criticism and developed a model of heterogeneity that best fit the accumulated data. By the 1980s, there is an emerging vision in which a laboratory style of reasoning will play a more active role in future research. Molecular techniques and brain imaging technologies will hopefully identify and isolate biological markers, and test the statistical hypotheses of the polygenic system. In the gene-mapping era of the 1980s, a new configuration of clinical, statistical, and laboratory styles takes shape around methods of 'genetic linkage'. The proponents of a laboratory style of reasoning conducting linkage studies on small, complex family pedigrees would seek to reconfirm a Mendelian hypothesis. But the limited success of finding single dominant genes once again highlights the ambivalent relationship between the laboratory style of molecular genetics and statistical style of genetic epidemiology. Rather than view these different programmes as competing or incommensurable 'paradigms' (Kendler 2005), we see more evidence of knowledge accumulating and mixing in the life sciences. In later chapters, we show that large-scale psychiatric genetics has become a multidisciplinary infra-structure in which clinical, statistical and laboratory styles of reasoning are once again reorganized. The scale of this enterprise has established a relatively stable domain of tractable problems as well as new forms of ambivalence and uncertainty.

Conclusion

In the first decades of the twentieth century, psychiatric genetics was a small network of investigators with an empirical vision of estimating the inheritance of severe psychoses. A new science of heredity took shape around developments in nosology, scientific genealogy and methodological diversity. However, Rüdin's disturbing legacy reminds us that European biopolitics was constitutive of empirical programmes for testing Mendelian inheritance: genetic prognosis jus-tified the means of removing the 'burden' of mental illness from German society. Attempts to disentangle science from politics are strategies to preserve a sense of continuity and decency between past and present. Whether or not critics were motivated by ideological concerns over eugenic science, or by exposing its methodological flaws, the field of psychiatric genetics has been inexorably shaped by controversy.

The ensemble of family, twin and adoption study methods emerged from a dialectics of radical and moderate criticism, which led to decisive modifications and improvements in design, execution and interpretation. But this is not to say that growing awareness of bias and error ended the controversy. Our concern is not to establish whether the classical methods of psychiatric genetics are intrins-ically flawed, but to draw attention to the efforts of researchers to 'authenticate' and 'stabilize' their style of reasoning (Hacking 1992). We have seen how the literature of twin and adoption studies is a pliable resource to cast an impression of uniformity and validity. Various practices of 'curating' discordant findings are not cynical attempts to conceal flaws, but rhetorical and statistical strategies for stabilizing its core findings. The fact that modern papers routinely cite the cred-ibility of this literature (see Chapter 3 for modern examples) is testament to the field's durability of maintaining a stable narrative of progress which has, for the most part, outlived its critics.

Psychiatric genetics entered a period of enlightenment in the early 1980s that crystallized into a theoretical synthesis of heterogeneity, Mendelian theory and environmental factors. An important factor that contributed to this enlightenment was adoption studies. Adoption studies were an 'event' that substantially altered the tide of opinion. They demonstrated in a way that was far more congruent with cultural opinion that environmental factors modified genetic transmission. The consolidation of a polygenic theory of inheritance provided a common ground and a 'looseness of fit' (Hacking 1985) between the clinical and statisti-cal styles of reasoning that cultivated a theoretical imagination about future research. The 1980s produced a concise statement of aetiology that has changed little today. The theoretical retreat from simple Mendelism is not consistent with

Kuhnian 'paradigms'. Instead, we find a gradual modification and preservation of theoretical models that coalesced into a distinctly flexible system. The polygenic multifactorial threshold model transformed the profound uncertainty of clinical and genetic heterogeneity into a promising vision that anticipated many of the developments of twenty-first-century genomic psychiatry.

Notes

1 Shorter (1997) tells us that professional psychiatry had reached a 'dead end' by the end of the nineteenth century. In the absence of any major advances in pathological anatomy, asylums had become warehouses and 'factories' of incurable patients (Dowbiggin 1991).
2 As Berrios and Hauser (1988: 817) explain, Kraepelin 'used deterioration as a *research or methodological criterion* in order to search for a predictive clinical picture, which would in turn become a *clinical criterion*'.
3 Kraepelin describes his discovery as follows:

> What convinced me of the superiority of the clinical method of diagnosis (followed here) over the traditional one, was the *certainty with which we could predict (in conjunction with our new concept of disease) the future course of events.* Thanks to it the student can find his [*sic*] way more easily in the difficult subject of psychiatry.
>
> (1896: xx)

4 Following Kraepelin's famous splitting of psychotic illness into affective and non-affective components, dementia praecox was characterized by flattened affect, defects in volition, disordered cognitive functioning and early onset illness with poor prognosis. Rüdin also systematically excluded the group of 'paraphrenias' consisting of non-deteriorating, paranoid hallucinatory syndromes with relatively better outcomes (Kendler and Zerbin-Rüdin 1996).
5 The term concordance usually refers to the presence of the same trait in twin-pairs, though the precise definition is more probabilistic than discrete. In a strict sense, it refers to the probability that a pair of individuals will both have a certain characteristic, given that one of the pair has the characteristic.
6 In the 1920s and 1930s, Germany was the world centre of twin research. Much of the biology of twins had been established by Weinberg (1909a, 1909b). It was Weinberg who inferred that monozygotic or identical twins result from the splitting of a single egg sharing 100 per cent genetic similarity, and dizygotic or fraternal twins result from the simultaneous fertilization of two separate eggs sharing 50 per cent genetic similarity. Hermann Siemens first used the twin study design in 1924 to investigate the inheritance of skin moles. Consistent with the views of degeneration theory, Siemens warned of the collapse of European civilization and the need for voluntary sterilization of 'pathological persons'. Like Siemens, Luxenburger had also supported the 1933 sterilization law and insisted on the sterilization of schizophrenic patients. In 1934, he wrote that being the identical twin sibling of an affected person was a criterion for being subject to racial hygienic measures.
7 Gottesman and Shields had worked under Eliot Slater using the twin registry at the Maudlesy and Bethlem Royal Hospital. Their 1966 study (published in 1972) was based on 16 years of consecutive admissions.
8 Boyle (1990) argues it is impossible to gauge similarity among concordant twins across studies, and impossible to establish similarity to a parent concept of schizophrenia which is itself ill-defined. The concept of schizophrenia spectrum over-extends the similarity of symptoms to establish concordance across studies. Boyle

uses some compelling analogies to make her point but does not ground her argument in the diagnostic criteria (because she rejects such criteria).

9 Since the 1970s, geneticists and twin researchers have preferred calculating concordance using the *probandwise* method, which expresses the percentage of proband subjects found independently with the same trait; this includes the possibility that a proband will be the others co-twin. It is assumed that the issue of 'double ascertainment' (counting twins twice) in a hospital sample will be balanced by pairs in which neither twin is ascertained as an index case (Allen *et al.* 1967). The pairwise method applies to *twin pairs*, while the probandwise method applies to *individuals*; it is calculation of the latter that enables risk rates to be reported for population prevalence (McGue 1992). But as a measure of concordance, the probandwise method is dependent on the accuracy of sampling a population. The problem, as Boyle (1990) sees it, is that one can never be sure that a sample *is* representative of the population because the parameters of *the* population are unknown. In the case of twin studies, there is no guarantee that the proportion of MZ and DZ twins is representative of the population of schizophrenia, especially if twins are sampled from hospital populations, which tend to inflate the concordance of MZ twins with schizophrenia.

10 There is also the issue that double ascertainment is perhaps more likely to occur among MZ twins for precisely the same reasons cited by early critics of twin research, i.e. they are more likely to come to the attention of researchers, they are treated more similar by others, and they tend to live closer together.

11 Researchers such as Crittenden (1961), Falconer (1965, 1967), Reich and colleagues (1972, 1975) and Gottesman and Shields (1967) began to develop multifactorial threshold models to explain the data on schizophrenia prevalence in relatives. The problem that divided researchers was that modified monogenic models explained the data equally well. By the 1970s, researchers had engaged in statistical modelling and theory-testing using Kallmann's original family data. At first, a single locus model was shown to be adequate in explaining patterns of variation (Elston and Campbell 1970), but was later rejected in favour of multifactorial models (Elston *et al.* 1978).

References

Allen G, Harvald B and Shields J (1967) Measures of twin concordance. *Acta Genetica et Statistica Medica* 17: 475–481.

Berrios GE and Hauser R (1988) The early development of Kraepelin's ideas on classification: A conceptual history. *Psychological Medicine* 18: 813–821.

Böök JA (1953) A genetic and neuropsychiatric investigation of a North Swedish population. *Acta Genet Stat Med* (Basel) 4: 1–100.

Boyle M (1990) *Schizophrenia: A Scientific Delusion?* New York: Routledge.

Brockington IF and Leff JP (1979) Schizo-affective psychosis: Definitions and incidence. *Psychological Medicine* 9(1): 91–99.

Craddock N and Owen MJ (2005) The beginning of the end for the Kraepelinian dichotomy. *The British Journal of Psychiatry* 186(5): 364–366.

Craddock N and Owen MJ (2010) The Kraepelinian dichotomy: Going, going ... but still not gone. *The British Journal of Psychiatry* 196(2): 92–95.

Crittenden LB (1961) An interpretation of familial aggregation based on multiple genetic and environmental factors. *Annals of the New York Academy of Science* 91: 769–780.

Damerow H (1865) Zur Statistik der Provinzial-Irren-Heil- und Pflege-Anstalt bei Halle vom 1. November 1844 bis Ende December 1863. *Allgemeine Zeitschrift für Psychiatrie* 22: 219–251.

Davenport CB (1911) *Heredity in Relation to Eugenics.* New York: Henry Holt and Co.

Dowbiggin IR (1991) *Inheriting Madness: Professionalization and Psychiatric Knowledge in Nineteenth Century France*. Berkeley: University of California Press.

Elston RC and Campbell MA (1970) Schizophrenia: Evidence for the major gene hypothesis. *Behavior Genetics* 1: 3–10.

Elston RC, Namboodiri KK, Spence MA, *et al.* (1978) A genetic study of schizophrenia pedigrees. II. One-locus hypotheses. *Neuropsychobiology* 4: 193–206.

Engstrom EJ, Burgmair W and Weber M (2016) Psychiatric governance, *völkisch* corporatism, and the German Research Institute of Psychiatry in Munich (1912–26). Part 2. *History of Psychiatry* 27(2): 137–152.

Essen-Möller E (1941) Psychiatrische Untersuchungen an einer Serie von Zwillingen. *Acta Psychiatrica et Neurologica* (Suppl. 23). Copenhagen: Munksgaard.

Falconer DS (1965) The inheritance of liability to certain diseases, estimated from the incidence among relatives. *Annals of Human Genetics* 29: 51–76.

Falconer DS (1967) The inheritance of liability to diseases with variable age of onset with particular reference to diabetes mellitus. *Annals of Human Genetics* 31: 1–20.

Foucault M (1972) *The Archaeology of Knowledge*. London: Tavistock.

Foucault M (2008) *Psychiatric Power: Lectures at the College De France, 1973–74*. Edited by J Lagrange and translated by G Burchell. Basingstoke: Palgrave Macmillan.

Galton F (1876) A theory of heredity. *Journal of the Anthropological Institute* 5: 329–348.

Gausemeier B (2008) *Pedigree vs. Mendelism. Concepts of Heredity in Psychiatry before and after 1900*. Preprint 343 [Conference: A Cultural History of Heredity IV: Heredity in the Century of the Gene]. Max Planck Institute for the History of Science, pp. 149–162.

Gausemeier B (2015) Pedigrees of madness: The study of heredity in nineteenth and early twentieth psychiatry. *History and Philosophy of the Life Sciences* 36(4): 467–483.

Gejman PV (1997) Ernst Rüdin and Nazi euthanasia: Another stain on his career. *American Journal of Medical Genetics* 74: 455–456.

Gershon ES (1997) Ernst Rüdin, a Nazi psychiatrist and geneticist. *American Journal of Medical Genetics* 74: 457–458.

Gilbert GN and Mulkay M (1984) *Opening Pandora's Box: A Sociological Analysis of Scientists' Discourse*. Cambridge: Cambridge University Press.

Goddard HH (1914) *Feeblemindedness: Its Causes and Consequences*. New York: Macmillan.

Gottesman II (1979) Schizophrenia and genetics: Towards understanding uncertainty. *Psychiatric Annals* 9(1): 54–78.

Gottesman II (1991) *Schizophrenia genesis*. New York: W.H. Freeman & Company.

Gottesman II and Bertelsen A (1996) Legacy of German psychiatric genetics: Hindsight is always 20/20. *American Journal of Medical Genetics* 67: 317–322.

Gottesman II and Gould TD (2003) The endophenotype concept in psychiatry: Etymology and strategic intentions. *American Journal of Psychiatry* 160: 636–645.

Gottesman II and Shields J (1966) Schizophrenia in twins: 16 years' consecutive admissions to a psychiatric clinic. *British Journal of Psychiatry* 112: 809–818.

Gottesman II and Shields J (1967) A polygenic theory of schizophrenia. *Proceedings of the National Academy of Sciences* 58(1): 199–205.

Gottesman II and Shields J (1972) *Schizophrenia and Genetics: A Twin Study Vantage Point*. New York: Academic Press.

Gottesman II and Shields J (1982) *Schizophrenia: The Epigenetic Puzzle*. Cambridge: Cambridge University Press.

Grassmann K (1896) Kritischer Ueberblick über die gegenwärtige Lehre von der Erblichkeit der Psychosen. *Allgemeine Zeitschrift für Psychiatrie* 52: 960–1022.

Hacking I (1985) Styles of scientific reasoning. In J Rajchman and C West (eds). *Post-Analytic Philosophy*. New York: Columbia University Press, pp. 145–165.

Hacking I (1992) 'Style' for historians and philosophers. *Studies in the History and Philosophy of Science* 23(1): 1–20.

Hagen FW (1876) *Statistische Untersuchungen über Geisteskrankheiten. Nach den Ergebnissen der ersten 25 Jahre der Kreis Irrenanstalt zu Erlangen unter Mitwirkung von deren Hülfsärzten*. Erlangen: Besold.

Hedgecoe A (2001) Schizophrenia and the narrative of enlightened geneticization. *Social Studies of Science* 31(6): 875–911.

Heston LL (1966) Psychiatric disorders in foster home reared children of schizophrenic mothers. *British Journal of Psychiatry* 112: 819–825.

Hippius H, Möller HJ, Müller N and Neundörfer-Kohl G (2008) *The University Department of Psychiatry in Munich: From Kraepelin and His Predecessors to Molecular Psychiatry*. Heidelberg: Springer.

Jackson DD (1960) A critique of the literature on the genetics of schizophrenia. In D Jackson (ed.). *The Etiology of Schizophrenia*. New York: Basic Books, pp. 37–87.

Joseph J (2003) *The Gene Illusion: Genetic Research in Psychiatry and Psychology under the Microscope*. Herefordshire: PCCS Books.

Joseph J (2013) Ernst Rüdin: Hitler's racial hygiene mastermind. *Journal of the History of Biology* 46: 1–30.

Jung W (1866) Noch einige Untersuchungen über die Erblichkeit der Seelenstörungen. *Allgemeine Zeitschrift für Psychiatrie* 23: 211–257.

Kallmann FJ (1946) The genetic theory of schizophrenia: An analysis of 691 schizophrenic twin index families. *American Journal of Psychiatry* 103: 309–322.

Karlsson JL (1968) Genealogic studies of schizophrenia. In D Rosenthal and S Kety (eds). *The Transmission of Schizophrenia*. New York: Pergamon Press, pp. 85–94.

Kendler KS (1997) Reply to Gejman, Gershon, and Lerer and Segman. *American Journal of Medical Genetics* 74: 461–463.

Kendler KS (2005) Psychiatric genetics: A methodologic critique. *American Journal of Psychiatry* 162: 3–11.

Kendler KS (2015) A joint history of the nature of genetic variation and the nature of schizophrenia. *Molecular Psychiatry* 20(1): 77–83.

Kendler KS and Zerbin-Rüdin E (1996) Abstract and review of 'Studien über Vererbung und Entstehung Geistiger Storungen. I. Zur Vererbung und Neuentstehung der Dementia praecox' [Studies on the Inheritance and Origin of Mental Illness: I. To the Problem of the Inheritance and Primary Origin of Dementia Praecox]. *American Journal of Medical Genetics* 67: 338–342.

Kety SS, Rosenthal D, Wender PH, *et al.* (1968) The types and prevalence of mental illness in the biological and adoptive families of adopted schizophrenics. In D Rosenthal and S Kety (eds). *The Transmission of Schizophrenia*. New York: Pergamon Press, pp. 345–362.

Kevles DJ (1985) *In the Name of Eugenics: Genetics and the Uses of Human Heredity*. Berkeley: University of California Press.

Kidd KK and Cavalli-Sforza LL (1973) An analysis of the genetics of schizophrenia. *Social Biology* 20: 254–265.

Knorr-Cetina K (1999) *Epistemic Cultures: How the Sciences Make Knowledge*. Cambridge, MA: Harvard University Press.

Kraepelin E (1896) *Psychiatrie. Ein Lehrbuch für Studirende und Ärzte.* Leipzig: Barth.

Kraepelin E (1899/1902) *Clinical Psychiatry: A Textbook for Students and Physicians, 6th Edition.* Translated by AR Defendorf. New York: Macmillan.

Kraepelin E (1962) *One Hundred Years of Psychiatry.* New York: Philosophical Library.

Krafft-Ebing R (1869) Ueber die prognostische Bedeutung der erblichen Anlage zum Irresein. *Allgemeine Zeitschrift für Psychiatrie* 26: 438–456.

Kringlen E (1967) *Heredity and Environment in the Functional Psychoses: An Epidemiological-Clinical Study.* Oslo: Universitetsforlaget.

Kringlen E (1976) Twins: Still our best method. *Schizophrenia Bulletin* 2: 429–433.

Kuhn TS (1962) *The Structure of Scientific Revolutions.* Chicago: University of Chicago Press.

Lerer B and Segman RH (1997) Correspondence regarding German psychiatric genetics and Ernst Rüdin. *American Journal of Medical Genetics* 74: 459–460.

Lewontin RC (1991) *Biology as Ideology.* New York: Harper Perennial.

Lorenz O (1898) *Lehrbuch der gesammten wissenschaftlichen Genealogie.* Berlin: W. Hertz.

McGue M (1992) When assessing twin concordance, use the probandwise not the pairwise rate. *Schizophrenia Bulletin* 18(2): 171–176.

Meehl PE (1966) The compleat autocerebroscopist: A thought-experiment on Professor Feigl's mind-body identity thesis. In K Feyerabend and G Maxwell (eds). *Mind, Matter, and Method: Essays in Philosophy and Science in Honor of Herbert Feigl.* Minneapolis: University of Minnesota Press, pp. 103–180.

Mellon CD (1996) *Hereditary Madness: The Evolution of Psychiatric Genetic Thought.* New Mexico: Genetics Heritage Press.

Myers G (1991) Writing biology: Texts in the social construction of scientific knowledge. *Journal of the History of Biology* 24(3): 521–527.

Neale JM and Oltmanns TF (1980) *Schizophrenia.* New York: John Wiley & Sons.

Neel JV and Schull WJ (1954) *Human Heredity.* Chicago: University of Chicago Press.

Nilsson-Ehle NH (1909) Kreuzungsuntersuchungen an Hafer und Weizen. *Lunds Univiversitets Årsskrift* Ns sec 2, 5(2): 1–122.

Price B (1950) Primary biases in twin studies: A review of prenatal and natal difference-producing factors in monozygotic pairs. *The American Journal of Human Genetics* 2(4): 293–352.

Proctor RN (1988) *Racial Hygiene: Medicine Under the Nazis.* Cambridge, MA: Harvard University Press.

Reich T, Cloninger CR and Guze SB (1975) The multifactorial model of disease transmission: I. Description of the model and its use in psychiatry. *British Journal of Psychiatry* 127: 1–10.

Reich T, James JW and Morris CA (1972) The use of multiple thresholds in determining the mode of transmission of semi-continuous traits. *Annals of Human Genetics* 36: 163–184.

Ritter HJ and Roelcke V (2005) Psychiatric genetics in Munich and Basel between 1925 and 1945: Programs-practices-cooperative arrangements. *Osiris* 20(1): 263–288.

Rosanoff AJ and Orr FI (1911) A study of insanity in the light of the Mendelian theory. *American Journal of Psychiatry* 68(2): 221–261.

Rosanoff AJ, Handy LM, Plesset IR, et al. (1934) The etiology of so-called schizophrenic psychoses. *American Journal of Psychiatry* 91: 247–286.

Rose S, Lewontin RC and Kamin LJ (1984) *Not in Our Genes: Biology, Ideology and Human Nature.* London: Pantheon.

Rosenthal D (1962a) Familial concordance by sex with respect to schizophrenia. *Psychological Bulletin* 59: 401–421.

Rosenthal D (1962b) Problems of sampling and diagnosis in the major twin studies of schizophrenia. *Journal of Psychiatric Research* 1: 116–134.

Rosenthal D (1970) *Genetic Theory and Abnormal Behavior*. New York: McGraw-Hill.

Rosenthal D (1972) Three adoption studies of heredity in the schizophrenic disorders. *International Journal of Mental Health* 1: 63–75.

Rourke DH, Gottesman II, Suarez BK, *et al.* (1982) Refutation of the general single-locus model for the etiology of schizophrenia. *American Journal of Human Genetics* 34: 630–649.

Rüdin E (1911) Einige Wege und Ziele der Familienforschung mit Rücksicht auf die Psychiatrie. *Zeitschrift für die gesamte Neurologie und Psychiatrie* 7: 487–585.

Rüdin E (1916) *Studien über Vererbung und Entstehung geistiger Störungen, Bd. 1: Zur Vererbung und Neuentstehung der Dementia Praecox*. Berlin: Springer.

Schulze TG, Fangerau H and Propping P (2004) From degeneration to genetic susceptibility, from eugenics to genethics, from Bezugsziffer to LOD score: The history of psychiatric genetics. *International Review of Psychiatry* 16(4): 246–259.

Shields J, Gottesman II and Slater E (1967) Kallmann's 1946 schizophrenia twin study in the light of new information. *Acta Psychiatrica Scandinavica* 43(4): 385–396.

Shorter E (1997) *A History of Psychiatry: From the Era of the Asylum to the Age of Prozac*. New York: Wiley.

Slater E (1958) The monogenic theory of schizophrenia. *Acta Genetica Sinica* 8: 50–56.

Sommer R (1901) *Diagnostik der Geisteskrankheiten für praktische Ärzte und Studierende*. Berlin: Urban & Schwarzenberg.

Sommer R (1912) Bericht über den II. Kurs mit Kongreß für Familienforschung, Vererbungs- und Regenerationslehre in Gießen vom 9. bis 13. April 1912. *Klinik für psychische und nervöse Krankheiten* 7: 150–342.

Strömgren E (1993) Fini Schulsinger's contribution to psychiatric research in genetic epidemiology. *Acta Psychiatrica Scandinavica* (Suppl. 370): 11–13.

Sullivan PS, Kendler KS and Neale MC (2003) Schizophrenia as a complex trait: Evidence from a meta-analysis of twin studies. *Archives of General Psychiatry* 60(12): 1187–1192.

Waddington CH (1966) *Principles of the Development and Differentiation*. London: Macmillan.

Weber MM (1991) Psychiatrie als Rassenhygiene. Ernst Rüdin und die Deutsche Forschungsanstalt für Psychiatrie in Munchen. *Med Gesellschaft Geschichte* 10: 149–169.

Weber MM (1993) *Ernst Rüdin: Eine kritische Biographie*. Berlin: Springer.

Weber MM (1996) Ernst Rüdin, 1874–1952: A German psychiatrist and geneticist. *American Journal of Medical Genetics* 67: 323–331.

Weinberg W (1903) Pathologische Vererbung und genealgischklinische Statistik. *Deutsches Archiv für Klinische Medizin* 78: 521–540.

Weinberg W (1908) Über den Nachweis der Vererbung beim Menschen. *Jahreshefte des Verein für vaterlandische Naturkunde zu Württemberg* 64: 369–382.

Weinberg W (1909a) Die Anlage zur Mehrlingsgeburt beim Menschen und ihre Vererbung. *Arch Rass-u Ges Biol* 6: 322–339, 470–482, 609–630.

Weinberg W (1909b) Über Vererbungsgesetze beim Menschen. *Zeitschrift für Induktive Abstammungs- und Vererbungslehre* 2(1): 276–330.

Weinberg W (1913) Auslesewirkungen bei biologisch-statistischen Problemen. *Archiv für Rassen Gesellschaftsbiologie* 10: 417–451, 557–581.

Zerbin-Rüdin E and Kendler KS (1996) Ernst Rudin (1874–1952) and his genealogic-demographic department in Munich (1917–1986): An introduction to their family studies of schizophrenia. *American Journal of Medical Genetics* 67: 332–337.

3 The rhetoric of complexity

In the previous chapter, we examined how a polygenic model of schizophrenia emerged as a relatively stable explanation of common disease. Rival monogenic theories were not discounted as such but absorbed and modified within the polygenic system. By the mid-1980s, the search for single dominant genes was resurrected as the prospects of using genetic linkage maps entered a new phase of optimism and competition. Following the retraction of several prominent discoveries, scientists working within the field of psychiatric genetics began to adopt a highly reflexive narrative of caution and responsibility. Conditions such as schizophrenia and bipolar disorder were reconsidered as *complex* traits. Such models of genetic complexity have gained significant ground, leaving few psychiatric traits or conditions without a putative biological explanation.

In the context of these, and other controversies that have dogged this field, we suggest that the turn to complexity accomplishes more than merely a description of the natural world, it also performs rhetorical work. Biomedical scientists are engaging in the management of intellectual responsibility. Among their accounts of past failure and future progress, notions of complexity provide theoretical coherence and respectability to an otherwise ambivalent relationship between genetic and non-genetic factors.

In this chapter, we show the ways in which narratives of psychiatric genetics employ a variety of invocations of complexity to present psychiatric genetics research as a cautious, flexible and responsible science. Accounts of complexity do not so much replace a simple, reductionist genetic hypothesis than provide a means to rescue research programmes from the failures of the past. The development of a vision of post-genomic complexity is accomplished through strategies and techniques of persuasion and fact-construction. Psychiatric genetics provides a case study of the defence of a controversial science: in this case, narratives drawing on complexity account for past failures and neutralize criticisms of genetic determinism by incorporating both the unknown and 'non-genetic' factors within their theoretical models.

Failure of linkage studies

Technological developments in the 1970s and 1980s set the foundations for great optimism in human molecular genetics. Recombinant DNA techniques and advances in chromosomal mapping allowed researchers to construct genetic linkage maps to identify the relative positions of mutations. A precursor to the HGP, linkage maps led to 'highly competitive races' (Cook-Deegan 1994) to identify genetic mutations *for* diseases. But it was not the gene hunting per se that precipitated these advances, it was the systematic analysis of reference families with well-defined pedigrees from whom DNA was readily available. In North America, for instance, the pedigrees of Mormon and Amish families provided the bedrock for collaborative efforts to construct genetic linkage maps.

Amidst the high-profile successes of this period – including the identification of the 'genes for' cystic fibrosis in 1985 (Tsui *et al.* 1985; Wainwright *et al.* 1985; Knowlton *et al.* 1985) and Huntington's disease in 1993 (The Huntington's Disease Collaborative Research Group 1993) – psychiatric genetics was inspired to apply the same techniques to locate genes for common psychiatric disorders. A raft of highly visible papers reported successes in using linkage studies to identify, amongst others, 'genes for' schizophrenia (Sherrington *et al.* 1988), bipolar disorder (Baron *et al.* 1987; Egeland *et al.* 1987) and alcoholism (Blum *et al.* 1990). But success soon turned to disappointment when other teams failed to replicate the findings for schizophrenia (Kennedy *et al.* 1988), manic depression (Detera-Wadleigh *et al.* 1987; Hodgkinson *et al.* 1987) and alcoholism (Gelernter *et al.* 1991, 1993). Authors of two of the 'successful' linkage studies that had claimed to find a single dominant gene for manic depression published retractions in *Nature* (Kelsoe *et al.* 1989; Baron *et al.* 1993). And as one commentator has noted, published retractions in high-impact journals are 'unusual and embarrassing events among scientists' (Berkowitz 1996: 43).

Our post-mortem of one linkage study highlights the difficulties in claiming simple genetic causation. Egeland and colleagues chose an Amish pedigree in Pennsylvania for their linkage study of manic depression. In 1987, they published their findings in *Nature*, confidently asserting that 'a dominant gene conferring a strong predisposition to manic depressive disease' (Egeland *et al.* 1987: 783) had been found on chromosome 11. However, in the same issue, two related studies found no linkage between the genetic markers identified and manic depression in three Icelandic families (Hodgkinson *et al.* 1987) and three North American families (Detera-Wadleigh *et al.* 1987). While *Nature* was careful to report these discrepancies, the Egeland study clearly occupied the spotlight, with the editor asserting that 'the use of DNA markers has shown that manic-depressive illness can be caused by a single gene' (Robertson 1987: 755).[1]

In a later issue of the same year, Baron *et al.* (1987) reported close linkage between manic depression and a region of DNA on the X chromosome. The researchers concluded: '[t]hese results provide confirmation that a major psychiatric disorder can be caused by a single genetic defect' (Baron *et al.* 1987: 289).

Despite the difficulties of replication and genetic heterogeneity, there was clearly a resurgence of support for a simple model of genetic causation for manic depression. However, by 1989, readers of *Nature* would have detected a tidal change in the waves of retraction and re-evaluation of the single gene hypothesis. For instance, Egeland's group published a re-evaluation of their own findings (Kelsoe *et al.* 1989) based on a change in diagnosis for two family members as well as new data from additional families. Two members of the Amish pedigree received a diagnosis of manic depression in the absence of the putative markers and an examination of an additional branch of the original pedigree found evidence against linkage. This reversal suggests that a theoretical model of genetic heterogeneity cannot, in itself, explain away or defend the single gene hypothesis.

In acknowledging this 'false start on manic depression', the editor of *Nature* conceded that the hypothesis of 'a gene on chromosome 11 could predispose to manic depression was calculated on a delicate balance of uncertainties' (Robertson 1989: 222). In hindsight, such failures to replicate, it was argued, 'highlight many of the problems that can be anticipated in genetic linkage studies of common and complex neuropsychiatric disorders' (Kelsoe *et al.* 1989: 242). In both articles, the term 'complex' signals an aetiological reversal allowing scientists to impute the inadequacy of linkage analysis and defer hope to new technologies on the horizon. An admission of aetiological complexity amounted to an explanation for failure.

In light of such problems, the field of psychiatric genetics reverted to a complex model of disease, recapitulating the statistical style of reasoning of the early biometric and epidemiological studies (see Chapter 1). Psychiatric disorders were now understood to be the product of several genes, which may be interacting non-additively, each with only a small effect, with different variations in each family (Gershon and Cloninger 1994). Technological developments derived from the HGP in the late 1990s and 2000s, such as high-density Single Nucleotide Polymorphisms (SNP) maps and high-throughput genotyping introduced the possibility of new ways of combining laboratory and statistical reasoning, which renewed optimism in the potential to genetically dissect complex disease. The articles analysed in this chapter are drawn from the bloom of review articles that provide accounts of this optimistic turn. However, the advent of complexity within this field is not a 'paradigm shift'. The shift from 'genes for' to 'susceptibility genes' involves a scaling up of gene identification programmes without necessarily incorporating notions of *nonlinear* complexity.

Rhetoric in scientific writing

We define 'rhetoric' broadly as the everyday organization of descriptions and explanations for managing candidates of truth and falsehood in scientific discourse. It also lends itself to the analysis of scientific controversies insofar as constructions of fact subtly or explicitly counter alternative descriptions (Dillon 1991). Scientific controversies can be analysed in similar ways to evaluate the techniques of rendering factual accounts robust and persuasive. Descriptions of fact are reworked and reframed to undermine competing accounts, and protected or insulated from counter-claims. For the purposes of our own analysis, in this chapter, we suggest that the activity of formulating scientific accounts of reality take on both an *action* and an *epistemological* orientation (Potter 1996).

While research interviews are interesting in their own right for showing how scientists' claims are subtly undermined by the contingency of their own verbal accounts (Gilbert and Mulkay 1984), written accounts of science have broader rhetorical reach. We maintain that journal articles provide an important site for evaluating the rhetorical dimension of language, the analysis of which helps us to understand the stability of psychiatric genetics in terms of the 'self-authenticating character of styles of reasoning' (Hacking 1992: 14). For this reason, we focus our rhetorical/discursive approach on the analysis of review articles.

The review article has surfaced as an important form of writing in the sciences, especially where there have been steady increases in published information and rapid developments in research (Virgo 1971; Bazerman 1988). Analysing these articles is constructive for two reasons. First, they can be considered the 'official' descriptions of scientific activity; their credibility as exemplary statements of the field is sanctioned by processes of peer review and publication. Second, these articles reveal a relatively stable genre of professional writing. Myers (1991) has argued that writers of review articles give the literature of a field a narrative form, inviting readers to extend and continue the story. As the narrative of the field is developed, key events and controversies are routinely cited (or omitted) in ways that provide coherence and stability. Sinding (1996) has also noted that review articles can be treated as a literary genre that provide opportunities for constructing and reconstructing knowledge claims. Review articles are important not only because they provide information but because they engage in multiple activities such as popularization (Hilgartner 1990), fact-construction (Myers 1992) and narrative reconstruction (Hedgecoe 2001). Indeed, it is the 'performative' (Brown and Michael 2003) nature of speculative and programmatic claims that seek to bridge disciplinary boundaries, gather allies and sanitize the past. Our work extends this tradition of textual analysis, taking the review article as a clearly emerging genre of scientific accountability.

From our reading of the literature of psychiatric genetics, we noticed a particular of genre of review writing. These articles are neither research papers nor reviews of research, but locate the field in a wider narrative of development. Taking the period of 1999–2008, the decade preceding our entry into the field, we narrowed down our sample to 35 articles and then selected ten articles for close analysis. In the following analysis, we describe the main rhetorical themes in these articles, and present key extracts to demonstrate the devices and techniques used to construct the narrative of the field.

Accounting for complexity

A common element of the narrative of psychiatric genetics is the emergence of complexity in accounting for past failures, justifying 'delays' in gene discovery, and justifying new methods. We identify two temporal strategies through which a narrative of psychiatric genetics is organized (Arribas-Ayllon *et al.* 2010):

- *Retrospective accounting*: in which accounts are oriented to manage the failures of genetic linkage studies. This strategy involves the routine citation of twin studies as evidence to defend the genetic hypothesis.
- *Prospective accounting*: in which accounts are oriented to the careful construction of the future, invoking the technical difficulties of complexity to moderate optimistic expectations.

All the articles examined contain these temporal strategies that navigate a narrative of problems, progress and potential. In this section, we show that descriptions of complexity are composed of competing assertions about the progress of psychiatric genetics. The emerging view of complexity is one that attributes increasing significance to polygenic, multifactorial causation, distancing the field from a simple Mendelian model of inheritance. Yet, as we shall see, this view has retained an interest in searches for single genes with medium-to-large effects associated with psychiatric disorders.

One way to accommodate the 'mixed findings' of previous studies into a coherent model of complexity is to construct these descriptions as 'factual' accounts. We found that the authors within our sample used a number of rhetorical techniques to direct attention away from speculations within the field and towards the 'objective' mechanisms of disease. An early example from within our sample of such a process can be found in the high impact journal *Molecular Psychiatry*:

> However, common illnesses pose much greater challenges for geneticists because, in the majority of cases, they result from the combined action of a number of different genes (each of which may result in only a modest increase or decrease in liability) as well as environmental influences; a witches' brew termed polygenic, multifactorial causation. Further complexities include the possibility of non-additive genetic effects, including gene–gene interactions (epistasis), and also potential gene–environment interactions.
>
> (Owen *et al.* 2000: 22)

We found that authors who presented the most circumspect accounts of progress were often collaborators in the new generation of GWAS. Working up complexity into a 'fact' provides justification for the collection of large samples to identify small-effect genes for common psychiatric disorders. Making this case requires distancing common illnesses from the study of large-effect genes. This is accomplished by contrasting rare, monogenic disorders ('However ...') from 'common illnesses', which 'pose much greater challenges for geneticists'. The transformation of speculation into factual descriptions is accomplished by casting complexity of common illnesses as the primary 'complicating' agent (e.g. 'they result from the *combined action*'). Complexity is described as the effects of multiple gene interactions and 'potential gene-environment interactions'. While this offers a more definite description of complexity than some accounts, there is a tension between uncertainty and object-reality. Various markers of modalization (*'may* result in', *'possibility of'* and *'potential'*) suggest that the nature of disease action is provisional and uncertain, which transfers speculation and uncertainty from the field to the disorders. Complexity becomes a constitutive part of the phenomena being studied. These processes of reification and ambivalence are recurrent features of descriptions in which new methods are proposed. Below is another example, published in the journal *Human Molecular Genetics* during the same year:

> The transmission patterns of psychiatric disorders are undeniably complex. It is likely that a variety of genetic as well as environmental pathways can increase one's susceptibility to a given psychiatric disorder. This is the concept of equifinality, where different initial conditions can lead to the same endpoint ... it is anticipated that to increase risk for many complex disorders, multiple deleterious genetic variants are required in combination. This is called multiplicative, epistatic, oligo- or multigenic inheritance.
>
> (Stoltenberg and Burmeister 2000: 927)

Addressing an audience well-versed in methodological issues but not specialist in psychiatric disorders, this description forms part of the growing realization that many susceptibility alleles will be common variants rather than rare mutations. Again, the existence of complexity appears to justify new methodological approaches of psychiatric genetic studies. Claiming that psychiatric disorders 'are undeniably complex' orients to an apparent consensus in the field. Markers of modalization ('It is likely that ... can increase') mitigate commitment to the provisional assertion of gene–environment interaction as an explanation for increased susceptibility. This is formalized by the propositional statement: 'This is the concept of equifinality.' Impersonal constructions ('it is anticipated that') produce a similar effect. They allow authors to distance themselves from conjecture when describing epistatic inheritance. Any sense of conjecture or interpretation is glossed by the propositional statement that follows ('This is called multiplicative ... inheritance'). These formal descriptions of complexity succeed in transforming 'disease complication' into a reified phenomenon.

All the articles in our sample employed this multifactorial model of complexity to make claims about promising new strategies and methods. This approach has the benefit of confirming the genetic hypothesis while at the same time eschewing reductionism by enrolling non-genetic factors. However, such descriptions of complexity were frequently accompanied by ambivalence and moderation, which points to a curious relationship between simple Mendelian and multifactorial models. If psychiatric disorders are 'undeniably' complex, why do authors need to *routinely* account for non-Mendelism?

To answer this question, we turn to two articles that illustrate competing accounts of methodological directions within psychiatric genetics. The first article, in the high impact journal *Trends in Genetics*, presents a methodological argument to a broad audience of geneticists. Evans *et al.* (2001) describe how linkage studies can overcome phenotypic heterogeneity (poorly defined diagnostic boundaries) by carrying out analyses under several diagnostic definitions. In the case of schizophrenia and bipolar disorder, diagnostic complexity may account for the clinical similarity of these disorders. Linkage studies of large family sets have produced 'mixed results', confirming that psychiatric disorders 'cannot entirely be accounted for by one or a few major loci' (Evans *et al.* 2001: 36). However, rather than dismissing linkage approaches, Evans *et al.* argue for combining linkage analysis with models of 'complex inheritance':

> Although linkage analysis has failed to detect loci in a number of study sets, it is striking that several genome-wide scans, in both single extended pedigrees and large sets of families and sibling pairs, have identified loci showing highly significant linkage. It seems probable, therefore, that susceptibility to psychiatric illness reflects a mixture of the two genetic models.
>
> (Evans *et al.* 2001: 36)

Notions of complexity are usually invoked to distance the new generation of research from monogenic theories, but this passage describes how genome-wide scans, designed to detect genes of small effect, can be used to identify genes of large effect. The methods used to explore complex genetics also detect Mendelian-like ('highly significant linkage') genes. This mixing of simple and complex models seems at odds with claims that complex genetics incorporates environmental factors, claims which neutralize criticisms that genetic psychiatry is reductionist (Rose *et al.* 1984; Rose 1995, 1998). In fact, this is precisely the strategy that Evans *et al.* employ towards the end of their article:

> Do genetics and genomics hold all the answers? Some commentators challenge the whole reductionist approach of genetics applied to psychiatry, dismissing it as a distraction from the importance of social and cultural influences. In truth, studies of genetic modulation and/or genetic variation are perfectly well suited to explore environmental influences, and to move beyond mere description towards a mechanistic and mathematical understanding of biological connectivity and emergent properties.
>
> (Evans *et al.* 2001: 39)

The accusation that psychiatric genetics is a 'distraction' from research into socio-cultural factors is countered by attributing agency to '*studies* of genetic modulation and/or genetic variation'. For Evans and colleagues, critics need not press for studies into 'social and cultural influences' because genetic research itself is 'perfectly well suited to explore environmental influences'. This move from 'mere description towards a mechanistic and mathematical understanding' may not satisfy the critics if 'social and cultural influences' are reduced to an algorithm.

While Evans *et al.* (2001) are excited about the prospects of combining linkage and association studies, Kendler (2006) offers a more circumspect account of progress. Writing in the *American Journal of Psychiatry*, the most widely cited psychiatric journal, Kendler is unconvinced by the nosological validity of family studies, suggesting that family aggregation has a tendency to produce *false positives* because it assumes that affected members have the same single dominant mutation. He suggests that rather than studying one disorder at a time, it may be more useful for nosologists to see if family aggregation occurs across or within diagnostic boundaries. But even if such studies confirmed that two disorders shared genetic risk factors, what explanatory value does this provide? Kendler is sceptical whether molecular genetics will provide the same clarity to classifications in psychiatry as it has for other fields of medicine. He asks whether psychiatry is at risk of adopting a 'gene-centred' approach that inflates the diagnostic value of individual genes of 'modest effect sizes'.

Kendler's critiques are unusual for a key scientist who speaks from *within* psychiatric genetics. He observes that the optimism of the field is closely linked to an 'essentialist model' that assumes an underlying genetic basis for psychiatric categories. Such models are attractive and simple to teach:

> They fit well into the traditional medical model, thereby supporting the status of psychiatry as a medical discipline ... they provide support for an organic disease model where psychiatric disorders are understood as resulting from pathological processes in the brain.
>
> (Kendler 2006: 1141)

Outlining the progress of the field, Kendler questions whether the way forward is to identify genes and then 'work our way back' to ground diagnostic categories on the foundation of a gene:

> By 2004, it had become clear to everyone in the field that no 'Mendelian-like' genes for psychiatric disorders were likely to be found. Nonetheless, there is continued hope that advances in psychiatric genetics and particularly the identification of individual susceptibility genes will alter, in fundamental ways, our approach to psychiatric diagnosis. If we are able to find a 'gene for' a particular psychiatric disorder, then we can work our way back up and – as predicted by the EGM [Essentialist Gene Model] – ground our diagnostic category on the firm foundation of a gene.
>
> (Kendler 2006: 1142)

This extract employs a number of techniques that disrupt accounts of progress. Descriptions of the recent past ('By 2004 ...') build a consensual account:

'it had become clear to *everyone* in the field'. The failure to find 'Mendelian-like genes' is presented as historical fact. Furthermore, the avoidance of impersonal constructions does not impute agency to theoretical models or empirical evidence, but to the responsibility of individuals who seek to ground diagnostic categories on a genetic foundation (*'our* approach', *'we* are able to', *'we* can work', *'our* diagnostic category'). Another strategy is to establish a correspondence between 'Mendelian-like genes' and 'the identification of *individual* susceptibility genes'. Kendler argues that while 'susceptibility genes' draw on notions of complexity to acknowledge the multifactorial dimension of psychiatric disorders, the lingering hope of seeking 'individual' genes is consistent with the essentialist model.

Kendler's account of the complexity of psychiatric disorders exercises far greater caution than other typical descriptions of complexity. 'Gene sharing', where the same gene can contribute to the production of widely different phenotypic effects, frustrates attempts to isolate genetic causation: the functional boundaries of the gene are 'blurred' by processes that alter the structure of expressed proteins. Further, the physical boundaries of the gene are obscured by the role of regulatory and control regions (i.e. 'promotors'), which play an important, yet under-described, role in gene expression. Rather than discrete entities, genes are seen as being 'dynamic parts of biological systems of immense complexity' (Kendler 2006: 1144). In Kendler's view, it makes little sense to search for the specific genes involved in the aetiology of psychiatric disorders because it is unlikely that these can offer the basis upon which to build a discrete categorical model of psychiatric diagnosis.

As we have seen, descriptions of complexity appear within key journals, providing not only an explanation for the failure of Mendelian inheritance, but also a justification for employing new generation GWAS. The reification of complexity as a coherent theoretical account cements methodological support for studies designed to find multiple genes of small effect. Despite the stability offered by such theoretical descriptions, there is considerable ambivalence about the nature of complexity in psychiatric disorders. This ambivalence permits 'interpretive flexibility' (Pinch and Bijker 1984). The continuing focus on finding single genes could reflect a practical preference for lingering methods, or explanations that more easily permit genetic tests and therapeutic interventions, rather than a lingering commitment to Mendelian ways of thinking. No matter the degree to which a multifactorial model proposes a complex relationship between genetic and non-genetic factors, the dominant essentialist view always allows single genes to play some role in the complex aetiology of psychiatric disorders.

Retrospective accounting

In this section, we show how authors routinely invoke historical accounts of genetic research to accomplish a number of rhetorical strategies. These strategies can be understood if we consider the implicit charge that the field of psychiatric genetics had failed to demonstrate the genetic basis of psychiatric disorders. Retrospective accounting is a strategy for neutralizing such charges by defending and/or justifying the genetic hypothesis.

A common pattern of accounting, appearing in a wide range of journals from general medicine to specialist genetics, from clinical to molecular psychiatry, involved authors revisiting the findings of twin and adoption studies (as discussed in Chapter 2). If contemporary notions of complexity are characterized by the multiplication of ambiguous and confounding factors, the same cannot be said about the early studies of heritability, which are contrastingly simple and well-replicated. The following selection briefly illustrates this pattern of accounting:

> It is now clearly established, on the basis of results from family, twin and adoption studies, that genetic factors play a major role in the etiology of schizophrenia.
>
> (O'Donovan and Owen 1999: 587)

> Nevertheless, in contrast to some other complex disorder no susceptibility loci for psychiatric disorders have been unambiguously identified. This is especially disappointing given the overwhelming epidemiological evidence that susceptibility to psychiatric disorders has a substantial genetic component.
>
> (Stoltenberg and Burmeister 2000: 927)

> In relation to substance use, twin studies provide unambiguous evidence that genes play an important role in the development of alcohol dependence.
>
> (Dick *et al.* 2006: 224)

A characteristic of the above examples is their use of 'extreme case formulations' (Pomerantz 1986) to construct a factual account (by upgrading commitment and certainty) that psychiatric disorders have a genetic component. These claims of unequivocal certainty are curious: none of the articles mention the methodological flaws and biases of twin and adoption studies (discussed in Chapter 2), which is telling because some of these criticisms have been raised from *within* the field (Kendler and Diehl 1993). For instance, Hedgecoe (2001) has observed that in the genetics of schizophrenia, authors provide selective accounts of twin and adoption studies, which elide such criticisms and bring closure to an area of controversy.

The invocation of twin and adoption studies also provides a continuous history, connecting contemporary research with the successes of the past, by which *present* concerns about the ambiguity of genetic complexity can be moderated. We identify two kinds of formulation in which simple history and complex present are contrasted to achieve persuasive results. The two formulations differ in the strength of their assertion of the genetic hypothesis. The 'moderate' formulation consists of the following sequence of claims:

1 *Identifying genes for psychiatric disorders is difficult.*
2 *This is because psychiatric disorders are complex.*
3 *However, history shows that psychiatric disorders are heritable.*

The sequence begins with the assertion/concession that gene-identification for psychiatric disorders is difficult. This claim warrants an account ('This is because ...'), which is supplied as a contrast in the second part of the sequence: psychiatric disorders are characterized by complex causation. The second part raises ambiguity about the specific role of genetic factors, whether they are single genes of dominant effect or multiple genes of small effect. Environmental influences are also included as playing a 'complicating' role to account for these difficulties. The final part of the sequence introduces another contrastive statement that reconfirms the genetic hypothesis via historical evidence. Twin studies confirm high heritability rates for psychiatric disorders, providing estimations of the proportion of 'liability to a disorder' attributed to 'genetic effects' (see Table 3.1).

History is used to show that genetic factors are primary, moving environmental influences to the background, thus avoiding their potential to obscure the role of genetic transmission. As a demonstration of this formulation, consider the following extract: 'In spite of these difficulties [that genetic complexity is compounded by nosological complexity], genetic epidemiological studies based upon operational research diagnoses have shown that genes play a role in many of the syndromes defined by psychiatric nosology' (Owen *et al.* 2000: 22). The authors explain that common psychiatric disorders are complex, which is further 'compounded' by nosological complexities. The history of 'epidemiological studies' is introduced by contrast ('In spite of these difficulties') to moderate the implicit charge that complexity is an *excuse* for not identifying genes or that genes play *no* role in psychiatric disorders. Epidemiological research, of which twin studies are the gold-standard, are enrolled to reassert the genetic hypothesis ('have shown that genes play a role in many of the syndromes'),

Table 3.1 Heritability estimates for selected psychiatric disorders

Disorder	*Heritability estimate (%)*
Schizophrenia	80
Bipolar disorder	80
Major depression	40
Generalized anxiety disorder	30
Panic disorder	40
Phobia	35
Alcohol problem or dependence	60

Source: Owen *et al.* (2000: 22), Table 1.

Note
Heritability is the proportion of liability to a disorder accounted for by genetic effects. The heritability estimates are based on twin studies which employed DSM-III-R research diagnoses. NB: the heritabilities should be regarded only as approximations.

thereby defending *genetic* complexity while simultaneously allowing environ-mental influences to play a mitigating role. The contrastive role of history is used in these 'moderate' formulations to defend complex gene interaction and reduce ambiguity.

In the 'assertive' formulation, similar assertions are made but the order is changed, as is shown in the following sequence:

1   *History shows that psychiatric disorders are heritable.*
2   *However, psychiatric disorders are complex.*
3   *Therefore, identifying genes for complex disorders is difficult.*

Instead of defending genetic causation from past failures and present complexi-ties, the history of twin and adoption studies is used to assert from the outset the robust nature of the genetic hypothesis. This provides a stronger footing for jus-tifying current programmes of molecular research. Complexity is introduced to modify this assertion without casting doubt over the central assumption. Com-plexity is no longer framed as an excuse for a lack of progress, but warrants inevitable delays in gene-identification. The presence of 'the environment' as a possible causal factor occupies a mitigating role in the complexity of psychiatric disorders. This more assertive sequence of claims reflects the basic structural elements of this genre of scientific accounting. The following extract illustrates this formulation at work:

> Twin and adoption studies consistently demonstrate a genetic influence on all major psychiatric disorders, confirming work that started in the 1930s. In fact, estimated heritability for bipolar disorder, schizophrenia and autism (80% to >90%) is much higher than that of breast cancer (5% to 60%) and Parkinson's disease (13% to 30%), for which several genetic risk factors are now well established. In many respects, psychiatric disorders are similar to other complex traits that have been studied genetically: studies are compli-cated by locus heterogeneity, imprecisely specified traits, incomplete pene-trance and interaction with non-genetic factors, resulting in a low contribution of each individual risk allele (odds ratios <2).
>
> (Burmeister *et al.* 2008: 527)

In Chapter 2, we discussed how the literature of twin and adoption studies is a pliable resource to cast an impression of uniformity and validity. Here, the history of twin and adoption studies provides a similar foundation ('studies con-sistently demonstrate') applying to '*all* major psychiatric disorders'. History is cast as uniform and continuous ('confirming work that started in the 1930s') to provide a strong basis for justifying contemporary research. Another technique frequently used in review articles is *comparisons to medicine* (see also Chapter 7), which shore-up the resemblance between research into psychiatric disorders and more successful work carried out in medical genetics (e.g. 'breast cancer' and 'Parkinson's disease'). The higher estimates of the heritability of psychiatric disorders are compared with the much lower estimates of heritability in the case of other medical disorders. This not only confirms genetic causation, but implies the future success of psychiatric genetics. The second part of the sequence introduces complexity via the modalized expression, 'In many respects', to assert the strong resemblance between psychiatric disorders and 'other complex traits' with a respectable pedigree of genetic research. The last part of the sequence elaborates the difficulties of studying complex traits ('studies are complicated by ...') confirming the existence of multiple genes of small effect.

As we have shown, the history of twin and adoption studies is contrasted with accounts of complexity in two different ways. In the moderate version, history defends the genetic hypothesis from the criticism that genetic factors play no role, or that environmental factors play a stronger role, in the causation of psychiatric disorders. In the assertive version, history justifies the claim that psychiatric disorders have a strong genetic component, which, as is the case for some medical disorders, are confounded by complex factors. Formulations of certainty and continuity reconstruct a version of history that sidesteps the criticisms that are routinely levelled at twin and adoption studies in order to establish a solid empirical foundation and to connect contemporary research with a strong, successful tradition. However, this version of history also accounts for the present: it reconfirms the central hypothesis that genes *do* play a role in psychiatric disorders; it reduces ambiguity surrounding explanations of complexity; and it allows complexity to explain the difficulties of disease prediction in terms of *delay* rather than failure.

Prospective accounting

Prospective accounting is another aspect of this genre of scientific narrative. Its main features are characterized by reprise (revisiting accounts of success and failure), condensation (summarizing the main arguments) and recommendation (identifying future areas of progress and caution). As we show, prospective accounting engages in the careful reconstruction of expectations in order to realign a narrative of progress and moderated optimism with the difficulties of complexity.

Within the field of psychiatric genetics, appealing to the future is shaped by the controversies of the past. The failure of the 'gene for' paradigm in the 1980s and 1990s led to more cautious forms of accounting. This responsibility is often performed by explicitly recognizing what the field has *not* achieved. This is the sobering description offered by one group of authors in *Genetics in Medicine*, a journal devoted to clinical applications of genetics:

> Although psychiatric genetics is characterized by unprecedented efforts to identify the underlying genetic basis, very few candidates have been accepted as definite risk genes. No genes that explain a major portion of the respective psychiatric disorder have emerged. Genes with a major effect might not exist; rather, increased risk for psychiatric conditions could result

from a large number of small gene effects. The availability of new methods for genetic analysis on the genome level now allows for studies that were unimaginable a few years ago. It remains to be seen whether these new approaches will translate into real success.

(Züchner *et al.* 2007: 338)

The authors contrast a sense of commitment and technological progress ('unprecedented efforts to identify') with the ineluctable failure to find 'definite risk genes'. Risk genes are presumed to be genes of major effect which, the authors claim, 'might not exist'. This is consistent with scientists' discourse on 'complexity', marking a provisional break with some of the troublesome aspects of Mendelian theory. But it also orients our attention to the uncertain future of mapping a 'large number of small gene effects'. Optimism is invested in the 'availability of new methods' for genome-wide scanning that will enable staggering scales of investigation that 'were unimaginable a few years ago'. In this 'update' to clinicians of what can be expected from the future, the passage explicitly avoids promise and adopts a more cautious 'wait and see' approach.

As much as responsibility entails the reluctance to make promises, it also involves highly publicized criticism of 'false' promises. This is clearly evident in the relatively recent and ongoing controversial case of genetic testing. The following extract appears in one of the highest impact journals in genetic research, *Nature Genetics*, wherein a fully mobilized account of complexity warrants caution about the predictive capabilities of genetic tests:

> Given the small individual effect sizes of the few identified risk variants and the complexities of overlapping genetic risk factors, phenotypes and environmental factors, it seems unlikely that genetic tests for diagnosing psychiatric disorders at an individual level will be informative any time soon – the launch of a test for a single unconfirmed rare variant seems premature. If large numbers of rare mutations are involved in the majority of cases, we might need to wait for cheap individual re-sequencing – the '$1,000 genome', which is on the horizon.

(Burmeister *et al.* 2008: 537)

A full description of complexity is contrasted with the simplicity of a Mendelian test for 'a single unconfirmed rare variant'. It is interesting to note that the kinds of criticism that have hampered the field more generally are now directed towards this untimely ('premature') development. The availability of a controversial, commercial genetic test allows the authors to present themselves as responsible commentators on the field by implying that they adhere to more rigorous standards of what constitutes a 'confirmed' risk gene. Even if rare mutations are involved in psychiatric diagnoses, this cautious account defers 'promising' until 'cheap individual re-sequencing' is available to scan the genome for 'a large number of rare mutations'. A common technique of prospective accounting is the deferral of promise until the advent of future technological developments, which are located perpetually 'on the horizon'. Earlier accounts of complexity were more radically sceptical about the possibilities for genetic testing:

> Indeed, even when all susceptibility genes for a given disorder have been identified, it will still not be possible to predict the development of disease with certainty until the relevant environmental risk factors have also been identified and the nature of the various interactions understood. Such interactions may be as complex as chaotic systems like the weather, which is notoriously unpredictable over even the relatively short term.
>
> (Owen *et al.* 2000: 29)

To the readers of *Molecular Psychiatry*, which positions itself at the interface of pre-clinical and clinical research, radical scepticism is maintained by contrasting the complicatedness of polygenic susceptibility with the non-linear complexity of disease prediction. The authors break from the reductionist model where prediction follows mechanistically from identifying 'all susceptibility genes'. Responsibility is manifest in the identification of the role of 'relevant environmental risk factors' and in the underscoring of the complexity of gene–environment interactions. The non-linear complexity of 'chaotic systems like the weather' introduces a qualitatively different description of multifactorial interactions to cast *extreme* doubt over disease prediction.

While some authors foreground complexity with moderate optimism, others consolidate the field's potential by foregrounding recent technological achievements. Systems biology, GWAS and the recent turn to 'endophenotypes' are all frequently cited as new directions for recasting promise. The completion of the HGP, for instance, affords more efficient methods of gene-identification according to psychiatrists writing in the *American Journal of Medical Genetics*:

> Psychiatric genetics is coming to a period of great promise as the means to identify susceptibility genes is becoming easier. With the completion of the Human Genome Project, the knowledge of the HapMap, and the imminent possibility of genome-wide association studies to complement genome-wide linkage studies, the ability to find the genes that cause psychiatric disorder becomes more and more likely.... With the acceptance that the DSM diagnoses may not be the most informative and that it is important to decompose those diagnoses into their component parts, once again the field is experiencing a resurgence of enthusiasm. The use of informative phenotypes that take into account measurement error and confounding has great potential to become the basis of a new strategy to find susceptibility genes for complex psychiatric disorders. We hope that as the field becomes more and more technical and statistical, it remembers that its roots are ultimately in clinical research.
>
> (Szatmari *et al.* 2007: 586)

Accounts of promise are less constrained when focusing on technological advances as opposed to the inherent difficulties of complexity. It is easier to speak of 'great promise' when the 'means to identify genes' represent a *quantitative* increase in the capacity to investigate more genes at any given time. The probability of finding susceptibility genes is invested in new molecular techniques of linkage and association ('knowledge of the HapMap, and the imminent possibility of genome-wide association studies to complement genome-wide linkage studies'). But these technical achievements must also be informed by recent innovations at the clinical level. Prospective accounting seeks to establish a new alignment between genotype-phenotype by moving away from the largely subjective and non-quantitative criteria of the DSM IV. The authors achieve this move by asserting consensus in the field ('the acceptance that') and by reporting the apparent 'resurgence of enthusiasm' with which researchers have turned their attention to endophenotypes: biomarkers that lie closer to the genetic underpinnings of disease (Gottesman and Gould 2003). The 'great potential' of this 'new strategy' of gene-identification seeks to redefine the terrain of psychiatric nosology by establishing stable phenotypes with a clear genetic connection. However, the authors imply that as the field becomes increasingly reliant on a statistical style to interpret the huge volumes of data generated by genome-wide scans (see Chapter 5), there is a danger that the field may drift from its 'clinical' foundations. This warning comes at a time when psychiatric genetics is increasingly characterized as a multidisciplinary enterprise. The size and shape of multidisciplinary collaborations involve managing a perceived imbalance between statistical and clinical styles of reasoning. The article, directed at both clinicians and geneticists, can be seen as maintaining clinical control by arguing that the future success of finding susceptibility genes relies on developing informative phenotypes.

Concerns about incorporating other specialties within the field often warrant appeals to integration. Expectations of progress are highlighted to mitigate organizational and disciplinary concerns, such as disputes between clinicians and statisticians or geneticists and neuroscientists. Neuroscientists claim that genome-wide scans of large samples are untargeted, and are likely to uncover weakly associated genes that may have no relevance to functional biology (*Nature* 2008). Geneticists, however, are not persuaded by the statistics on a few candidate genes whose functional links are poorly established; they opt instead for statistical power across much larger case-control studies (Wellcome Trust Case Control Consortium 2007). Such disciplinary disputes over the choice between targeting a few genes of biological relevance or searching through many genes for statistical significance, allows authors to underscore the 'political' obstacles of progress. Appeals to cross-disciplinary integration made in high profile journals, such as *Nature Genetics*, attempt to rally the field by incorporating disciplines with relevant expertise, by building large collaborations, and by establishing datasets amenable to common analysis. In contrast to the clinicians who warn of psychiatric genetics drifting from its clinical foundations, the following extract challenges bioinformaticians to identify ways of integrating styles of reasoning across relevant disciplines:

Currently, the fields of neuroscience, proteomics, gene expression analysis and genetics operate largely independently of each other. Once the functional pathways that are involved in psychiatric disorders and their associated traits of interest are identified, statistically sound combined analysis of genetics with gene expression and pathway analysis will be needed. Testing biologically plausible candidate genes for genetic association surely falls into this category, but this approach ... has led to many false positives and irreproducible reports, probably owing to a combination of genotyping error, publication bias and insufficient correction for multiple testing.... Merging different data types from separate fields into a common analysis that results in a joint statistical probability is a bioinformatic and statistical challenge.

(Burmeister *et al.* 2008: 537)

The lack of integration of the different research programmes working on the biology and genetics of psychiatric conditions is cast in terms of numerous fields that 'operate *largely* independently of each other'. Possible tensions arising from such divisions are glossed as technical and disciplinary. The authors accommodate the views of neuroscientists who advocate 'testing biologically plausible candidate genes for genetic association', but the form of responsible accounting we saw earlier suggests that attempts to do so have failed in the past ('this approach ... has led to many false positives and irreproducible reports'). The mention of such failures also warrants an explanation ('probably owing to a combination of genotyping error, publication bias and insufficient correction for multiple testing') upholding the geneticists' view that larger studies would not only find the variants of small effect but would also avoid false positives. The prospective strategy of overcoming the boundaries that separate these fields, notably the tensions between neuroscientists and geneticists, is a matter of 'triaging association studies' to incorporate 'analysis of genetics, with gene expression and pathway analysis'. Responsibility for taking up this 'challenge' is assigned to bioinformaticians, who are central to integrating the knowledge of these separate fields (see Chapter 5 for more).

Appeals to integration also coincide with the logics of interdisciplinarity which are often framed in terms of accountability and innovation (Strathern 2004; Barry *et al.* 2008). Interdisciplinarity promises a more accountable science, responsive to user needs while forming closer ties with economies of innovation. Breaking down the barriers of scientific specialization and thus promising greater interaction and the creation of unforeseen synergies has clear rhetorical value. In the life sciences especially, where problems are constructed in terms of their complexity, the development of solution strategies often justify increasingly complex forms of social organization. This is implied by Burmeister *et al.* (2008) who view the multiple levels of complexity as requiring equally complex strategies of investigation: 'It is unlikely that a single strategy will allow the identification of all genetic risk factors, but this complexity will have to be attacked from many different angles' (2008: 537). Thus, complexity in psychiatric genetics is central to justifying novel social arrangements in large-scale biological research.

Rebuilding the narrative

Hacking (1992: 13) reminds us that styles of scientific reasoning have a 'self-authenticating' character that maintain their stability: 'The remarkable thing about styles is that they are stable, enduring, accumulating over the long haul.' Similarly, by giving the literature of a field a narrative form, review articles can also be viewed as techniques that reconstruct key events and controversies so as to provide coherence and stability. A feature of the articles we have examined is the retrospective and prospective framings of an existential present: they reconstruct a history of disappointments and a future of hope, and incorporate criticisms, while at the same time erasing or minimizing the controversies from which they are derived. This has the effect of producing a history of continuity and internal reflexivity, rather than a history of contingency and human error; past failures are recast as technical errors of a methodology informed by flawed assumptions about Mendelian inheritance; twin and adoption studies are routinely cited to provide evidence supporting the central genetic hypothesis; accounts of failure are converted into success as the field comes to recognize the underlying complexity of psychiatric disorders.

In the narrative of simple-to-complex, complexity emerges as an explanation for the failure of linkage studies, later solidifying into a theoretical model of multifactorial and polygenic interaction. This web of genetic and non-genetic factors, the so-called 'witches brew' of psychiatric genetics (Owen *et al.* 2000; Arribas-Ayllon *et al.* 2010), constitutes a rescaling and reordering of the way in which psychiatric pathology is genetically constituted. It no longer makes sense to say that there is a 'gene for' a disorder. As Rose (2007: 204) has noted:

> the claim is now that mutations associated with increased susceptibility can be identified in precise loci in the base sequence of the genes that control the synthesis of the proteins involved in the production and transportation of neurotransmitters, receptors, enzymes, cell membranes or ion channels regulating the activity of neurons.

The emphasis on 'susceptibility' is indicative of a new gaze in which the molecularization of psychiatric pathology is continuously distributed and multiplied.

As much as the post-HGP view of complexity constitutes a new way of seeing and speaking about psychiatric disorders, the focus of this chapter has been to show that 'complexity' performs rhetorical work in order to preserve hope for a research programme. This analysis demonstrates the ways in which a particular genre of scientific accounting accomplishes a number of strategic objectives:

- it exonerates the failure to identify genes for psychiatric disorders by suggesting a *slowing down* of progress as the science comes to grips with the sheer scale of susceptibilities throughout the human genome;
- it allows scientists to incorporate non-genetic factors, in theory, which insulates the field from criticisms of determinism by according these factors an indeterminate role;
- it presents susceptibility as being complex in nature, allowing scientists to engage in moderated forms of promising that explicitly avoid hype and thus appear cautious and responsible;
- it allows the field to attribute progress to processes that can address complexity via increased speed of production (e.g. cheaper and faster sequencing) and organizational reordering (e.g. multidisciplinary integration, large-scale collaborations and data sharing);
- it allows gene-identification programmes to continue under the hypothesis that multiple genes are implicated in disease susceptibility;
- it confers a kind of respectability to biological psychiatry by adopting the same rhetoric of complexity as that of the much larger and less controversial programmes such as those investigating diabetes and heart disease.

The rise of complexity explanations within psychiatric genetics is a story not just of changes in scientific ideas, but also of the incorporation and neutralization of controversies. Complexity is cast as a sophisticated realization of the further work needed in the field; the simple-to-complex trope extends this narrative, generating hope by directing attention to 'rapid advances' that will convert complexity into models of prediction and drug discovery.

However, the ambivalent descriptions of complexity found in many of the review articles not only imply uncertainty about the precise aetiology of psychiatric disorders, but also suggest ways of resolving tensions between different methodological viewpoints. The instability of the simple–complex boundary is sufficiently vague enough to incorporate Mendelian *and* polygenic models, which, rather than generating tensions at an ontological level, may actually relieve tensions between competing research practices. In appealing to non-Mendelian patterns of inheritance, complexity is neither a straightforward negation of monogenic theory nor a revolutionary 'paradigm shift', but a shift in focus. Hedgecoe (2001) has noted that multifactorial models allow single genes some role in the aetiology of schizophrenia. This is because 'enlightened' models of molecular analysis employ the same methods used to detect single genes of major effect.

The appeal of the 'essentialist gene model' (Kendler 2006) describes much of the old generation of molecular genetics, such as linkage and association studies. The problem with this explicitly laboratory style of reasoning is that research often assumes a one-to-one relationship between genes and diagnostic categories; it is more committed to extending the 'parts list' of molecular biology than understanding the interactions among the parts. Essentialism reduces complexity via traditional methods of nomenclature and resemblance, assuming that disease categories are reliable entities. But pleiotropy (the idea that single genes are implicated in multiple traits) suggests that the essentialist view does not capture the multidimensionality of gene function. Advances in molecular biology are undermining the simple definition of the gene. The complexity of 'gene sharing' would suggest that the boundaries and functions of genes are fuzzy and unpredictable. Kendler argues:

> Genes are not discrete entities like atoms of gold and silver. They are dynamic parts of biological systems of immense complexity. The discovery of specific genes that are involved in the aetiology of psychopathology will not likely prove to be the basis on which to build an essentialist and categorical model of psychiatric diagnosis.
>
> (2006: 1144)

These strong versions of complexity challenge the assumption that genes are natural kinds, and thus unproblematic units of investigation. More seriously, these accounts, which see complexity as something qualitatively different from the quantitative expansion of 'simplicity', are sceptical towards the foundation upon which the field builds its economies of hope. The prospects of anchoring psychiatric categories to a gene-centred approach drives the development of pharmaceutical interventions.

The appearance of genetic tests for neuropsychiatric disorders is an example of how different versions of complexity are more or less amenable to commercial exploitation. Genetic testing for neuropsychiatric disorders is a major goal for translational medicine, the so-called push 'from bench to bedside'. The view that common psychiatric disorders are complex suggest that genetic tests are unlikely to be offered to the public any time soon. And yet, in 2008, just before we entered the field, three companies (Psynomics™, NeuroMark Genomics Inc. and SureGene™) began offering genetic testing for major psychiatric disorders. It is perhaps unsurprising that in a sector of the personal genomics industry known for its volatility and failure, only Psynomics™ and SureGene™ survive at present offering mainly pharmacogenomic testing (predicting patient metabolism of antidepressants). Other flagships of the personal genomics industry such as Navigenics and deCODEme have ceased trading since the FDA crackdown on direct-to-consumer genetic testing in 2015; while other companies such as 23andMe have adapted by moving offshore to countries with less stringent regulations. Nevertheless, scientists within the psychiatric genetics community had raised, and continue to raise, strong concerns about the poor predictive value of genome tests; that the burden of recognizing their limited predictability falls onto clinicians and patients (Couzin 2008; Braff and Freedman 2008; Burmeister *et al.* 2008; Mitchell *et al.* 2010; Appelbaum and Benston 2017). However, increasing 'complexity' by adding more genes is not an assurance of more accurate information – pleiotropy and complex gene interactions are likely to increase the difficulty of interpretation. Braff and Freedman (2008) argue that, since the reduced complexity offers limited or spurious predictability, the 'simplicity' of the direct-to-consumer model may even be harmful to patients.

When scientists contribute to the historical narrative of psychiatric genetics they often foreground the complexity of the field to work up professional responsibility. Foregrounding complexity, especially in controversial areas of science, accepts responsibility for unknowns, displays flexibility towards present problems and moderates future promises (Brown and Michael 2003). A discourse of professional responsibility is rhetorically organized via elaborate sequences of 'hedging' or contrast structures – i.e. juxtaposing areas of potential development with methodological uncertainty and limitation. These contrastive formulations produce the distinctive 'cautiously optimistic' framing of progress, often anticipating future problems while avoiding accusations of 'genohype'. It is worth asking to whom are these accounts of complexity directed? The range of publications indicates a multidisciplinary focus directed at scientists and clinicians across various disciplines: medicine, biology, genomics and psychiatry. The fact that this genre of accounting is not found within the home journal *Psychiatric Genetics* is indicative of the outward focus of the genre. Contrasting formulations of complexity also perform different rhetorical functions. For instance, strong versions of complexity that foreground nonlinear causation emphasize 'extreme caution', while moderate versions of complexity that foreground 'complicatedness' emphasize 'moderate optimism'. Mainstream descriptions of 'complicatedness' are more inclined to justify exploring multiple gene models while retaining a focus on single gene approaches. Such descriptions are likely to appease opposing methodological camps and establish connections with wider professional communities.

If foregrounding complexity is a means of performing responsibility when engaging other professional communities, does complexity have this effect when engaging publics? Depending on the recipient, complexity can be a platform for authority, caution and competence, or an effacing admission of partial authority, uncertainty and confusion. Given the peculiar history of psychiatric genetics with its narrative of success, failure and moderated optimism, a reader is unlikely to infer a loss of scientific authority and control from these invocations of complexity. An admission of complexity that serves as a reason for integrating different models, methods and specialties can be seen as performing responsibility to a 'lurking public', which includes the interested readers of the scientific literature who are not psychiatric geneticists (see more in Chapter 7). In the case of the commercialization of genetic testing for psychiatric disorders, there are different stakes at risk on either side of the public/professional boundary. When commercial actors seek to profit from the results of molecular research the public are sold simple genetics, not the complexity so meticulously constructed in review articles. The way the professional community has responded to such recent developments illustrates the rhetorical power of complexity: they describe the complexity of psychiatric disorders in order to stress the poor predictive value of tests based on the simplicity of single 'genes for'. Within this genre of scientific accountability, genetic testing is presented as scientifically and clinically irresponsible, a 'bridge too far too soon' (Braff and Freedman 2008).

Conclusion

This chapter demonstrates that scientific accounts of complexity are not merely descriptions of 'complicated' or 'complicating' factors in the aetiology of psychiatric disorders; they also perform professional responsibility. This illustrates an important aspect of the reflexivity of scientists as molecular biology grapples with the volume of information generated by high-throughput technologies in the post-genomic era. For some, it is tempting to pronounce a 'paradigm shift' to denote a move from simple to complex gene models. However, the discourse on complexity does not entail a straightforward shift from simple to complex. In addition to exonerating the field from past failures, complexity appears to offer a justification for new social arrangements and combining different styles of reasoning under the banner of 'psychiatric genetics'. Complexity is not simply a responsible admission of uncertainty, but a call for multidisciplinary integration: it seeks to assemble a multidisciplinary domain of tractable (or 'doable') problems (Fujimura 1987). The broad range of high impact journals in which this genre appears suggests a strategy of developing closer links between genetics, neuroscience, psychiatry and molecular biology. Furthermore, as the field becomes increasingly inundated with data, it relies on bioinformatics to resolve complexity. In the empirical chapters that follow, we explore how one research site copes with this multidisciplinary reorganization. Our analysis suggests that, for psychiatric genetics, complexity and reductionism are not mutually exclusive categories, but coexist at the interstices and uncertainties of molecular biology. Descriptions of complexity are rhetorically organized justifications for marshalling new resources and reconstructing promises. We argue that this particular pattern of scientific accounting is not unique to scientists nor the field of psychiatric genetics, but forms part of the everyday resources for managing uncertainty.

Note

1 It worth noting that the discrepancies between the Egeland study and those reported in the same issue of *Nature* (Detera-Wadleigh *et al.* 1987; Hodgkinson *et al.* 1987) have three possible explanations: any one of these studies could have been 'wrong'; manic depression could have been attributed to a single gene in the Egeland study and to polygenic factors in the other studies; manic depression might have been caused by a single gene in a different location with no linkage to chromosome 11. Only the third possibility was considered by the editor of *Nature*, which indicates the 'great eagerness to support a hypothesis of simple genetic causation for manic depression' (Berkowitz 1996: 44).

References

Appelbaum PS and Benston S (2017) Anticipating the ethical challenges of psychiatric genetic testing. *Current Psychiatry Reports* 19: 39.

Arribas-Ayllon M, Bartlett A and Featherstone K (2010) Complexity and accountability: The witches' brew of psychiatric genetics. *Social Studies of Science* 40(4): 499–524.

Baron M, Risch N, Hamburger R, *et al.* (1987) Genetic linkage between X-chromosome markers and bipolar affective illness. *Nature* 326 (25 March): 289–292.

Baron M, Nelson FF, Risch N, *et al.* (1993) Diminished support for linkage between manic depressive illness and X-chromosome markers in three Israeli pedigrees. *Nature Genetics* 3: 49–55.

Barry A, Born G and Weszkalnys G (2008) Logics of interdisciplinarity. *Economy and Society* 37(1): 20–49.

Bazerman C (1988) *Shaping Written Knowledge: The Genre and Activity of the Experimental Article in Science.* Madison: University of Wisconsin Press.

Berkowitz A (1996) Our genes, ourselves? *BioScience* 46(1): 42–52.

Blum K, Noble EP, Sheridan PJ, *et al.* (1990) Allelic association of human dopamine [D sub.2] receptor gene in alcoholism. *Journal of the American Medical Association* 263: 2055–2060.

Braff DL and Freedman R (2008) Clinically responsible genetic testing in neuropsychiatric patients: A bridge too far too soon. *American Journal of Psychiatry* 165(8): 952–955.

Brown N and Michael M (2003) A sociology of expectations: Retrospecting prospects and prospecting retrospects. *Technology Analysis & Strategic Management* 15(1): 3–18.

Burmeister M, McInnis MG and Zöllner S (2008) Psychiatric genetics: Progress amid controversy. *Nature Reviews Genetics* 9: 527–540.

Cook-Deegan RM (1994) *The Gene Wars: Science, Politics and the Human Genome.* New York: W.W. Norton.

Couzin J (2008) Gene tests for psychiatric risk polarize researchers. *Science* 319 (18 January): 274–277.

Detera-Wadleigh SD, Berrettini WH, Goldin LR, *et al.* (1987) Close linkage of c-Jarvey-ras-1 and the insulin gene to affective disorder is ruled out in three North American pedigrees. *Nature* 325 (26 February): 806–808.

Dick DM, Rose RJ and Kaprio J (2006) The next challenge for psychiatric genetics: Characterizing the risk associated with identified genes. *Annuals of Clinical Psychiatry* 18(4): 223–231.

Dillon GL (1991) *Contending Rhetorics: Writing in Academic Disciplines.* Bloomington: Indiana University Press.

Egeland JA, Gerhard DS, Pauls DL, *et al.* (1987) Bipolar affective disorder linked to DNA markers on chromosome 11. *Nature* 325 (26 February): 783–787.

Evans KL, Porteous DJ, Muir WJ, *et al.* (2001) Nuts and bolts of psychiatric genetics: Building on the Human Genome Project. *Trends in Genetics* 17(1): 35–40.

Fujimura JH (1987) Constructing 'doable' problems in cancer research: Articulating alignment. *Social Studies of Science* 17(2): 257–293.

Gelernter J, Goldman D and Risch N (1993) The A1 allele at the D2 dopamine receptor gene and alcoholism: A reappraisal. *Journal of the American Medical Association* 269: 1673–1677.

Gelernter J, O'Malley S, Risch N, *et al.* (1991) No association between an allele at the D2 dopamine receptor gene (DRD2) and alcoholism. *Journal of the American Medical Association* 266: 1801–1807.

Gershon ES and Cloninger RC (1994) *Genetic Approaches to Mental Disorders.* Washington, DC: American Psychiatric Press.

Gilbert GN and Mulkay M (1984) *Opening Pandora's Box: A Sociological Analysis of Scientists' Discourse.* Cambridge: Cambridge University Press.

Gottesman II and Gould TD (2003) The endophenotype concept in psychiatry: Etymology and strategic intentions. *American Journal of Psychiatry* 160: 636–645.

Hacking I (1992) 'Style' for historians and philosophers. *Studies in the History and Philosophy of Science* 23(1): 1–20.

Hedgecoe A (2001) Schizophrenia and the narrative of enlightened geneticization. *Social Studies of Science* 31(6): 875–911.

Hilgartner S (1990) The dominant view of popularization: Conceptual problems, political uses. *Social Studies of Science* 20: 519–539.

Hodgkinson S, Sherrington R, Gurling H, *et al.* (1987) Molecular genetic evidence for heterogeneity in manic depression. *Nature* 325 (26 February): 805–806.

The Huntington's Disease Collaborative Research Group (1993) A novel gene containing a trinucleotide repeat that is expanded and unstable on Huntington's disease chromosomes. *Cell* 72 (26 March): 971–983.

Kelsoe JR, Ginns EI, Egeland JA, *et al.* (1989) Re-evaluation of the linkage relationship between chromosome 11p loci and the gene for bipolar affective disorder in the old order Amish. *Nature* 342 (16 November): 238–243.

Kendler KS (2006) Reflections on the relationship between psychiatric genetics and psychiatric nosology. *American Journal of Psychiatry* 163: 1138–1146.

Kendler KS and Diehl SR (1993) The genetics of schizophrenia: A current, genetic-epidemiologic perspective. *Schizophrenia Bulletin* 19(2): 261–285.

Kennedy JL, Giuffra LA, Moises HW, *et al.* (1988) Evidence against linkage of schizophrenia to markers on chromosome 5 in a northern Swedish pedigree. *Nature* 336 (10 November): 167–170.

Knowlton RG, Cohen-Haguenauer O, Van Cong N, *et al.* (1985) A polymorphic DNA marker linked to cystic fibrosis in located on chromosome 7. *Nature* 318 (28 November): 381–382.

Mitchell PB, Meiser B, Fullerton J, *et al.* (2010) Predictive and diagnostic genetic testing in psychiatry. *Psychiatr Clin N Am* 33: 225–243.

Myers G (1991) Stories and styles in two molecular biology review article. In C Bazerman and J Paradis (eds). *Textual Dynamics of the Professions: Historical and Contemporary Studies of Writing in Professional Communities.* Madison: University of Wisconsin Press, pp. 45–75.

Myers G (1992) 'In this paper we report …': Speech acts and scientific acts. *Journal of Pragmatics* 17(4): 295–313.

Nature (2008) Editorial: An unnecessary battle. *Nature* 454 (10 July): 137–138.

O'Donovan MC and Owen MJ (1999) Candidate-gene association studies of schizophrenia. *American Journal of Human Genetics* 65(3): 587–592.

Owen MJ, Cardno AG and O'Donovan MC (2000) Psychiatric genetics: Back to the future. *Molecular Psychiatry* 5: 22–31.

Pinch T and Bijker W (1984) The social construction of facts and artefacts: Or how the sociology of science and the sociology of technology might benefit each other. *Social Studies of Science* 14(3): 399–441.

Pomerantz A (1986) Extreme case formulation: A way of legitimizing claims. *Human Studies* 9(2–3): 219–229.

Potter J (1996) *Representing Reality: Discourse, Rhetoric and Social Construction.* London: Sage.

Robertson M (1987) Molecular genetics of the mind. *Nature* 325 (26 February): 755.

Robertson M (1989) False start on manic depression. *Nature* 342 (16 November): 222.

Rose N (2007) *The Politics of Life Itself: Biomedicine, Power, and Subjectivity in the Twenty-First Century*. Princeton: Princeton University Press.

Rose S (1995) The rise of neurogenetic determinism. *Nature* 373 (2 February): 380–382.

Rose S (1998) Neurogenetic determinism and the new euphenics. *British Medical Journal* 317: 1707–1708.

Rose S, Lewontin RC and Kamin LJ (1984) *Not In Our Genes: Biology, Ideology and Human Nature*. London: Pantheon.

Sherrington R, Brynjolfsson J, Petursson H, *et al.* (1988) Localization of a susceptibility locus for schizophrenia on chromosome 5. *Nature* 336 (10 November): 164–167.

Sinding C (1996) Literary genres and the construction of knowledge in biology: Semantic shifts and scientific change. *Social Studies of Science* 26(1): 43–70.

Stoltenberg SF and Burmeister M (2000) Recent progress in psychiatric genetics: Some hope but no hype. *Human Molecular Genetics* 9(6): 927–935.

Strathern M (2004) *Commons and Borderlands: Working Papers on Interdisciplinarity, Accountability and the Flow of Knowledge*. Wantage: Sean Kingston.

Szatmari P, Maziade M, Zwaigenbaum L, *et al.* (2007) Informative phenotypes for genetic studies of psychiatric disorders. *American Journal of Medical Genetics* 144(5): 581–588.

Tsui L-C, Buchwald M, Barker D, *et al.* (1985) Cystic fibrosis locus defined by a genetically linked polymorphic DNA marker. *Science* 230 (29 November): 1054–1057.

Virgo JA (1971) The review article: Its characteristics and problems. *The Library Quarterly* 41(4): 275–291.

Wainwright BJ, Scambler PJ, Schmidtke J, *et al.* (1985) Localization of cystic fibrosis locus to human chromosome 7cen-q22. *Nature* 318 (28 November): 384–385.

Wellcome Trust Case Control Consortium (2007) Genome-Wide Association Study of 14,000 cases of seven common diseases and 3,000 shared controls. *Nature* 447 (7 June): 661–684.

Züchner S, Roberts ST, Speer MC, *et al.* (2007) Update on psychiatric genetics. *Genetics in Medicine* 9(6): 332–340.

4   Inside 'Big Biology'

In the last chapter, we showed how the rhetoric of complexity is deployed in scientific writing to pave the way for large-scale biological research on psychiatric conditions. Complexity is not merely an ontological description of an elusive phenomenon, but a means of enrolling visions and resources to assemble large multidisciplinary programmes of genomic research. In this chapter, we draw on ethnographic observations and research interviews with scientists to examine the manifestation of large-scale biological research at a leading UK research centre. In a field that has adopted high-throughput technologies to study correlations between genotype and phenotype, we make the case that psychiatric genetics has become 'Big Biology' (Davies *et al.* 2013; Hilgartner 2013). More than a simple quantitative description of increasing speed, scale and production, we use this category to highlight epistemic and social changes in the way work is done, careers are understood and scientific questions are answered. By taking a closer look 'inside' the laboratories of Big Biology, we will see that what counts as 'scale' and 'biology' is ambiguous and fluid.

Large-scale biology

The HGP was an obvious precursor to *-omic* large-scale biology, of which contemporary psychiatric genetics is an example. It created a socio-technical apparatus for imagining and organizing biological research on an industrial scale (Bartlett 2008). Those who advocated the early vision of mapping and sequencing the human genome claimed that it was biology's first opportunity to become a 'Big Science' (see Cantor 1990). In their retrospective of the HGP, Collins *et al.* (2003: 286) also used the term 'Big Science' to describe not vast, expensive, centralized apparatus, in the way that Big Physics is built around objects such as particle accelerators and gravity wave detectors, but rather 'a remarkable collection of scientists' across different countries, disciplines and levels of seniority. In this sense, Big Biology was unlike Big Physics; the key object of aggregation is seen to be people, not machines. Indeed, it should be noted that there was some resistance to the idea of labelling large-scale biology 'Big Science' at all because it implied a form of scientific organization that many molecular biologists were keen to avoid (Hilgartner 2013).

Balmer (1996) notes a similar ambivalence among scientists involved in the earlier UK Human Gene Mapping Project (HGMP). The commonplace view was that gene mapping was intensely tedious and, essentially, not scientific. The sheer scale, routinization and industrialization of the project had created a division between 'mapping for mapping's sake' and the 'rest of biology', implying that mapping was a 'pre-biological'[1] exercise. The 'real' biological work of characterizing and interpreting gene function would only come after the mapping had been completed. Gene mapping imposed a division between different 'styles' of research; with the new 'DNA jocks' contrasted with 'human geneticists' (Balmer 1996: 538). One style was characterized by geneticists as dull, menial and repetitive, with some going so far as to liken it to 'stamp collecting' and 'fishing expeditions', while the other style was 'biologically-minded' lab work, involving experimentation and creative thinking.[2] Mapping was not Big Science in the sense of the HGP, nor the subsequent large-scale *-omic* programmes, but it did demonstrate many of the *qualitative* changes in the style of biological work that we see in Big Biology today. The opposition to diverting resources to gene mapping (and later, sequencing) on an industrial scale was that it was technical work emptied of 'real' biological work. In this sense, the concerns that scientists had regarding Big Biology show a commonality with earlier concerns about Big Science in physics (see Weinberg 1961); that the small-scale excellence of biology would be left behind as the scale of research programmes increased.

The HGP introduced a socio-technical infrastructure that allowed biological research programmes to re-enter the discovery phase with increased statistical power. For psychiatric genetics, this was seen as a panacea for the limited success of earlier research programmes based on methods such as family-based linkage studies. The availability of high-throughput technologies revitalized the earlier vision of a common disease-common allele model first proposed by researchers in the 1980s (see Chapter 2). By the mid-1990s, the accessibility of 'diallelic polymorphisms' was widely considered a tractable solution for detecting common variants of small to moderate effect (Risch and Merikangas 1996). Early visions of GWAS were appealing because they promised to transcend the limitations of studying small numbers of families with highly penetrant, heritable forms of psychiatric disorders. Researchers had been faced with the gloomy prospect that family studies would never provide sufficient statistical power to detect gene variants that play a casual role in psychiatric disorders. The technical possibility of genotyping very large samples of unrelated individuals for common markers opened up new territories of scale. Characterizing thousands of SNPs for thousands of cases and controls was a *technical* solution to a statistical problem. Hailed as 'a powerful tool for human genetic studies' (Wang *et al.* 1998: 1077), SNPs were less informative than existing genetic markers, but more abundant and their characterization had greater potential for rationalization, standardization and automation. In other words, genetic markers of common variation were attractive because they were *scalable*, and the development of high-density marker maps of SNPs provided the technological conditions to embark on a new phase of *mass inscription* (we say more about these processes in Chapter 5).

The absence in contemporary large-scale biology of vast, expensive apparatus (like that of Big Physics such as CERN, LIGO or the VLT) often elides the fact that there is an expensively and skilfully assembled material core of 'big' psychiatric genetics: the biological and phenotypic samples collected for GWAS. The first published GWAS examined 65,761 SNPs in a sample of 94 (Ozaki *et al.* 2002). This was large-scale in historical terms (Burton *et al.* 2009), but in less than a decade, the number of SNPs genotyped increased nearly 20-fold and the acceptable sample size rose to the tens of thousands. The 'brute force'[3] method of increasing the statistical power of GWAS requires a dramatic increase in sample sizes. By 2009, just as we entered the field, the argument was that for common psychiatric conditions, 'good or excellent power requires samples of *circa* 8,000 to 20,000 case subjects (plus comparison subjects) ... (i.e. larger than any sample collected by a single research group to date)' (Psychiatric GWAS Consortium Coordinating Committee 2009: 544). To do 'good science', psychiatric genetics had little alternative but to scale up the collection of DNA samples and rich phenotypic data to attain what had always seemed to elude the field: sufficient statistical power. The potential and possibilities of GWAS ushered in an era of Big Biology in psychiatric genetics. As we show, much of the scale of this enterprise is hidden from the casual observer by processes that not only displace menial and repetitive functions but also the 'laboratory style' of reasoning.

Inside the Centre

The bulk of the fieldwork for this chapter was conducted between 2008 and 2011, consisting of regular observations and interviews with a group of biomedical scientists working on large-scale studies of psychiatric genetics (with GWAS being the dominant method). The 'Centre' is a leading international research group in the field of psychiatry, neurology and clinical psychology. The original hospital campus site (see Introduction) where much of the laboratory and clinical work was conducted accommodated approximately 150 biomedical scientists, including 30 faculty, 100 postdoctoral researchers/research associates and 20 PhD students. In recent years, as we stepped away from the field, these numbers have grown after winning a major research council grant to expand facilities. This includes not only a move to a new building but the expansion of large-scale studies of the genetics of psychiatric disorders as well as multidisciplinary integration of molecular biology, cell biology, neuroscience, animal models, clinical psychiatry and psychology, epidemiology and epigenetics. Scholars have argued that a characteristic of Big Biology is the designation of 'projects' as practical units of organization and value creation (Davies 2013; Lezaun 2013). In this case, projects are organized with regard to major disease groups, such as schizophrenia, bipolar disorder, major depression, attention deficit hyperactivity disorder (ADHD), Alzheimer's and Parkinson's disease.

Though Principal Investigators, postdocs and PhD students are assigned to these projects in a formal sense, the organization of the Centre is characterized by a degree of movement between disease-focused projects. In this section, we briefly describe our initial impressions of being *inside* Big Biology.

The rhetorics of scale can be misleading. It would be easy to read the scientific literature that we reviewed in Chapter 3 and see the claims to Big Biology as giving the impression of monolithic scale. Indeed, much like the commentaries following the HGP, this new arrangement of psychiatric genetics research was imagined via two master metaphors: 'scale' and 'mobility'. Statements read that large-scale multidisciplinary research would reveal the 'genetic architecture' of psychiatric disorders, giving way to 'translational research' and the development of 'novel therapies'. From the descriptions that stressed the escalating scale of the research, it would be easy to assume that the production of biological value was conducted by industrial scale assemblages. The numbers of collaborating authors on high-impact papers and the exponential increase of reported sample sizes had cast the impression of a large infrastructure, the kind of scale that would immediately impress itself on the senses. But when we visited the laboratories at the Centre, we found a scene similar to that of 'traditional', 'small science' biology. There were no obvious signs of large-scale labour, no rows of machines, no overt signs of bureaucratic top-down surveillance, and no clear sense of how value was created. In short, there were no obvious signs of Big Science.

The laboratories looked like any other. Long benches divided the main room, with storage over and under for glass and plastic-ware. There were a few pieces of kit; the ordinary apparatus of molecular biology. Fridges were filled with tube after tube of DNA samples, hand-written codes corresponding to phenotypic data stored electronically. There were a handful of other smaller rooms: a genotyping room, a room filled with Polymerase Chain Reaction (PCR) machines, a small, cramped room in which DNA was extracted from blood samples of research participants, and a room containing a liquid-handling robot. These rooms also contained the recent history of molecular biology; obsolete machines, stored on benches, superseded and pushed to one side. In these 'wet' labs only a handful of people were seen to be at work. Indeed, visiting the laboratories to call on scientists taking part in large-scale projects, it was not uncommon to find that these teams had no one doing 'wet' work. Though GWAS evidently involved vast amounts of repetitive laboratory labour, it was nowhere to be seen. That is, labour *was* being conducted, but not *here* at the Centre.

The offices were busier, corridor-like rooms containing two rows of computers with scientists working back to back. It was striking that these workspaces contained few, if any, books, aside from some handbooks on computer programming and statistical software. Even the literature and the reading practices of science were *in silico*. At desktops, people browsed spreadsheets, genome databases, electronic journals, and conducted statistical analysis; this was clean, 'dry' science. It seemed the building's design priorities were set when laboratory space was of greater importance, thus office space was limited at the hospital campus. In fact, these offices were now overflowing; only the most senior scientists had their own office space, with most sharing a room with half a dozen others, or 'hot desking' at shared work stations.

If scale was not an overt feature of the laboratories nor was it a property of the office space of the fieldworkers who collected the raw material of blood samples and phenotypic data for each project. Graduate psychology students, mostly young women, occupied a separate office from which they planned and reviewed their work. As the projects have grown in size (and funding), so have the number of fieldworkers. Once, this kind of work had been conducted by scientists or clinicians with an extensive knowledge of psychopathology, collecting relatively small numbers of samples from interesting family pedigrees. When we visited the Centre, the interviews had been standardized and the fieldworkers were trained specifically to collect data. As the scale of psychiatric genetics has grown, fieldwork was becoming increasingly 'rationalized', creating an acute division between 'analysis' and 'data collection'. The most valuable work of the fieldworkers was conducted 'on the road', driving to the homes of research participants, conducting lengthy phenotypic interviews and taking blood samples (we describe these practices at length in Chapter 6). Their work was dispersed by necessity, that is, by the distribution of living participants from whom DNA was extracted, disassembled as 'data' and later reassembled by statistical, computational methods.

Much of the increasing scale of psychiatric genetic has been accommodated by processes of distribution and displacement. The growth of the productive power of laboratory work is the result of the combination of collaboration, the subdivision of labour within research 'projects', the outsourcing of repetitive labour, the flexible specialization of knowledge work, and the automation and miniaturization of laboratory processes. These processes accommodate some of the increasing scale of psychiatric genetics and distribute much of the rest, leaving the research laboratories of psychiatric genetics to appear as 'small science'. Unlike the massification of instruments found in Big Science, Big Biology involves (indeed, depends upon) the miniaturization of 'high-throughput' technologies. In the next section, we examine how the consortium-based collaboration has changed the nature of scientific collaboration and, more acutely, the conduct and management of work in the laboratories.

Consortium-based collaboration

In psychiatric genetics, the move to Big Biology has produced institutional changes in the individual research sites that operate within an international consortium. To understand the scale of activities at the Centre, we need to understand its location within the Psychiatric Genetics Consortium (PGC). The rise of consortium-based collaboration in post-HGP *-omic* biology is an indication of how large-scale biological research operates across diverse locations and through a variety of material practices.

The PGC was born during a telephone conference in March 2007 when senior scientists leading separate GWAS projects agreed to create a consortium for the joint analysis of results. In the pursuit of statistical power (and in engaging in collaborative competition with the larger groups), the overarching purpose was to conduct 'mega-analyses'[4] of GWAS. By 2010, the PGC included 160 investigators from 65 institutions in 19 countries (Sullivan 2010).[5] The framework of ethical governance was designed to be inclusive, democratic, transparent and rapid: ensuring that 'no single individual or group dominates' (2010: 5). The PGC adopted a model of balancing the 'rights' of 'states' with the 'federal' coordinating committee, which is described as 'non-intrusive and facilitating'. Data are stored on a cluster farm in the Netherlands for warehousing and analysis. On this neutral and secure platform, data harmonization and quality control is applied to each step of the GWAS process: ascertainment of subjects, diagnostic procedures, genotyping, removal of unconfident data, etc. Raw data are de-identified and restricted. Each group can access these data and conduct analyses, but they cannot download it on to their own servers. One of the managers of the consortium described it as a 'circle of trust' '[where] no one has got our data'. However, exchanging data on this scale was a not a mode of activity that these scientists were used to. The director of the Centre describes the transition to 'consortium-based' collaboration as follows:

> Well, in the past, collaborations have formed around a real kind of mutual benefit and convenience, but also you know they're based on liking the other people really, and getting on well and trusting them and so on, but what's happened more recently is the technology's moved into this very large-scale genome wide studies that require very large numbers that are beyond the ability of just one or two groups to do together, there's been an increase in the scale and the drivers have changed slightly … so one of the drivers [has] been really the money to do the genotyping so what we've had is a set of groups that have been collecting samples um have the expertise but don't have the money … ah well that don't have enough samples to do meaningful work themselves and then it becomes … the problem is how do you get the money to genotype several thousand people and several thousand controls and that's what's driven it.
>
> (Centre director of neuropsychiatric genetics)

Psychiatric genetics has always involved an element of collaboration and yet a striking characteristic of Big Biology is an emphasis on the 'imperative to share' (Lezaun 2013). The adoption of GWAS has changed the structure of collaboration from what the director describes as 'convenience' (involving trust and other personal, tacit, contingent factors) to the implied inconvenience of collaborating within explicit bureaucratic constraints with competing laboratories. An important consequence of consortium-based collaboration is therefore the institutionalization of trust. Economies of scale drive scientific collaborations inasmuch as larger consortia allow the parcelling out of the genotyping of several thousand cases and controls into manageable portions, distributing the material, machinery and labour in ways that are unlike the kind of concentration of resources that typify archetypal Big Science projects. In the extract above, the director implies that large-scale collaboration is not a preferred system of scientific organization. Yet, in a field comprising many smaller laboratories and a few, larger dominant ones, collaboration is seen as not only a technical, scientific necessity, but also as sensible *realpolitik*.

> Yeah, but, you know, when you're competing with the Broad MIT [Massachusetts Institute of Technology], you know, who are working on ... and that's just the psychiatry, they've also got big programmes on diabetes and cancer and, you know, that's fairly tough and they ... so we think ... you know, you have to collaborate to compete with groups that big.
>
> (Centre director of neuropsychiatric genetics)

Thus, collaboration is not simply an economic necessity, but also a survival strategy for smaller groups to continue to do 'meaningful work' by combining samples; 'collaborating to compete' and 'competing by collaborating' with larger US laboratories. Some laboratories, such as the Broad, are so large that their psychiatric genetics research is complemented by world-leading programmes dedicated to cancer genomics and infectious disease. Some of the expertise and infrastructure of these programmes are transferable, providing a competitive advantage. While there is an element of concern that collaboration has become a precondition of survival, others working at the Centre took a more optimistic view. In the following extract, one senior scientist explains the steep increase in collaborative work in terms of fulfilling the need for increased statistical power:

> And therefore that's promoted collaboration between various groups ... although you collaborate you're still in competition, so it's an interesting balance, but by and large it seems to have worked ... everybody comes together to do a large study, and that's largely because funding bodies will only fund the large studies, funding bodies have promoted this ... and that has worked well, and then we all go our separate ways after the collaboration and then start competing against each other again, and that's healthy enough and that's how it should be really.
>
> (Senior lecturer in neuropsychiatric genetics)

Collaboration and competition is not a zero-sum game between groups. This fits with what Atkinson *et al.* (1998) call the 'trajectory of collaboration and competition', which describes a continuum ranging from full cooperation to intense competition. Flexibility within this continuum is considered 'healthy'. However, this kind of cooperation with competitors does not arise 'naturally'. In this case, it is not the product of the independent volition of various actors, but rather is instigated by funding bodies who incentivize (and even demand) collaboration. Why are some groups hesitant or wary to collaborate? Moreover, if sharing larger samples is a technical imperative, a necessary condition of good science, and if the pressure to compete with larger groups demands greater collaboration, why would funding agencies need to incentivize? We might naively expect 'good science' to surely drive itself. As the director explains below, collaboration in science is also mediated by 'classic' concerns, such as trust and reputation:

> I mean we're just at the moment waiting to hear on a paper where we think, in fact we're sure, we've found a novel risk gene for schizophrenia where we've managed to persuade groups, you know, from at least … I can't count them all up, but at least six other groups to work with us to prove this stuff, and I think that's a measure that, you know, we trust them but also that they kind of like us enough to do it for us cos there's not a lot in it for them. I mean they'll be on our paper but it's not their finding and then of course we have to … we'll do that for them and we do and they trust us to do it back, so, you know, I think we have a reputation of being reasonably trustworthy people and that's what you're … I mean it's a classic kind of social setup isn't it, you've got to be trusted.
>
> (Centre director of neuropsychiatric genetics)

Often the group seeking collaboration is the one that stands to benefit the most, in this case by aggregating the samples of other groups to find novel genetic risk variants. The fact that other groups need to be persuaded implies a risk, principally a loss of potential reward. The reward system in science is such that not everybody can share the spoils of success when a significant discovery is published at a collective level. Beaver (2001) described the contemporary rise of 'fractional scientists', whose individual share of the symbolic rewards of science have fallen as scientific projects have grown larger. In these kinds of distributed projects, the erosion of symbolic reward even begins to impinge on groups as well as individuals. This is because reward cannot be distributed to groups equally, especially when scientific capital is asymmetrical. It can also entail an uncomfortable delay in sharing rewards over time. As the director indicates above, groups who rotate success with their partners are those who accrue respect.

Consortium-based collaboration is probably the single most important mechanism for facilitating the transition to Big Biology. It involves reorganizing psychiatric genetics into what Collins (2003) calls 'federal' Big Science – a field comprising multiple temporary cores. In the extract below, one senior scientist describes the tension between group autonomy and federal collaboration that sits at the heart of this transition:

> … and so people have come from a different background, [and with a] range of ideas of what they thought was reasonable, people vary in what they want and what they think their entitlement is or what they'll accept … I feel it's a highly undesirable situation that a group's work would just get swallowed into some big whole and they wouldn't really be able to have any you know

... I don't mean personal reward but group specific recognition, but on the other hand I think being part of the consortium in itself is, you know is it really important to them? I mean to my mind that's actually a much better use of data than publishing it in a way that it can't be easily put into the bigger group but it's just at the moment the field's transitioning from where it was possible to sort of, for a group to think they could do something really important on its own to the stage where actually the really big samples are needed ... but it'll take people a while to adjust.

(Professor in bipolar research)

As someone involved in the high-level management of large-scale consortia, this senior scientist is all too aware that these forms of scientific collaboration come with different expectations and investments. This complicates the superordinate goal because there is a risk that a laboratory's resources (and interests) will 'just get swallowed into some big whole'. One of the problems with federal big science, in this context, is that the reward system either privileges the more powerful members of the collaboration (those whose names appear at the beginning or the end of a publication) or attributes reward to an abstract category ('the collaboration'), which makes it harder for any specific individual or group to extract symbolic capital.

While most of the senior members of the Centre talked about tensions in collaboration at the collective level, other members of the Centre felt the effects of collaboration at the level of the laboratory. One postdoc, for example, described the changes in laboratory practice in terms of a loss of mobility and visibility:

We did a linkage analysis about five years ago ... so it was published in, I think, about 2003, and at the time it was one of the biggest ones that had ever been done, and we worked ... that was two years' worth of work going into it, it was a big project and we ... when you look for the effect sizes of the genes that you expect for diseases like this [schizophrenia], we were always thinking, well we had so much power to detect the genes of certain effect sizes, when you now look at the effect sizes that we actually think are operating in diseases like schizophrenia we found that we probably had about 20 per cent power to find something in the sample, so that means that basically that whole project was deemed a failure ... I mean some people haven't got the facilities to do that and that's why it's changed, and that's where you need collaborations and that's why it's a bit of a muscle game at the moment, the guys with the bigger samples, you know, and the best facilities are out muscling those groups that haven't got it.

(Postdoctoral researcher, schizophrenia team)

And how does this affect you?

That's probably the biggest downside of the way that it's going in one respect is that you've got two choices, I mean, you can either set up a big group, and you can say, well I'm actually happy because I'm not leading the project, I'm not able to get the number of first authorship papers that I may be used to be able to get, but I'm actually part of the group that's actually pushing, really really pushing the frontiers of science forward, and it's been something that's … been a grievance for the last few years, but I'm starting to sort of fit more into it, I mean, I haven't … there's no opportunity in my world at the moment to get any funding myself … and it's not encouraged to do that sort of thing, if I said I wanted a grant for something, I don't think they'd encourage me to do it, I really don't, and the reason being is because they don't want me deviating my time from what they want me to do, so you lose a lot of control.

(Postdoctoral researcher, schizophrenia team)

The first project conducted 'five years ago' was not intrinsically flawed, but rather was *superseded* by the view that the genetic contributions to psychiatric disorders comprise multiple genes of small effect. The project was 'deemed a failure' retrospectively because it lacked statistical power. All this amounts to a justification for the necessity of collaboration, as psychiatric genetics moved into a phase in which it can be described as a 'muscle game', with the inference being that the need for power is highly competitive and asymmetrical. These changes have had a direct impact on the career trajectory of the postdoc. Socialized in the idea that a scientific career involved a succession of small projects from which they might publish as first author, the move to GWAS means that the postdoc occupies a largely *in situ* role within a network geared towards high-throughput production. In these interviews, there is a sense of oscillation between 'grievance' and acquiescence as the mobility to do creative work is framed as 'deviation' from the group's core activities. In Big Biology, where research is both data-driven and necessarily collaborative, the orientation is towards group rather than individual success. The pursuit of group success may justify the decreased mobility of junior researchers, but it also results in the symbolic rewards accruing to the senior scientists at the apex of these collectivities of large-scale biological research.

Genotyping and outsourcing

GWAS are 'observational' (Lambert and Black 2012) studies of genome-wide variants associated with a trait. They adopt a classic case-control design of comparing the DNA of participants with (cases) or without (controls) a disease trait. The approach is not without its limitations and criticisms (see Chapter 8 for a discussion). The process known as 'genotyping' occurs *after* participants have been classified as presenting with or without disease (an approach known as 'phenotype-first' as opposed to the 'genotype-first' strategy of many genetic epidemiological studies). Classification of the phenotype is paramount in psychiatric GWAS because, more so than other disease types, psychiatric disorders are difficult to diagnose accurately (we discuss this further in Chapter 6).

Although GWAS involve multiple processes of transforming DNA from one state to another (for example, via cellular extraction, purification and hybridization), high-throughput genotyping is essentially a process of *mass inscription* in which thousands of genetic variants are 'read' using high density microarrays. Following Latour and Woolgar (1986), we can say that microarrays are 'inscription devices' that transform the properties of a participant's DNA into a system of inscriptions, such as 'DNA profiles', 'Manhattan plots' and scientific publications. But the inscription devices involved in genotyping have other effects as well; their high density and high-throughput design also divest and displace the material labour of manually producing inscriptions of scientific value. In this section, we discuss how the material practices of genotyping – which are constitutive of the *laboratory style* of reasoning – are increasingly displaced and distributed, creating an acute (and acutely *felt*) division of labour at the Centre.

On our early visits to the laboratories of the Centre, we noticed rows of large fridges filled with DNA samples but little evidence of the material processes required to extract its value. Speaking with the scientists and technicians working at the Centre, we were told that in the past, DNA extraction had been conducted on site, by scientists working in these laboratories on relatively small-scale projects. However, for large-scale projects, blood samples were sent away to commercial laboratories. In fact, much of the 'wet' laboratory work of contemporary psychiatric genetics, not just DNA extraction, but also genotyping and other repetitive labour-intensive tasks, was outsourced, either to Contract Research Organizations (CROs) or to 'genetics factories' (the term used by one senior scientist) such as the Sanger Institute. These concentrations of machines and technicians – a legacy of the HGP and the subsequent growth of the biotechnology sector – provided their own incentive to outsource. Outsourcing displaces the scale of psychiatric genetics from the site of the research laboratory, minimizing the visibility of routinized labour, and allowing biological research to appear as the kind of small-scale laboratory science examined by Knorr-Cetina (1999). But outsourcing also creates an 'epistemic vacuum' that displaces a laboratory style of reasoning.

> Any genomics laboratory has seen huge changes and it is seeing huge changes over the next few years in that most of the work we actually can't do ourselves, both for practical reasons and economic reasons we have to actually outsource to large centres such as the Sanger Centre ... so we would have our postdocs that previously would be getting interesting research papers out, they would now be just sending DNA to a company and then they would come back and they would be analysed by statisticians, and molecular postdocs have a lot less to do these days, I mean essentially they've had to change their skill base and become analysts and that's quite daunting if you are a molecularly skilled postdoc, and the other problem as well is that these projects are huge therefore ... authorship has to change because if it's a large collaboration for example it could be, you know, fifty plus authors and if you're a postdoc who did a significant amount of your two year tenure in that project you will be somewhere in the middle of this

cast of thousands if you like and you're not noticed and sometimes it doesn't even appear on PubMed so obviously some of these searches it doesn't often appear because it might just appear as *The Collaboration*, and that's becoming a challenge you know we all have to be assessed at some point and we all have to help be recognized for um promotion committees grant committees everything and that's becoming difficult.

(Senior lecturer in schizophrenia and ADHD)

By reducing costs and removing much of the manual work of genotyping, the logic of outsourcing creates new kinds of manual and technical work, which are seen as less scientifically rewarding than the creative application of 'wet' laboratory skills. Rather than writing 'interesting research papers' based on their laboratory work, postdocs were spending part of their time 'just sending DNA to a company'. The molecular biology postdoc has 'a lot less to do these days', because most of the craft skills that typified their material expertise has been automated and outsourced, and the demand for these skills have been superseded by the requirements of analysing vast amounts of incoming data. The expertise of the molecular biologist, including the tacit knowledge involved in laboratory work, is displaced by a *statistical style* of reasoning. As noted above, this creates problems for the postdoc in terms of accruing rewards that have become, to borrow a previous expression, 'swallowed into some big whole'. Outsourcing sustains an informational and collaborative regime in which at-the-bench biological skills, and the rewards for using these skills, are diminishing.

As we have described, the ante-rooms of the research laboratories at the Centre were lined with large freezer units, each containing polystyrene trays holding ranks of hand-labelled tubes. These stores of the base material of genetic research extend back through years of collection. Each tube contains the extracted DNA of a case – a person – whose blood was drawn by fieldworkers. While above we heard an account from a senior scientist of the way in which the Centre has come to rely on outsourced laboratories, below we have the perspective of a technician whose role has also changed:

So before I was very much involved in extracting DNA from the blood but now it is changing more and more towards outsourcing the bloods so it can be extracted by a company … because we are getting more and more patients. So at the moment we have this big project and we will have to get blood from around 4,000 people, so regarding my work, this has changed towards supervising and [the] coordination of the … logging of the bloods in the lab because there are at least five people who are collecting bloods and some of them are from [place] so obviously they send the bloods to here and we have to be very careful … not to get blood mixed up … and after that, when we have the DNA, we genotype it and I'm the only person in my team who is blood-based so basically I use different platforms to genotype the DNA and after that is the analysing of the results and I participate in that as well.

(Research technician, part-time PhD student, schizophrenia team)

This is a first-hand account of the way in which the biological work of measuring and manipulating materials, a 'green fingered' (Keating *et al.* 1999) practice often compared to 'household cooking' (Lynch 2002), is replaced by new skills that resemble accounting and stocktaking. Rather than performing the DNA extraction herself, the research assistant now acts as a coordinating contact with commercial bioscience laboratories. References to 'supervising and coordination' and 'logging of the bloods' describes labour that is essential but involves little knowledge of biology. The shift from wet lab work to the management of thousands of incoming and outgoing samples is consistent with existing characterizations of Big Biology (Davies 2013). The apparent deskilling of the role of technicians corresponds to a shift from the centrality of biological objects to a focus on the management and analysis of large-scale datasets. Big Biology is an information science, and the management of outsourcing large samples changes the types of labour to be found in the laboratories of the Centre.

Not all the genotyping is outsourced though: a small proportion continues to be conducted in-house. While this may mean that basic skills are preserved to some extent, there have been significant technological changes to accommodate the massive increase in scale. The issue of scale here not only relates to the size of the sample to be genotyped, but also the number of markers genotyped for each case. Laboratories use machines that enable this process to be miniaturized and automated. Miniaturization reduces reagent costs, and means that even small laboratories can conduct high-throughput research. This produces a concomitant reduction in the amount of physical space and labour required to increase the size of biological datasets (see Oliver 2002, and more radically, King *et al.* 2009). Two technologies that have substantially increased the scale of psychiatric genetics are the gene chip and the liquid handling robot. A senior postdoc was asked to give 'a sort of snapshot, an overview' of the technological changes that have affected the way research is conducted:

> Yeah, so a lot of work now involves robots, liquid handling robots … instead of having a plate that's got space for 96 samples, you now have plates that have 384 wells in them, and the volume that you're pipetting is a very small volume, and to get that, to perform that level of accuracy and consistency can only be done by a robot, so that's something that we do now as an absolute standard and when we set up our reactions, unless you're doing some optimization stage where you're doing a very few samples, well it's all done on robot. So that's removed a lot of the pipetting at the bench.
>
> (Postdoctoral researcher, schizophrenia team)

Miniaturizing the platform on which the reactions are conducted is one way of coping with the scale of genotyping. During our fieldwork, the scaling up of reactions from plates with 96 wells to 384 was achieved, in part, by decreasing the volumes of liquid involved. This requires increasing automation since 'the level of accuracy and consistency can only be done by a robot'. Automation has become 'an absolute standard' not only because it has become routine practice to use robots, but because the precision of mechanization allows a greater degree of standardization.[6] Some of the craft skills of liquid handling are retained for 'optimization' purposes, but robots have essentially removed the manual work of 'pipetting at the bench'. While the transfer of skills from the menial and routine to setting up genotyping platforms may seem to be a triumph of automation, it also introduces new burdens:

> A lot of the work that goes on in a lab now is quite high-throughput, and is why we need all the robots and why we have machines that can analyse so many samples, but it's a lot more ... I don't know, you have to be good at what you do in order not to make mistakes. It's difficult, it's actually very taxing for the people who do that.

And what about compiling the data from different batches?

> Each plate will have 30 markers for 400 people, and you have to go through and genotype and then you have to get that data and compile it with another ten, 12 plates you have to do, the amount of QC [quality control] and just manual handling of the data is ... I think one of the biggest differences to what we had before is just physical size, because it's so easy to make mistakes nowadays ... that's the biggest, you know, they're such big experiments, if anything goes wrong you could lose thousands of pounds in just one day.
>
> (Postdoctoral researcher, schizophrenia team)

In large experiments the potential for error and the costs of failure are amplified by the sheer scale of production. This places additional pressure on practices of quality control. So, while machines are able to miniaturize and automate genotyping, producing a high-throughput laboratory, the work of checking, cleaning and aggregating incoming data has increased exponentially. The stocks of raw material must also be maintained. This relates to earlier descriptions of the increase in the labour of 'stocktaking', in which postdocs are responsible for ensuring that the lab does not 'run out of sample':

> Even with just the whole management of your sample, looking out, making sure you don't run out of your sample. If you do run out of your sample ... have you got (enough) DNA which is a massive issue at the moment, because you can do so much genotyping you've got a danger of actually using your whole sample up, so you can't do any more. But yeah it's not easy to do all these things in the lab, it's quite stressful, it's a very stressful job at the moment, when you talk of such scales and when you're genotyping.
>
> (Postdoctoral researcher, schizophrenia team)

A rather complicated picture emerges in which displacement of biological work through outsourcing, and the technical handling of raw materials, is changing the division of labour within the laboratory. Stocktaking, data-checking and tending to high-throughput machines have replaced traditional craft skills, while at the same time increasing the management of error and risk. The rhetoric of the fully automated laboratory (King *et al.* 2009), delivering freedom from laborious routines, is offset by laboratory scientists describing the 'dangers' and 'stresses' of high-throughput genotyping, especially with regard to the management of finite resources. In fact, what Big Biology conceals within the apparent ease of scaled-up production is the intensification of the management of biological resources. The premium placed on collaboration and circulation of data to create new kinds of biological value also creates new kinds of labour, which are, by contrast relatively immobile and *in situ* (Lezaun 2013).

These figures of immobility appeared from time to time during our visits at the laboratories – the technicians working at CROs whose labour is conducted somewhere over the horizon, the bioinformaticians whose work is often 'lost in the middle' (see Chapter 5), and the fieldworkers whose work 'on the road' is largely unseen (and unstated) by geneticists and clinicians (see Chapter 6). But there were also imagined figures who served as reminders of what a scientific life without these means of ameliorating the scale of psychiatric genetics might look like in the laboratory. On one occasion, a senior postdoctoral researcher explained that although they have the machines and expertise that would be necessary in order to do the work in-house, it would require a member of the laboratory staff working in 'a dark room for a year'. A junior postdoc researcher working nearby interjected to agree: it would mean sending that person to a 'dark place'. The imagined abyss of repetitive, uninspired wet lab work served as a reminder that, without the distributed management of resources, those doing laboratory work at the Centre would be intolerably immobile and invisible.

Doing biology?

Participants in our interviews, especially senior scientists, expressed a curious longing for the return to the laboratory style of reasoning that had preceded Big Biology. Neither explicitly nor implicitly, no one at the Centre described the adoption of GWAS as involving a 'paradigm shift' – a permanent change in the way that psychiatric genetics was organized and conducted. Rather, there was a sense, or at least a hope, among some that Big Biology was an uncomfortable interlude, a temporary phase of 'discovery science', before returning to the small-scale excellence of experimental biology. While the hope of 'doing biology' was a steady vision, it was frequently deferred by new technologies on the horizon:

> Absolutely that's what we're hoping. That's what I'm certainly hoping because I'm a molecular biologist at heart, but it's difficult to see that for the next phase of grants though, the next phase of grants are very much large-scale, and very much in discovery again and you discover things by

doing large-scale genetic studies such as sequencing, and then you do unparalleled analysis packages. At the moment nobody knows how to analyse the data that we'll be generating over the next few years.

So you're producing data that you don't know how to analyse?

No, no, no, that's correct yes it's going to be of a scale which is unprecedented ... so we would previously be looking at half a million data points in each individual now we'll be sequencing so we'll be looking at 30 million data points ... I would say for the foreseeable future there's a large-scale genetics projects which will be largely outsourced because you cannot do a lot of these in-house but the analysis you'll have to do yourself and that's where we will have to focus on and then after that I would hope that we will identify genes which are worthy of follow up ... worthy of molecular approaches etc. I guess one of the changes perhaps I'm referring to with this lab [which] means genotyping and sequencing effectively, and the pieces of kit the approaches and the skills we've developed to do association studies have now been superseded and that's the point. So the skills that we have are just not needed anymore. I would say it's just not cost-effective to do it yourself, you outsource and then you do other things yourself, so there's quite a different shift so I would say that postdocs will be preparing samples for the outsourcing and then trying to interpret the samples as they come in now whether the same individuals will have the appropriate skills to prepare the samples and also do analysis the samples is another thing. Not many people will have both those skills I think ... it's changing it's tough it's a tough time to be a postdoc you have to choose wisely I think.

(Senior lecturer in Parkinson's disease)

While we were conducting fieldwork at the Centre, genome sequencing was set to be a controversial leap forward in the field of psychiatric genetics as some were coming to believe that SNP-based genotyping had not delivered the 'low-hanging fruit' that people had been expecting (Hardy and Singleton 2009; Goldstein 2009; Manolio *et al.* 2009; Turkheimer 2012). While consortium-based GWAS maintain the conviction that 'common' polygenes for psychiatric disorders will be detected by SNP genotyping (Psychiatric GWAS Consortium Coordinating Committee 2009), sequencing offers the opportunity to read 'everything' in the hope of finding 'rare' variants. However, as scientists revealed to us in interviews, the decision over which approach a group takes, the pursuit of rare or common variants, the use of sequencing or genotyping, does not lie solely with scientists based on their expertise, but also with funders. There was no 'foreseeable' end to high-throughput research; next-generation sequencing is an intensification of the 'data deluge'. Outsourcing will continue and the transition to computationally focused biology will accelerate. How laboratories will cope with these changes and what form their skill base will take is uncertain:

I've been very worried about outsourcing for a while because I didn't ... you know some groups and my competitors in the States are really ... they really do not have a lab, I mean they might have a technician who can aliquot DNA and a freezer, but they don't, you know just everything is outsourced and I never wanted that, I wanted us to be able to do some biology afterwards and do some of the sort of, the smaller scale experiments which often are the most interesting ones.

(Centre director of neuropsychiatric genetics)

As some of those at the Centre see it, several US laboratories maintain their competitive edge by outsourcing 'everything', investing very little in the 'biology afterwards'. Here, the director gives this distinction a moral cast since heavy reliance on outsourcing leads to an erosion of laboratory skills. By seeking to avoid this scenario, the director suggests that 'doing biology' is more than the constituent requirements of doing good science, but is actually the core style of psychiatric genetics. GWAS are not about identifying associations between genetic variants and disease for its own sake, but about using these associations as signposts to understand the underlying biology of psychiatric disorders. This point was made emphatically by a senior lecturer:

We're not stamp collecting, and we're not just trying to get a bunch of significant hits and then just list them and say, hey we've identified X number of genes for schizophrenia, we want to realize why they cause the illness.

The hope of 'doing biology' is a reason for enduring Big Biology:

I mean the hope is you know the reason you do it, is that it moves you past the blockage in the science. You know, I think there's a feeling now that we're all fed up looking for risk genes we need to find some stuff and move on and do the imaging and the mouse models and then you know ... and a feeling that you know your field has been a success. I mean I personally I have played quite a large role in establishing this as a field so I want, you know, I get a lot of pleasure out of it moving forward and satisfaction out of that ... I'm not saying it's a terrible problem but you certainly think about it and it's uncomfortable, but it's better to sort of ... you know it's much better that we move past the blockage really and we need to harness all these groups and resources together to do that.

(Centre director of neuropsychiatric genetics)

Conclusion

In this chapter, we have argued that contemporary large-scale psychiatric genetics is 'Big Biology'. We use this category to distinguish the distributed management of GWAS from the intensive aggregation of labour and resources typical of 'Big Science' in physics. Inside the laboratories of the Centre, we found that high-throughput genotyping does indeed conform to an amplification of research efforts. But we found nothing resembling the centralization or visibility of Big Physics. In ways that are quite distinct from supercolliders, gravity wave detectors, or indeed, the 'industrialized' genomics of the HGP, scale is a property of highly distributed processes. In fact, these processes conceal the scale of the labour so efficiently that they challenge the meaningfulness of attributing an 'inside' to Big Biology. Many of the activities at the Centre are externally oriented to sharing and transforming raw materials into objects that are intended to circulate among networks while, internally, the actual labour of adding or creating value to these objects is rendered fractional and invisible.

The reorganization of psychiatric genetics into consortium-based GWAS has facilitated the circulation of biological samples and, more importantly, data between remote laboratories and various technology providers. Laboratories that once competed with one another are now incentivized by funding councils to collaborate by assembling ever-larger samples to increase statistical power in order to compete with larger, well-funded programmes. Psychiatric genetics has become a so-called 'muscle game' in which competition over limited resources produce conditions that incentivize economies of scale. The pressure to reduce research costs and to collaborate with competitors does afford a degree of flexibility, described by some as a 'continuum' between cooperation and competition (Atkinson *et al.* 1998), whereby trust and reputation are essential mechanisms for negotiating rewards. A key tension in this federation of research laboratories is balancing autonomy of group-specific recognition with the benefits of cooperation. As the imperative to share biological samples creates denser and more numerous collaborative infrastructures, there is a sense in which the 'outside' of Big Biology is 'diminishing' (Davies *et al.* 2013) as the inside becomes more distributed (we return to this point in Chapter 8).

The transformation of psychiatric genetics into consortium-based GWAS was, of course, a response to a key technology of post-genomic biomedicine: microarrays. Data-driven research is facilitated by high-throughput processes of genotyping that produce mass inscriptions of biological value. The transformation of raw material into symbolic forms of scientific capital are not merely processes of *revealing* biological value, but processes of *creating* value by giving them a form amenable to statistical styles of reasoning. The so-called 'technologization of vitality' (Rose 2013) in the life sciences – greatly assisted by the automation and miniaturization of machines – implies that objects acquire value by virtue of their circulation (see Rose's 2007 comments about circulation being a characteristic of the 'bioeconomy'). But Lezaun (2013: 481) argues that in data-driven infrastructures, data stripped of their material parts become radically *de-valued*: 'It is only when these data are reinstated into specific forms of labour and care – when data are collated, curated, interpreted and otherwise acted upon – that such a thing acquires the status of meaningful and valuable asset.' Our concern is not whether data itself is devalued – indeed, our empirical work suggests that data are one of the most important forms of scientific capital in the kind of collaborations that characterize contemporary psychiatric genetics – but whether scientific practices are themselves devalued. From our observations, the problem of Big Biology is not the circumstances by which data acquire the properties that allow them to circulate as 'weightless' inscriptions, but the *devaluation* of the labour required to create and generate their value. At the Centre, the distributed management of genotyping displaces laboratory work, which further reduces the mobility and visibility of junior members. It also obscures the contributions of individuals who face the problem of becoming fractional scientists: 'invisible, in a formal sense, to the larger research community ... just "names" on a paper ... essentially anonymous' (Beaver 2001: 370).

In regimes that involve the distributed management of biological resources, molecular biologists and technicians are consigned to being custodians of biological materials. This involves the curation and coordination of biological objects dispatched to specialized sites for disassembly, inscription and then reassembly as usable genomic data. The efficiencies of displacing material work outside the Centre has changed the division of labour and the allocation of scientific reward. In some respects, these flexible regimes parallel the developments of post-Fordist techniques of cost and scale reduction. However, distributed processes such as 'outsourcing' also create 'a *sharpened* division between mental and manual labour and a *strengthening* of the hierarchical relation between labour of the "head" and "hand"' (Vallas 1999: 91). The molecular biologist socialized in the laboratory style finds that the craft skills that underpin her style of reasoning have been displaced from the centres of Big Biology, and her share of the distribution of rewards diminished. Big Psychiatric Genetics has become increasingly dominated by a statistical style of reasoning, in which the scale of data-driven research is measured in megabytes rather than square feet of laboratory space. This arrangement has created new networks of production in which biologists find themselves working alongside statisticians, mathematicians and computer scientists. In the next chapter, we consider how the statistical style of *bioinformatics* has become epistemically central to psychiatric genetics, and yet institutionally peripheral to multidisciplinary collaboration.

Notes

1 'Pre-biological' in the sense that the work that was being done was not so much science as the preparation for doing science. An analogy could be drawn with the difference between assembling a scientific instrument and using that instrument to 'do science'.
2 Interestingly, 'stamp collecting' was the phrase used by a scientist we interviewed to stress that data-driven research was not only the kind of work being done at the Centre. Writing about similar developments in cancer genomics, Keating and Cambrosio (2012) argue that at the turn of the twenty-first century we find a 'hybridization' of data-driven and hypothesis-driven research as complementary styles of reasoning.
3 The terminology of 'brute force' often refers to the 'hypothesis-free', data-driven method of detecting genetic variations of small effect which, in the case of psychiatric genetics, are believed to be the genetic components of psychiatric disorders. However, Leonelli (2012) has argued that 'hypothesis-free' is a misunderstanding of the epistemology of these projects.

4 Mega-analyses are different to meta-analyses: the former combines individual-level genotype and phenotype data from all subjects in each study, while the latter combines 'summary results' across multiple studies.

5 Of course, the numbers representing the scale of the PGC do not include the uncounted research technicians, both in-house and through CROs, the invisibility and remoteness of whom are characteristic of Big Biology.

6 Keating *et al.* (1999: 125) suggest that 'molecular biology as a whole has been singled out as ripe for automation partly because of the lack of routine' that is a result of the 'green-fingered' character of the craft techniques of laboratory work. In fact, the automation of molecular biology introduces a level of 'accuracy and consistency' that systematically eliminates repetitive human labour from the bench.

References

Atkinson P, Batchelor C and Parsons E (1998) Trajectories of collaboration and competition in a medical discovery. *Science, Technology & Human Values* 23(3): 259–284.

Balmer B (1996) Managing mapping in the Human Genome Project. *Social Studies of Science* 26(3): 531–573.

Bartlett A (2008) *Accomplishing Sequencing the Human Genome*. PhD Thesis, Cardiff University.

Beaver DD (2001) Reflections on scientific collaborations (and its study): Past, present and future – feature report. *Scientometrics* 52(3): 365–377.

Burton PR, Hansell AL, Fortier I, *et al.* (2009) Size matters: Just how big is BIG. Quantifying realistic sample size requirements for human genome epidemiology. *International Journal of Epidemiology* 38(1): 263–273.

Cantor C (1990) Orchestrating the Human Genome Project. *Science* 248(4951): 49–51.

Collins F, Morgan M and Patrinos A (2003) The Human Genome Project: Lessons from large-scale biology. *Science* 300(5617): 286–290.

Collins HM (2003) LIGO becomes big science. *Historical Studies in the Physical and Biological Sciences* 33(2): 261–297.

Davies G (2013) Arguably big biology: Sociology, spatiality and the knockout mouse project. *Biosocieties* 8(4): 417–431.

Davies G, Frow E and Leonelli S (2013) Introduction: Bigger, faster, better? Rhetorics and practices of large-scale research in contemporary biology. *Biosocieties* 8(4): 386–396.

Goldstein DB (2009) Common genetic variation and human traits. *New England Journal of Medicine* 360: 1696–1703.

Hardy JH and Singleton A (2009) Genomewide Association Studies and human disease. *New England Journal of Medicine* 360: 1759–1768.

Hilgartner S (2013) Constituting large-scale biology: Building a regime of governance in the early years of the Human Genome Project. *Biosocieties* 8(4): 397–416.

Keating P and Cambrosio A (2012) Too many numbers: Microarrays in clinical cancer research. *Studies in History and Philosophy of Biological and Biomedical Sciences* 43: 37–51.

Keating P, Limoges C and Cambrosio A (1999) The automated laboratory: The generation and replication of work in molecular genetics. In M Fortun and E Mendelsohn (eds). *The Practices of Human Genetics*. Dordrecht: Kluwer Academic Publishers, pp. 125–142.

King RD, Rowland J, Oliver SG, *et al.* (2009) The automation of science. *Science* 324 (3 April): 85–89.

Knorr-Cetina K (1999) *Epistemic Cultures: How the Sciences Make Knowledge.* Cambridge, MA: Harvard University Press.

Lambert CG and Black LJ (2012) Learning from our GWAS mistakes: From experimental design to scientific method. *Biostatistics* 13(2): 195–203.

Latour B and Woolgar S (1986) *Laboratory Life: The Construction of Scientific Facts.* Princeton: Princeton University Press.

Leonelli S (2012) Introduction: Making sense of data-driven research in the biological and biomedical sciences *Studies in History and Philosophy of Biological and Biomedical Sciences* 43: 1–3.

Lezaun J (2013) Commentary: The escalating politics of 'Big Biology'. *Biosocieties* 8(4): 480–485.

Lynch M (2002) Protocols, practices, and the reproduction of technique in molecular biology. *British Journal of Sociology* 53(2): 203–220.

Manolio T, Collins FS, Cox NJ, *et al.* (2009) Finding the missing heritability of complex diseases. *Nature* 461: 747–753.

Oliver B (2002) Fly factory. *Genome Research* 12: 1017–1018.

Ozaki K, Ohnishi Y, Lida A, *et al.* (2002) Functional SNPs in lymphotoxin-alpha gene that are associated with susceptibility to myocardial infarction. *Nature Genetics* 32(4): 650–654.

Psychiatric GWAS Consortium Coordinating Committee (2009) Genome Wide Association Studies: History, rationale, and prospects for psychiatric disorders. *American Journal of Psychiatry* 166: 540–556.

Risch N and Merikangas K (1996) The future of genetics studies of complex human diseases. *Science* 273: 1516–1517.

Rose N (2013) The human sciences in a biological age. *Theory, Culture & Society* 30(1): 3–34.

Sullivan PF (2010) The psychiatric GWAS consortium: Big science comes to psychiatry. *Neuron* 68(2): 182–186.

Turkheimer E (2012) Genome wide association studies of behaviour are social science. *Philosophy of Behavioural Biology* 282: 43–64.

Vallas SP (1999) Rethinking post-Fordism: The meaning of workplace flexibility. *Sociological Theory* 71(1): 68–101.

Wang D, Fan JB, Siao CJ, *et al.* (1998) Large-scale identification, mapping, and genotyping of single-nucleotide polymorphisms in the human genome. *Science* 280(5366): 1077–1082.

Weinberg AM (1961) Impact of large-scale science on the United States. *Science* 134(3473): 161–164.

5 Drowning in data

Once upon a time, biology was *simple*. Its practitioners cultivated things in Petri dishes and flowerpots, or studied them through fieldglasses. They might count them, measure their lengths or even weigh them. But the numbers – and the crunching needed to interpret those numbers – rarely taxed their mathematical skills beyond a level that they would have learned at school. That is, however, changing fast. Biological data are flooding in at an unprecedented rate.

(*Economist*, 24 June 1999)

Biology was never actually 'simple', but as the HGP neared completion, some anticipated that an increasingly data-intensive biology was entering a new and potentially troubling phase. According to this horticultural image of biology presented above, biologists had used numbers to represent the physical and observable properties of objects in laboratories. However, the volume of high-density data generated by post-HGP techniques – not just sequencing but also the array of *-omic* sciences that have followed in its wake – required a different relationship to mathematics, statistics and computer science. The problem was not merely the *quantity* of data, but that the nature of biological data was changing, to the extent that the physical traces of the biological system were no longer available for reasoning; increasingly biology was moving from the 'wet' laboratory to the 'dry' laboratory of the computer. The unprecedented flood of genomic data has created a widening gulf between inscriptions produced by biology and the objects to which they refer. To access biology, those trained in the laboratory style of reasoning inculcated by molecular biology and genetics are required to cooperate with those trained in a statistical style of reasoning of other disciplinary specialisms. In this chapter, we argue that the move to 'Big Biology' in psychiatric genetics is concomitant with a network of production in which *bioinformatics* plays a central role. As we will see, the social and epistemic organization of this network at the Centre has generated tensions and asymmetries between different styles of scientific reasoning.

A coalition of expertise

In their retrospective essay on the impact of the HGP, Collins *et al.* (2003: 286) explained that the 'mind numbing scale' of mapping and sequencing the genome required more than 'new technologies, new approaches to automation, and new computational strategies'. At the Sanger Institute, John Sulston recalled that 'at first everyone did everything' (Sulston and Ferry 2002: 90), which followed the earlier tradition of manual sequencing. However, they soon realized that the best method of organization was to transition to an increasingly acute division of labour, recruiting staff of varying skills from sequencing technology to computer analysis. Indeed, some were recruited without any prior scientific experience to do just one small part of the job of producing finished sequence data (Bartlett 2008). As Collins *et al.* (2003) recall, organizing 'large-scale biology' required the development of a new network of national laboratories-cum-sequencing factories, each with their own area of scientific expertise.

The director of the Centre conveyed a similar vision of organizing an ensemble of expertise to accomplish large-scale biology.

> I suppose one definition [of the Centre] is also the fact that each study depends upon a kind of coalition of expertise, you know. Whereas a small science study is one where the investigator might use a number of helpers or postdocs – basically it's one set of skills that kind of designs the experiments and analyses the data and interprets the results. Whereas we bring together skills required from the technical side, the genetic skills, the statistical skills and so on.
>
> (Centre director of neuropsychiatric genetics [interview])

In small-scale biology, the structure of the genetics laboratory can be understood as functioning to reproduce the expertise of the principal investigator (PI). Laboratory technicians, assistants, PhD students and postdocs often contribute to the productive capacity of the PI largely by way of contributing additional labour. Of course, psychiatric genetics has always involved contributions from different disciplines, with clinical psychiatrists, geneticists and statisticians combining their expertise. However, the move to Big Biology, in the form of GWAS, led to the Centre being incorporated into a 'federal' model of organization, not entirely dissimilar, though scaled down, to that of the HGP (see Chapter 4). The range of expertise required to accomplish large-scale psychiatric genetics had exceeded that of a lead researcher. There was now a requirement to not only multiply the supply of scientific labour, reproducing the efforts of the PIs, but also to bring new, specialist expertise, from outside the disciplinary domains of the PIs, to the network.

The director's rhetorical account of the Centre as a 'coalition of expertise' implies 'bottom-up' management of human resources (see Collins *et al.* 2003 for similar description of management in the HGP). Different kinds of expertise are combined and coordinated in 'projects' and 'work teams', led by research managers or PIs. However, one postdoc we spoke to, who had witnessed the 'massive' changes at the Centre, was forthcoming in describing the unique challenges of having to work in a different style of reasoning:

> If you work in the lab you are also expected to be able to run all these statistical programmes and do this and do that, and it was well, I've never trained for this, I'm a biologist or I'm a geneticist and I wouldn't expect ... if someone from upstairs who worked in the [bioinformatics unit], if they went, well I'm interested in this, now I wouldn't expect them to come down into the lab and spend a week generating their own results. And I think a lot of the times it never went in that direction. A lot of the times the PIs were a lot more, well you know, just do it. You know, you've got to do it, and the danger with that is that I think, you can generate the wrong results and it's very easy, it's so easy to do with statistics you know. Do you do an ANOVA, do you do a compare the means, do you do something with co-variants, how do you put your co-variants in? Does the programme you're actually working with allow you to do that, because you haven't got any means or ... there's so many that you need to know? You need to know a lot about statistics ... I'm not an expert on that and I don't pretend to be ... I'm happy to run some things but that's something that's, you know, changed massively since I first started here. Mind you it's not just lab work, it's a lot of statistics involved now.
>
> (Postdoctoral researcher in molecular biology [interview])

The postdoc, trained in molecular biology, describes the way in which routine laboratory work has been displaced by increasingly statistical and computational labour. There has been an expectation to assimilate statistical methods into their suite of expertise, but the collaborative arrangements at the Centre that have drawn together the laboratory and statistical styles of reasoning were asymmetrical and often remote. When we entered the field, the biostatisticians and bioinformaticians were located 'upstairs', in a separate part of the hospital campus, while molecular biologists, increasingly reliant on computational, statistical and mathematical expertise to conduct meaningful analysis, drew on this expertise at one step removed. In the background, the voice of the PI can be heard saying 'just do it' – an injunction that implies little tolerance for discussion between collaborating equals. The technical imperative is that laboratories *must* apply statistical methods to produce biological knowledge. The problem is that those socialized in a laboratory style of reasoning – who admit that they lack expertise in statistics – the choice of analytic technique, of computational method in the GWAS era, will always involve deference to those from a different disciplinary tradition. The postdoc's uncertain account conveys a sense of the broader changes occurring within the genomics laboratory; accessing 'biology' now requires the integration of objects and methods that belong to a statistical style of reasoning.

One of the reasons for this shift towards a statistical style is because GWAS involve material practices of 'mass inscription' (Lewis and Bartlett 2013, after

Latour and Woolgar 1986). High-throughput biology takes the material properties of blood, DNA and base pairs and abstracts them into a mass of *primary inscriptions*. The common variation of thousands of cases and controls appears as text files displaying the genotype and the accession numbers of specific SNPs. These inscriptions are 'primary' because they constitute the first phase of substituting molecular objects for a symbolic, representational form. *Secondary inscriptions* are the result of the further transformation of these primary representations – in the case of GWAS through statistical, bioinformatic techniques – into a new secondary order of symbolic forms. The volume of data produced by the Centre and its collaborators are primary inscriptions amenable to this statistical analysis. Molecular biologists found that they must integrate bioinformaticians and biostatisticians into their knowledge-making practices in order to deal with the influx of these primary inscriptions. Some of our interviewees stressed the differences between the styles of reasoning employed by those collaborating in this knowledge-making; highlighting that wet lab biologists had been trained in a science that was intimately connected to the material world, socializing them to value the descriptive, the tactile and the visual; whereas statisticians and informaticians are comfortable making inferences about biology without having to refer to its materiality. This situation was conveyed succinctly by a senior lecturer:

> So, for example, ten years ago we would be publishing studies with 100 to 500 individuals analysed, now it is greater than 5,000 and that requires a lot of management, and that's logically difficult and I think that is a challenge for some people. Even then interpreting the data, you can't open the files in Excel. You have to use specific tools, and often you can't visualize the files. Everything is command line-based. So, it's quite tricky. You're, analysing data without seeing what it looks like, and that's difficult. And so when you're molecular you tend to be quite visual, you tend to have a feel [but] when you're a mathematician or an epidemiologist, you're quite happy for these blackboxes of analysis, if you like. But a lot of people have to change and it's quite difficult for some people, including myself. But I quite like computers, I'm not that bad, but some molecular biologists are finding it quite difficult.
>
> (Senior lecturer [now professor] in psychiatric genetics [interview])

The increasing scale of psychiatric genetics that accompanied the move to GWAS-based research has not only intensified the quantity of data circulating throughout laboratory networks, but has also changed the nature of data. The abstracted properties of genomic data stored in text files and displayed via statistical software is not accessible to a laboratory style of reasoning, which gives the molecular biologist very little to see and feel. The abstraction of the biological to digital data means that, from one point of view, it is not so much that statistical techniques have been 'black-boxed' for use by biologists, but that biology itself has become a 'blackbox' within a statistical style of reasoning.

In a world of data flows, automated laboratory robots and outsourced laboratory labour, it can appear that there is very little for molecular biologists at the Centre to do. As we saw in Chapter 4, even the work of producing primary inscriptions involves the routine, largely *non-biological* work of curating samples and preparing DNA for outsourcing. The traditional craft skills of the molecular biologist – the 'green-fingered' style of observing, studying and manipulating raw materials – are rationalized, reified into the workings of machines,[1] or outsourced to commercial laboratories. As one senior biologist stated: 'the skills that we have are just not needed anymore. It's just not cost effective to do it yourself, you outsource and then you do other things yourself'. What counts as biological work today requires new tools, interfaces and collaborations in order to imagine the function of living (and diseased) bodies.

A shotgun wedding?

Before the HGP era, gene-finding methods in psychiatric genetics were conducted using a predominantly laboratory style of reasoning. In contrast to contemporary, post-HGP approaches, the linkage era of molecular genetics was relatively small science; using small numbers of research participants, identified as part of family pedigrees, with research designed to identify chromosomal regions of interest. However, by the 2000s, advances in *-omic* techniques and technologies provided an opportunity to move away from an approach that grounded psychiatric disorders in an essentialist model of 'genes for' (Kendler 2006). The justification for a move to a 'hypothesis-free', 'discovery science' was that many variants of small effect were hypothesized to be the biological building blocks of psychiatric disorders, and the new technologies and expertise of the post-HGP era enabled a new style of multi-scale, integrative thinking to be imagined. Across the *-omic* sciences, this required new data-processing networks in which statistics and computer science played an increasingly central role. In what follows, we discuss the circumstances in which bioinformatics was institutionally 'wedded' to the 'wet lab' molecular biology at the Centre.

Bioinformatics has been described by some as the so-called 'shotgun marriage' between computer science and molecular biology (Spengler 2000; Marijuán 2002). Others note how it emerged from independent developments in computing and DNA sequencing in the 1960s and 1970s (Mackenzie 2003; Suárez-Díaz 2010; Garcia-Sancho 2012), and became increasingly central to the production of biological knowledge during and after the HGP. What we can agree on is that the HGP brought increasing stabilization to the field of bioinformatics and, with it, a growth of disciplinary trappings, including journals, funding, technologies, curricula and conferences (Bartlett *et al.* 2016). This marriage of computer science and molecular biology though has not been completely harmonious (Lewis and Bartlett 2013; Lewis *et al.* 2016). Indeed, the older alliance between mathematics and biology has a troubled history. In the early twentieth century, the biometrician/Mendelian controversy highlighted the deep antagonism between quantitative and qualitative biology (see Chapter 1). Ronald

Fischer maintained that statisticians should not only analyse the results of experiments, but should also have a hand in designing experiments. Fischer believed that statistics ought to be instrumental in guiding the objectives of science (MacKenzie 1981). In a similar vein, a professor of bioinformatics affiliated to the Centre suggested that mathematical and statistical principles needed to be imposed upon the research design of existing bioscience:

> One of the issues that we have, is historically, and even I would argue now as well, is that biology and biomedical research a lot of the time is a relatively descriptive science, whereas the other sort of pure sciences are a lot more analytical. So for me the interesting things is the mathematicians, the statisticians, the computing people imposing analytical quantitative research on a fairly descriptive area, relatively speaking.
>
> (Professor of bioinformatics [interview])

Calling science 'descriptive' can often be a pejorative reference to non-hypothesis-driven research (Grimaldi and Engel 2007). Biology is *merely* descriptive when reasoning is non-explanatory. Interestingly, the professor turns on its head the standard discussion of the epistemological changes that have accompanied the -*omic* sciences. While many describe -*omic* techniques such as GWAS as 'hypothesis-free', in contrast to the hypothesis-driven linkage studies of the pre-HGP era, the suggestion above is that the imposition of the styles of reasoning found in the quantitative sciences (or 'pure' sciences) to biological problems will transform a previously 'descriptive' science into an 'analytic' science. What the 'pure' sciences can do that 'descriptive' biology apparently cannot is transform the primary inscriptions produced by high-throughput genotyping into 'secondary inscriptions', which can be used not only to *describe* robust statistical relationships between phenotype and genotype, but can also *begin* to explain the function of genetic variants identified. However, there are institutional tensions involved in bringing a new style of reasoning to bear on biology; of imposing analytical constraints upon existing practices to which people have a disciplinary commitment. To give an illustration of these tensions, we discuss the relatively recent circumstances in which a bioinformatics unit was established in and around the Centre.

In 2003, a biostatistics and bioinformatics group, which we call 'the Hub', was established to provide bespoke advice, analysis and support to researchers at the Centre. The vision was to consolidate expertise for the next phase of large-scale psychiatric genetics, including GWAS. The team was formed by relocating people who were already embedded in existing projects at the Centre, as well as by recruiting new researchers from a variety of backgrounds. The ambition articulated by senior scientists at the Centre was that by creating a critical mass of statistical and computational researchers, the Hub would generate 'added-value' by acting as an efficient provider of 'outsourced' specialist expertise to other groups within the university. Physically, the Hub was located just 'outside the Centre', in another part of the building. By being physically, and to some degree intellectually distinct, a part of the Centre but also outside, the Hub presented an opportunity to establish disciplinary autonomy and identity.

> [The Hub] had great potential. It gave a name for bioinformatics as historically people would have been one person here and one person there. It should have brought everybody together under this one umbrella. They brought in the MSc course. Unfortunately what happened is that they weren't particularly interested in the service provision that everybody was expecting. Everybody thought they were going to do some research and they are going to do some service and all their collaborations got formed with one department. So what came in as a body that should have been helping everybody, giving a name to everything that we were all working on, just became another offshoot group of a department. I don't think it gained support across the institution that it could of if it had been a little bit more open and approachable of what it was doing.
>
> (Bioinformatician in medical genetics [interview])

The trade-off for giving bioinformatics a 'name' and a dedicated unit within which bioinformaticians can perform disciplinary autonomy is the expectation that they provide a 'service' to other academic groups, which, as we demonstrate in this chapter, is understood by some as adopting a subordinate position. But according to many of our interviewees, it seems that the Hub struggled to fulfil the promise of also providing outsourced services to those beyond the Centre. Tied into a service provider position vis-à-vis the Centre, we explore how the positioning of bioinformatics as a service was experienced by those working in psychiatric genetics when we consider the relationship between bioinformaticians and biologists at the Centre.

While we were conducting our fieldwork, the expertise provided by the Hub became a central strand woven through nearly all the Centre's work, with their bioinformatic capacity understood to have played a significant role in the capture of large research grants. By the time we revisited the Centre in 2013, the Hub was no longer a separate entity; bioinformatics and biostatistics were now integrated into the Centre as another one of several research themes. It was the awarding of one large grant in particular that led to the Centre moving to a new, purpose-built building, concentrating psychiatric genetics researchers in one place (see Introduction). After this move, bioinformaticians were situated within the Centre physically, beneath and besides the 'wet' laboratories of the new building. Members of this research theme now work in an open plan arrangement, with long rows of computer desks surrounded by a ring of offices. Indeed, molecular biologists, bioinformaticians, graduate psychologists and an assortment of PhD students sit at computers in the middle of the room together, while (mostly) senior scientists occupy the outer ring of offices – a floor plan reminiscent of Bentham's Panopticon (see Stevens 2011 for a similar description of the Broad Institute). Bioinformaticians conduct the practical work of 'dry' biology. This work comprises an assortment of desktop activities from routine database management to developing algorithms for data processing. Physically speaking, the spatial arrangement appears to be designed to facilitate integration and interaction, yet it conceals the asymmetry of collaboration.

> Our group is involved in producing statistical results that basically- really form parts of other people's research ... so basically we never prove any-thing, all we can do is quantify the evidence in favour of something and basically say it is very likely that such and such gene is involved in such and such a disease, we can't prove it for sure.
>
> (Professor of bioinformatics [interview])

The professor gives the impression that working on 'other people's research' is not exactly a fulfilling arrangement. This echoes the accounts found in the work of Lewis and Bartlett (2013), in which bioinformaticians often bristled at being characterized as service providers by their 'wet' biology collaborators, sometimes struggling to access the circuits of reward and recognition so important in a scientific career (Lewis *et al.* 2016). The mundanity of quanti-fying evidence in favour of gene associations bears little resemblance to the more extravagant claims that bioinformatics will be pivotal to 'untangling the networks of life' (Marijuán 2002: 111). Though bioinformaticians may want to impose analytical constraints on 'descriptive' biology or engage in creative, multi-scale thinking, in practice, and within institutions such as the Centre, bio-informatics is subordinated to the interests of the biologists who produce and 'own' the primary data.

Mixing styles of reasoning

The growing importance of bioinformatic methods and tools for understanding biological data – with some going so far to say that all biology now is computa-tional biology (Markowetz 2017) – has created a new hybrid scientist. On the one hand, the *field* of bioinformatics is an interdisciplinary bricolage of experts and expertise from various fields working on collaborative tasks and shared problems. On the other hand, the practitioners of bioinformatics fall into an 'anomalous' category with regard to the established order of traditional discip-linary boundaries, particularly in academia (Lewis *et al.* 2016). As a specialism bridging the 'wet' style of biology and the 'dry' style of computer science and statistics, bioinformatics represents a domain of interstitial knowledge. In this section, we consider the ways in which the statistical style of bioinformatics is positioned within the life sciences. Given that these are issues relating to Big Biology in general, we supplement our fieldwork with interview extracts from bioinformaticians working outside the Centre, and with statements from a UK-wide survey of academics working in and around the field of bioinformatics (reported in Lewis *et al.* 2016; Bartlett *et al.* 2016).

For some biologists, bioinformatics is a 'service', a set of tools and skills to be 'bought in' to a project, its existence only meaningful as an adjunct to biology

(Lewis and Bartlett 2013). For many bioinformaticians (and some scientists more closely acquainted with the field), bioinformatics is a discipline in its own right, while others see it as a 'bridge' spanning the disciplinary gulf between biology and computer science. However, many interviewees were acutely aware of the multiplicity of meanings applied to 'bioinformatics'.

> It depends on who you talk to and you can absolutely argue it both ways. I think that you can only define it as a discipline if you are really doing some cutting-edge research and you are using entirely new statistical computational or mathematical approaches in the area that haven't been used before and I think then it becomes a discipline. Otherwise, I think it is a service or a facilitator for knowledge. Whatever the definition of bioinformatics, it depends on who you talk to. For me it's the use of computers to facilitate biomedical research, but other people will have quite different definitions so I think it could be everything.
>
> (Senior lecturer based in biotechnology services [interview])

As Gieryn (1983) has observed, scientists regularly draw and redraw boundaries to justify their claims as to the value and legitimacy of their science. In the extract above, the senior lecturer at the biotechnology services unit is being tactful by implying that boundaries are relative: whether or not bioinformatics is a discipline depends on whom you speak to; there is no right or wrong answer. Having said this, they offer their own definition of what counts as a discipline, and the conditions are set quite high: 'disciplines' produce 'cutting-edge research' and use 'entirely new … approaches'. Disciplines then are defined by virtue of their autonomy and creativity, and without these virtues, we are told, bioinformatics is merely 'a service or a facilitator for knowledge'.

Biologists that we spoke with often engaged in 'boundary work' by drawing a distinction between biology as a science and bioinformatics as a 'non-science', a service, or an inferior *in silico* science. Bioinformaticians complain that these distinctions stem from ignorance regarding the interdependence of biological research and statistical expertise.

> [Biologists] need bioinformatics. Because bioinformatics is still called a new discipline it is viewed as IT … it is viewed as computer science by biologists whether it be lack of understanding or whatever, which is probably right actually because if you talk to biologists about an area that they are not familiar with, whether it be another area of genetics or whatever they won't want to talk about it. They either rubbish it or won't carry on with the conversation. That applies for bioinformatics because they don't understand it. It is either statistics to them, or it is computer science, and in that sense it hasn't been accepted as a discipline in its own right by biologists and has ended up as a service. In other words there are a number of geeks out there who can analyse data.
>
> (Associate professor in bioinformatics [interview])

Bioinformatics being likened to 'IT', and bioinformaticians as being seen as the 'geeks out there' reduces the field to external technical support, a service that has a tendency to 'blend into the background' (van Baren-Nawrocka 2013). This view of bioinformatics is not only a commentary on its invisibility but also its subordinate position in relation to the relatively powerful disciplinary identities of biologists. Attributing homogeneity to a field demotes its priority within collaborative networks.

From our own observations at the Centre and our research at other sites of post-HGP life science research across the UK, we found that bioinformatics is anything but homogenous. Some approach the challenges of their work from a computational perspective, others from a biological perspective; some are driven academically to develop new algorithms and lead research projects, while others *are* content to offer a 'service', applying existing approaches to support biologists. But few people working in bioinformatics claim to have the kind of deep understanding of both biological mechanisms and function *and* cutting-edge statistics and computer science that would be required to be 'individually' interdisciplinary (Calvert 2010).[2] Some of our respondents state that the different ways in which these 'home' disciplines think about the world are difficult to reconcile. In short, there are distinct styles of reasoning employed by these disciplines. They are not incommensurable (as would be the case with Kuhnian paradigms), but they are not straightforwardly complementary.

> It seems difficult for computer-mathematics-physics-etc.-based bioinformaticians to grasp the concepts and needs of biologists and medical scientists. Bioinformaticians with a biological background are often less comfortable developing complex algorithms.
>
> (Lecturer in medical department [survey])

> There is also a lack of knowledge of biomedical research culture on the part of computer scientists. There are fundamental differences in the logic of research in the two fields.
>
> (Postdoctoral researcher in computer science [survey])

> [The biggest challenge is] understanding each other's problems, requirements, difficulties and backgrounds.
>
> (Research fellow in computer science [survey])

Others have found similar differences between wet and dry scientists (Penders *et al.* 2008, 2009; Torgersen 2009). For instance, Penders *et al.* (2008: 748) observed that in nutrigenomics the wet and dry divide distinguishes different 'styles of scientific reasoning'. Styles are flexible and portable methods that overlap with disciplinary boundaries. Extending Galison's (1999) idea of the 'trading zone', Penders *et al.* argue that specific sites of cooperation and exchange between wet and dry practices converge in what they called the 'moist zone'. The exchange of methods and techniques often take place around 'boundary objects' such as gene pathways. Statistical methods of validating gene pathways establish the conditions for trade. However, despite their cooperative nature, 'wet and dry practices do not always mix very well' (Penders *et al.* 2008: 748) because styles have different histories, occupy different localities, have different priorities and value systems, and employ different vocabularies.

In Big Biology, the mixing of different styles of reasoning is shaped by the different priorities (disciplinary, individual and institutional) that are at work. At the Centre, for instance, psychiatric genetics involves similar trading zones of wet and dry research practices, but the conditions of trade are governed by scientists whose disciplinary hinterland is that of psychiatry and genetics. It is scientists from these backgrounds – who are often granted the core funding, and through that control the biological samples – who determine the priorities of the research programme, and accrue the symbolic rewards of individual and institutional prestige. To understand how these priorities work, consider the following account of a senior scientist describing their dependence on statisticians:

> Most of the data analysis that I do relates to transcriptional data, microarray data.... So I have the biological knowledge but I haven't really ever been taught to programme. So, at the moment, I'm kind of, teaching myself to programme using the 'R' language because that is what most of the microarray packages come in. I can do the standard analyses myself, that really isn't a problem. There are a number of standard packages that you can pull down. So, provided you know how to organize your data you can do, actually, even quite complicated analyses without actually having to programme very much. I could edit other peoples' scripts so that, effectively, once I've done something once then I can do it again and again and again, but there are a number of problems. Some of which will be alleviated by actually having a student who has more computational knowledge because there's a limit to how much you can get [done] yourself.... But when it comes to higher-level statistics where you, for instance, need permutations to organize, to decide the significance etc., or where you need models ... you actually need to fit models to your data ... then I can't do that and I would refer to a statistician. Even if I could programme it I think that I would probably refer it to a statistician because you would want to be sure that it was referee proof, you'd want to be sure it was right. Because, really, what you want is the truth and it can be really hard to pick that out of a huge wealth of data.
>
> (Reader in neuropsychiatric genetics [interview])

There are lot of things the scientist claims they can do. They can teach themselves to programme at a basic level; they can use 'standard packages' to analyse data and thus reduce the need to programme; they can also 'organize data' for analysis and even 'edit other people's scripts'. Whatever they cannot do is 'alleviated by actually having a *student* who has more computational knowledge'. Though we might say that styles of reasoning are exchanged in a cooperative manner, the conditions of exchange between supervisor and student are asymmetrical. Statistical and computational knowledge is appointed to the biologist, whose priorities are to ensure that their own work is 'referee proof'. In other words, within the Centre (and other bioscience institutions) the statistical style supplies a service to ensure that the clinical and laboratory styles can meet their own 'standards of objectivity' (Hacking 1992).

A service-oriented bioinformatics permits, among other things, the 'blackboxing' of artefacts and expertise. Its success is determined by rendering its own internal workings invisible (Latour 1999). To some extent, biologists need not understand these processes but can trust the socio-technical machine to produce reliable tools. It is a process synonymous with the outsourcing of work to dedicated, external facilities (whether commercial or not), or to in-house (physical or virtual) hubs offering technical services across institutions. But the apparent efficiency and flexibility of embedding services to support scientists is an arrangement which is viewed with some ambivalence, in a manner reminiscent of McNally's (2008) distinction between 'blackbox optimists' and 'blackbox pessimists'. Some celebrate the benefits of making bioinformatics a recipe-like exercise or a push-button tool, to be used by biologists without a deep understanding of the underlying principles. This frees up biologists to spend their time, energy and imagination formulating biological models and hypotheses. However, like the biologist who finds that the pull towards a statistical style reduces the ability to think biologically about statistical patterns, pessimists are concerned that blackboxing statistical operations results in a loss of cognitive authority over the production of laboratory knowledge:

> This [blackboxing] is a big problem.... One of the reasons for learning to programme yourself is because you want to know what's happening. I want to know what's happened to my data. I want to know what people have done to it. And I want to know that – because I want to know that the information coming out is as good as it can be, as representative of the truth as it can be. I don't want to spend my career chasing red herrings. I think there is a big problem because I think people genuinely need to understand how their data had been analysed, and I think there is an inclination to take their data and stick it in genes.... So I sit on the Post Graduate Research Committee and I find that a few students, now, since macros have become quite popular, who've got data but they haven't really ... if you ask them in detail they don't really understand how it's been analysed and they need to understand that. So I think it is a problem, yes.
>
> (Reader in neuropsychiatric genetics [interview])

Here, the problem of mixing styles is described as if it is a zero-sum game – the gain of one style is the loss of another. The blackbox pessimist is concerned about issues of control, expertise, ownership and trust: 'I want to know what's happened to *my data*. I want to know what *people have done to it*.' Rather than outsourcing being a practical substitute for skills and knowledge, the biologist wants to understand the underlying principles of analysis; they want to be *accountable* for the ways in which candidates of truth (or falsehood) are arrived at. In the politics of cooperation, the mixing of styles runs the risk of deskilling biologists and thus losing control of laboratory processes that may well produce 'red herrings'. Bioinformatics as a 'service' to biology is a bioinformatics that is blackboxed. The reader's desire for control and ownership can only be achieved by individual interdisciplinarity, or by collaboration with bioinformaticians that treats them not as a *service provider*, but as fully, trusted *scientific collaborators*.

Although the statistical style of reasoning is central to psychiatric genetics, institutionally its practitioners are often subordinate to other scientists working in established disciplines. To borrow and extend the analogy of 'trawling' often used in the field, bioinformaticians may fish the seas to land a catch of statistical significance, but biologists own the ships, the catch and, to some extent, the seas upon which they fish. In many situations, bioinformaticians are working *for* biologists, conducting their computational and algorithmic work on biological data under the direction of biologists, with the greater part of the scientific reward accruing to those who own and control the production of value. Psychiatric genetics requires highly skilled computational scientists but neither their methods, nor the centrality of their style of reasoning, are sufficient to guarantee an equal partnership or 'marriage'.

Value tensions

Unlike established disciplines that have relatively stable pathways of socialization through dedicated departments and undergraduate curricula, bioinformaticians often arrive at bioinformatics having travelled from a variety of backgrounds. They may come from a hinterland of training and work in biology, medicine, computer science, mathematics or information science. As we mentioned in the previous section, this has resulted in the formation of a heterogeneous group at the Centre and similar bioscience institutions. In this section, we explore the various kinds of 'value tensions' (Hackett 1990, 2005)[3] experienced by those working in and with bioinformatics at the Centre.

Part of the remit of setting up the Hub in 2003 was the launch of a new MSc programme that offered training in bioinformatics, statistics and information management. Distinct from previous generations, new cohorts of PhD students and postdocs were being trained *as* bioinformaticians. One PhD student we interviewed revealed an interesting division emerging within the group:

> If you speak to my supervisor, he would say there is a slight difference between a bioinformaticist and a bioinformatician … I think of myself as more of a developer than a service, so I am not necessarily the person you would come to [though] it might appear that I am. I actually have done that initially in my PhD and people come along and say I want to find this gene through an analysis of that. But it is an area I want to move away from and

to move towards a developing aspect, developing applications rather than using them and giving people the results. I want them to do that rather than me. So that is why there is a definition between a bioinformaticist and a bioinformatician because they seem to vary.

(PhD student in bioinformatics [interview])

In ways that may at first seem unusual to other established disciplines, the PhD student draws a boundary *within* bioinformatics between 'bioinformatician' and the apparently creative role of the 'bioinformaticist'. The bioinformatics group were creating their own endogenous categories[4] to distinguish those who, like *technicians*, provide services and support by applying existing techniques of data analysis, and those who, as *scientists*, conduct original research by developing new techniques. Having fulfilled a service role during the early stages of his PhD, the tensions between instrumental and intrinsic value resulted in the student consciously moving further towards the research pole of the service–research axis. For someone at the formative stages of their academic career, imagining a future in which his role involved the originality of 'developing applications' provides an insight into what the field values: autonomy and creativity are constitutive – indeed, are the entitlements – of those working as a scientist.

Not long after the Hub was established, a reader at the Centre agreed to be interviewed and asked us whether our work would have any influence on the availability of bioinformatics.

I think one of the big problems for people in bioinformatics is that everybody else regards them as a service and wants their service, so they don't get time to do their own research. I've employed two bioinformaticists, actually it was the same post but the first person left, both very good bioinformaticists, completely different. One of them was a career bioinformaticist, wanted to develop his own thing, and so they spend their time developing new resources. And when we have a PhD student, I expect that person to want to develop new things, different ways of looking at data, to survey what's around and see what can be done with that and what needs to be new. That's very different from someone who sits down and analyses other peoples' data. I do think there's a big divide here and I think that's [where] we run into trouble. I think, in this institute we've run into trouble because people don't recognize that the two are different things. So a service bioinformaticist is different to a bioinformaticist who does it at a research level … just doing their experiments but on their computer, just the same as we do ours, but on the bench.

(Reader in neuropsychiatric genetics [interview])

Aside from overestimating the power of sociology, the reader recognizes the distinction between the 'career bioinformaticist' and the 'service bioinformatician'. The career bioinformaticist left the post to 'develop his own thing', suggesting that it was difficult to realize his scientific identity and autonomy in this kind of post, while the technically minded bioinformatician had different expectations of 'reward'. The expectation that the Centre can recruit bioinformatic expertise into its projects, to hire 'someone who sits down and analyses other people's data' presents a problem. This kind of *immobile* role may not satisfy those who have spent years being socialized to expect the kind of symbolic reward and recognition – and personal satisfaction – upon which the 'economy' of academic science is built. As expertise for hire, service bioinformatics is institutionally devalued.

In describing her own work, the reader explains that she would like to see more blackboxed 'service bioinformatics', though acknowledges that some would see this as a waste of the talents of bioinformaticians.

> I think some of the things I do, it would be much easier to have someone technical in post and to say to them, please can you run this algorithm for me, or please can you code up this algorithm for me so I can try it out or, please can you pull this algorithm down from this website and see if it works, which I would find much more time consuming than they would. I think that it would be good to have more service bioinformatics. I think that would worry [the] College, perhaps they would not see these people being used as fully as they might be.
>
> (Reader in neuropsychiatric genetics [interview])

In most cases, the technical work of bioinformatics is epistemically distinct from that of the biologist. Biologists are usually dependent on bioinformatic support because traditionally they have not been trained to use bioinformatic software, never mind to 'code up' the algorithms required in order to analyse their data. However, the reader takes an instrumental view, implying that this kind of work is merely a 'time-consuming' technical task. From this perspective, service bioinformatics allows the biologist to pursue the more rewarding 'intrinsic value' (Hackett 2005) of developing biological models and publishing high-impact papers. Some of our participants identified that one of the problems with these kinds of service arrangements, in which postgrad students and postdocs are treated as technicians, is that those doing the 'time-consuming' technical work, learn to master techniques and to solve a set of well-defined technical problems rather than learn how to 'think' creatively within their own discipline. Among the bioinformaticians who see their work as belonging to an independent scientific discipline, what they intrinsically value is developing statistical methods that *inform* biological models. Along these lines, a research associate with a background in biology and affiliated with the Hub describes his PhD work in bioinformatics:

> The decision was made very early on that my skills were very much *in silico* rather than in the lab so let somebody else do that work they are better at it than me. The PhD was more about working out how to analyse the data. You have got very high throughput techniques which run in the regions of 40,000 to 50,000 experiments all in parallel. You then do that on only a few different

samples, so you have got some interesting sort of stats challenges of what is the interesting changes within a dataset. Really it was a case of going through looking at what cutting-edge stuff was, looking back at the more classical statistical type methods and then just assessing. There is more and more stuff coming out of the literature every week but nobody ever says this one is better than this one because of this so that is what a lot of work was centred on. There was another ... a bit which was the ok you have done your stats analysis, you have got a list of interesting findings, what can we then do to try to inform biologically without biasing things with the oh look I recognize that gene, I like that gene therefore this validates what I thought was going on. It was trying to look at the results as a whole and make sense of them.

(Research associate in bioinformatics [interview])

Faced with a choice of the lab or the desktop, the researcher decided to pursue a career based on his computational skills. Their PhD is described as a kind of critical literature review of statistical methods for analysing high-throughput data, the intrinsic value of which is oriented to solving statistical problems, synthesizing and assessing different approaches, and applying them in ways that produce 'interesting findings'. The researcher contrasts the voice of the biologist, who discerns patterns intuitively, with 'unbiased' methods that examine data holistically and at scale. The intrinsic reward of thinking and acting in a statistical style is to develop rigorous methods of validating gene findings.

On these terms, at least, biology and bioinformatics are capable of carving out a productive relationship. However, the problem of mixing styles of reasoning is not only an issue of discordant priorities and vocabularies (Penders *et al.* 2008), but a problem of discordant values. What one specialism considers scientifically valuable might be irrelevant or merely instrumental to another. From our survey data, we learned that the tensions between biologists and bioinformaticians were not unique to the Centre but endemic to *multidisciplinary*[5] research across the UK. Here is a sample of relevant statements:

To be good, bioinformatics has to be relevant to biology and answer real, testable questions. Too much bioinformatics is irrelevant and can be ignored.

(Research fellow in genetics department [survey])

[The challenge is] overcoming the attitude of many biologists that anything that requires computation is not really biology; changing the perception that bioinformaticians are support personnel.

(Research fellow in computer science department [survey])

Biologists often consider bioinformatics as being 'made up' or somehow not real ... I was told that I had to do real experiments to be successful despite the fact that my bioinformatics work had led to several *Nature/Science* publications.

(Scientific curator in bioinformatics research centre [survey])

Whatever organizations say, they do not like multidisciplinary research. In cross[ing] boundaries, you confuse people, and confuse systems. Worst, you get expected to sit on two or three committees. Finally, everybody thinks that their work is harder than everyone else's. So, if you work in two or three disciplines, people generally assume that your work is simple – you aren't doing real computer science of course, you aren't doing real biology.

(Reader in computer science department [survey])

This is only a small selection of what biologists and computer scientists have to say about each other (for a detailed and lengthy discussion see Lewis *et al.* 2016; Bartlett *et al.* 2016, 2017). These statements reveal the extent to which boundary work ascribes the limits of 'good' science within interdisciplinary and multidisciplinary research. A common complaint is that, conducted under the jurisdiction of biology, much bioinformatic work is seen as technical, scientifically uninteresting or even 'non-science'. Disciplinary collaboration is bound by tensions and contradictions between wet and dry cultures of research, which arise from contrasting value systems. Different styles of reasoning reflect 'epistemic cultures' (Knorr-Cetina 1999) that have their own ways of validating the worth of scientific work. The dynamics of these research groups move along axes that, as we will see in the final section of this chapter, centre on the question of who produces value and on what basis different groups can allocate or claim scientific reward.

Value, credit and reward

In this section, we consider how credit and reward is distributed among wet and dry researchers in post-HGP Big Biology. We draw mainly from survey data to illustrate our claims because bioinformaticians at the Centre were reluctant to speak 'on record' on this sensitive topic. Nonetheless, our observations and off-the-record conversations with researchers at the Centre confirm that these concerns are generalizable, and that while in post-HGP Big Biology bioinformatics is epistemically central, it is often institutionally peripheral (Lewis and Bartlett 2013).

Scientific reward and recognition can come at the personal, group, and institutional level. Indeed, there are many types of contribution to research for which people seek credit, with different disciplines valorizing different types of contribution and 'outputs'. But value systems do not travel well within distributed networks, which often clash in borderlands – in this case the 'moist zone' (Penders *et al.* 2008) between wet and dry research. A senior manager of a research council gives an overview of the incommensurability of value systems in this multidisciplinary borderland.

The other thing that causes [a] problem … is that biologists publish papers in journals and that is how they get credit. Computer scientists get credit for invited talks at computer science conference[s].… Whereas a biologist will have first author papers, computer scientists would have a series articles which have appeared at the proceedings of conferences and that is how they value each other. Bioinformaticists measure their worth in terms of open ware software, which is released to the rest of the community. That means if you are sitting there as a biology head of department or whatever and you have gone and got yourself a multidisciplinary team, half of them are going to be producing outputs that your biological community is going to regard as completely worthless. So, you have got a whole range of cultural change issues which are to do with the discipline silos and how they move about.

(Senior manager in research council [interview])

Biologists and bioinformaticians (with disciplinary backgrounds in computer science) simply have different reward structures. Biologists value first or last author publications in high-impact journals, while those socialized in computer science value a range of other outputs, such as conference proceedings and the development of software freely given to the community. Different measures of reward reflect the cultural values of their epistemic community. Drawing the hypothetical case of the 'multidisciplinary team', the senior manager illustrates the ways in which the outputs of the less powerful disciplines are devalued by the discipline that holds institutionalized power. For some scientists moving into bioinformatics, the fact that they are judged *as* biologists is a category mistake that confuses academic departments and frustrates career progress.

It is difficult to ensure one gets appropriate credentials to continue to make one's department happy. The conference-biased nature of the CS [Computer Science] collaborations I do has had my department actually entirely discount conference papers I've done. Additionally, the need to be 'first or last' author makes it very difficult for PIs with PhD students involved in collaborations – even if my PhD student ends up first author, the PI of the biological lab that collected the data is invariably last. And often there just isn't 'enough' to do one bio[logical] and one computer biased paper on each project.

(Senior lecturer in biology and mathematics [survey])

A point of commonality between the surveys and our informal, off-the-record conversations at the Centre is that the positioning of bioinformatics as a service has clear implications for the allocation of credit and reward. Although bioinformatics encompasses a range of essential activities at the Centre – from developing algorithms and standards, creating annotations and metadata – the artefacts of the dry lab have to fit within the established value system of biology. Others have noted that assigning and allocating credit is often a contested activity with 'debates about who, what, how, why and when to give credit for any form of scholarly contribution' (Borgman 2015: 241). Since bioinformatics is often incorporated into the structure of psychiatric genetics as a service subordinate to biology, practitioners struggle to have their contributions recognized. For instance, a professor of bioinformatics at the Centre indicates that what might have once been considered a cutting-edge technique, highly valued by colleagues in the 'wet' lab, is barely worthy of acknowledgement as the technique becomes more routinized.

> These people have had an intellectual influence on the project, they should be on the research papers and get due credit. If it is simply we send you a gel spot, tell us what it is then there isn't a great deal of intellectual input. Although, there is always this case when techniques are cutting-edge you are on paper but as it becomes routine and it becomes a service you get into the acknowledgements and ultimately not even that far.
>
> (Professor of bioinformatics in psychiatric genetics [interview])

The attribution of authorship on academic publications is a particular point at which 'value' is made manifest. Publishing papers is one of the primary rewards of scientific work. Although different disciplines have different ways of assigning authorship (Osborne and Holland 2009), traditionally, first and last authorship on the paper carries the greatest symbolic value, without necessarily reflecting levels of contribution. Until the 1950s, most academic publications were single-authored. Scientists designed their own experiments, collected and analysed their own data (Birnholtz 2006), so long as research technicians are carefully written out (Shapin 1989). In contemporary science, never mind in Big Science, a single author very rarely writes a scientific paper. The trend is towards multiple authors (Galison and Hevly 1992; King 2013), and in Big Biology there can be hundreds of authors on a single paper. These developments have created 'fractional' scientists (Beaver 2001), who might well feel that they are merely one of a long list of names on a paper, essentially anonymous in an economy of symbolic reward. A common complaint among bioinformaticians is that they are not afforded the opportunity to lead projects and papers, despite being central to the biological work.

> [The biggest challenge is] leading author on subsequent papers, where the bioinformatician/statistician has done most of the work.
>
> (Research associate in statistics department [survey])

This positioning of bioinformatics not only renders the contributions of bioinformaticians invisible, but it also impairs their chances of career mobility. This is reflected in the literal positioning of bioinformaticians as middle authors. The collective expertise of Big Biology is distributed throughout an acute division of labour whereby each scientist is taking on a narrow role within a project. Rather than receiving the symbolic reward of being named as first or last author, bioinformaticians find their authorial position mirrors their disciplinary position, bridging disciplines, situated in the middle (Lewis *et al.* 2016).

> The somewhat 'service-oriented' role of many bioinformaticians such as myself can make first-author papers difficult.... Bioinformaticians can be

stuck between 'collaborator' and 'service' roles. Combined, this makes winning independent funding difficult, and creates reliance on contributions from collaborators, and careful budgeting in their grants.

(Postdoctoral researcher in biology department [survey])

Bioinformatics lies in the interstices between biology and computer science. This invariably means that bioinformaticians occupy a liminal space in the academy, as they do in the Centre. The apparent 'middle-ness' between collaborator or service provider, afforded the space, at best, between first author and last author, can be understood as reflective of an odd kind of centrality, of the indispensability of bioinformatics to Big Biology. But as we have seen, middle-ness can also mean that bioinformaticians are not rewarded for their contribution in ways that can satisfy people socialized to expect to be part of the economy of symbolic reward in the sciences. Writing from a US context, Chang (2015: 152) makes a similar observation: 'The research system does not recognise bioinformaticians for doing what the scientific community needs most.' Though collaborative work is a core activity of the field, it is not captured on standard metrics because they are evaluated individually in terms of 'research' outputs. One respondent suggested that existing methods of accountability need to change.

If the bean counters used different performance metrics for assessing researchers (other than numbers of publications etc.), then this may help. This may place less emphasis on only finding things that can be easily published on paper.

(Reader in biology research centre [survey])

Although psychiatric genetics has seen significant changes over the past few decades, the reward mechanisms have not yet adapted to the new forms of social and epistemic organization of Big Biology. Bioinformaticians find themselves, to some degree, in an anomic situation.

Conclusion

In this chapter, we have shown that Big Biology relies on multidisciplinary arrangements, combining laboratory and statistical styles of reasoning to analyse and manage the large volumes of genome data produced by mass inscription devices. For psychiatric genetics, the move to GWAS has promised to deliver meaningful correlations between genotype and phenotype as key markers of functional pathways in the 'genetic architecture' of psychiatric disorders. In later chapters (especially Chapter 8), we will review the success of these programmes, but for now, our focus is to understand the impact of Big Data on scientific researchers at the Centre.

GWAS involve the efficient and intensive management of resources, which has changed the social and epistemic organization of scientific work at the Centre. Although GWAS seek to extract meaningful 'biology' from statistically significant associations, it is the statistical style of reasoning that dominates this iteration of psychiatric genetics rather than the laboratory style, in all its experimental, material, green-fingered craft. This has occurred because GWAS produce a mass of primary inscriptions that strip biological resources of their material properties. These processes of abstraction allow a greater number of data points to appear as freely circulating artefacts amenable to computational and statistical analysis. Data become *in silico* objects that *refer* to biological content – a single nucleotide, a protein sequence, an expression pathway – but they also have numerical properties for aligning, editing, testing and modelling this content. Without biology, these inscriptions have no functional meaning and without computational expertise, biology is blind. The conditions of cooperation between styles of 'wet' and 'dry' reasoning are opportunities to exchange methods in so-called 'trading zones' (Galison 1999), imposing analytic constraints on laboratory processes. This is the strong version of cooperation where bioinformatics 'informs' biology. The weak version (and the most prevalent at the Centre and many other UK institutions in which bioinformatics plays a role) is that in which bioinformatics provides generic or bespoke tools to 'help' others see and navigate biology through unfamiliar artefacts and devices.

While we were in the field, from 2008 to 2010, the Centre was in a state of rapid transition. From our own observations, the director's rhetorical description of bottom-up management, the so-called 'coalition of expertise', is in contrast with accounts of bioinformaticians being treated as service technicians to biologists. The rhetoric of investing in *expertise* is superficially persuasive, but conceals the old networks of senior scientists – the psychiatrists and geneticists – who secure collaborations and core funding, and thus maintain the steady supply of biological resources. The establishment of the Hub in 2003 represented an opportunity to invest in statistical and computational expertise, which had the outward-facing vision of providing support to other groups in the university, but eventually was absorbed into service work for the Centre. The 'Hub' is perhaps a misleading label that implies a central point around which others are organized; in fact, it became a virtual organization of embedding computational and information experts in projects led by senior geneticists and psychiatrists, and later a central strand of the Centre's work. The conditions of exchange in these trading zones are often unequal. The common refrain of 'working on other people's data' indicates that bioinformaticians occupy an ancillary role within multidisciplinary arrangements.

Rather than dissolving boundaries and jurisdiction, we find that a politics of multidisciplinarity re-inscribes new and acute divisions and valuations of expertise. Indeed, these divisions are symptoms of knowledge and power that expose the instabilities of the network. For example, those working in bioinformatics who want to 'develop applications' – and be rewarded *as scientists* for that work – or who want to 'do their own thing' in terms of exercising the degree of scientific autonomy they might have been socialized to expect, may have to leave the Centre and pursue other avenues of research. Alternatively, for senior biologists, there are concerns that an 'instrumental' approach to bioinformatics – blackboxing it either in technological or social boxes that remain unopened – means that biologists lose cognitive authority and oversight over the processes of production.

At this point, the question we might ask is: who is granted mobility and visibility within these processes of production and exchange? Among networks that privilege the increasing mobility and circulation of biological data, we argue that the curators and analysts of Big Data are contrastingly immobile and *in situ*. To borrow a phrase from Boltanski and Chiapello (2007), bioinformaticians are the 'stand-ins' of Big Biology.[6] As with the junior and mid-career biologists referred to in the previous chapter, many bioinformaticians find that their participation in these research collaborations marginalizes their ability to participate in the scientific economy of reward and recognition. The 'middle-ness' of authorship, the inability – excepting a few high-profile professors – to lead on grants and publications, and the demotion of symbolic reward for scientific labour – sometimes to as little as a mention in the acknowledgements section – indicate the ways in which vast quantities of scientific labour are rendered invisible in this 'federal', networked Big Biology. The biologist describes the (literally) *in situ* role of bioinformaticians as 'someone who sits down and analyses other people's data', who, by adding value to other people's data, create the conditions for biologists to increase their own value. Value systems do not travel well in collaborative research. In the Centre, the dominance of those trained in the science of the clinic or the science of the laboratory results in particular measures of contribution and distributions of reward which are not designed for Big Biology; they are not designed for epistemic organizations built on the scientific labour of people from other disciplines, working with other styles of scientific reasoning. Though bioinformatics is epistemically central to psychiatric genetics, it is institutionally peripheral to its structures of reward and recognition (Lewis and Bartlett 2013).

Notes

1 As Bartlett (2008: 75) wrote of the HGP, routinization is 'the material reification of rationalisation'.
2 This was exemplified during a presentation by a leading member of the Hub at a Centre 'retreat'. He presented the results of his bioinformatic research, highlighting various 'hits' across the genome associated with a particular phenotype. His presentation ended with him saying that he had no idea what the biological relevance of these hits might be, and that that was the job of the biologists.
3 Hackett (1990, 2005) argues that academic science is bounded by tensions between intrinsic versus instrumental value, independence versus dependence, and traditional-collegial versus legal-rational modes of authority. The ambivalence of scientific norms resembles 'axes of variation' that define potentials for cultural change as organizations respond to social, political and economic forces. Tensions between intrinsic and instrumental value are indicative of recent changes in 'science as a vocation' – a shift from treating scientists and their apprentices as intrinsic ends in themselves to expecting some utility from them (Hackett 1990). In so-called 'small science', scientists may be socialized to expect personal satisfaction, creativity and autonomy as intrinsic rewards

for doing science. In large-scale research, however, expectations are increasingly oriented to practical and measurable benefits that often serve funders and the wider scientific community.

4 Despite the distinction drawn by our interviewee, which is useful for understanding the types of work being done under the title of 'bioinformatics', we do not use these categories in a formal way as it is not at all clear that this nomenclature is widely used (see Lewis and Bartlett 2013).

5 We believe the tensions between established and emerging disciplines is a symptom of *multidisciplinarity*. Although interdisciplinarity and multidisciplinarity are often used interchangeably, Klein (2010) has shown that there are important differences between these terms. While 'interdisciplinarity' seeks to integrate and harmonize disciplines within a coherent whole, 'multidisciplinarity' recruits knowledge and skills from different fields but retains their disciplinary boundaries. The problem of multidisciplinary integration is not unique to the Centre, but consistent with how bioinformatics is embedded in other projects across the UK.

6 Drawing on Boltanski and Chiapello's (2007) analysis of contemporary capitalist production, Lezaun (2013) argues that where the creation of value in 'Big Biology' centres on increasing mobility, circulation and connectivity, the 'stand-ins' (*doublure*) are actors who become figures of exploitation:

> The 'stand-ins' are those actors who must remain *in situ* while others circulate, and are thus unable to capitalize on individual projects in order to enhance their own versatility and mobility. They care for all that is rooted and situated in the nodes that make up the network, and in so doing create the conditions for others to move and increase their own value.
>
> (Lezaun 2013: 483)

References

Bartlett A (2008) *Accomplishing Sequencing the Human Genome*. Unpublished PhD Thesis, Cardiff University.

Bartlett A, Lewis J and Williams ML (2016) Generations of interdisciplinarity in bioinformatics. *New Genetics and Society* 35(2): 186–209.

Bartlett A, Penders B and Lewis J (2017) Bioinformatics: Indispensable, yet hidden in plain sight? *BMC Bioinformatics* 18: 311.

Beaver DD (2001) Reflections on scientific collaborations (and its study): Past, present and future – feature report. *Scientometrics* 52(3): 365–377.

Birnholtz JP (2006) What does it mean to be an author? The intersection of credit, contribution, and collaboration in science. *Journal for the Association for Information Science and Technology* 57(13): 1758–1770.

Boltanski L and Chiapello E (2007) *The New Spirit of Capitalism*. London: Verso.

Borgman C (2015) *Big Data, Little Data, No Data: Scholarship in the Networked World*. London: MIT Press.

Calvert J (2010) Systems biology, interdisciplinarity and disciplinary identity. In JN Parker, N Vermeulen and B Penders (eds). *Collaboration in the New Life Sciences*. Farnham: Ashgate, pp. 201–219.

Chang J (2015) Core services: Reward bioinformaticians. *Nature* 520(7546): 151–152.

Collins F, Morgan M and Patrinos A (2003) The Human Genome Project: Lessons from large-scale biology. *Science* 300(5617): 286–290.

Economist (1999) Drowning in data, 24 June. www.economist.com/node/346020 [accessed 28 April 2016].

Galison P (1999) Trading zone: Coordinating action and belief. In M Biagioli (ed.). *The Science Studies Reader*. New York: Routledge, pp. 137–160.

Galison P and Hevly B (eds) (1992) *Big Science: The Growth of Large-Scale Research*. Stanford: Stanford University Press.

Garcia-Sancho M (2012) *Biology, Computing and the History of Molecular Sequencing: From Proteins to DNA, 1945–2000*. Basingstoke: Palgrave Macmillan.

Gieryn TF (1983) Boundary-work and the demarcation of science from non-science: Strains and interests in professional interests of scientists. *American Sociological Review* 48: 781–795.

Grimaldi DA and Engel M (2007) Why descriptive science still matters. *BioScience* 57(8): 646–647.

Hackett EJ (1990) Science as a vocation in the 1990s: The changing organizational culture of academic science. *Journal of Higher Education* 61(3): 241–279.

Hackett EJ (2005) Essential tensions: Identity, control and risk in research. *Social Studies of Science* 35(5): 787–826.

Hacking I (1992) 'Style' for historians and philosophers. *Studies in the History and Philosophy of Science* 23(1): 1–20.

Kendler KS (2006) Reflections on the relationship between psychiatric genetics and psychiatric nosology. *American Journal of Psychiatry* 163: 1138–1146.

King C (2013) Single-author papers: A waning share of output, but still providing the tools for progress. *ScienceWatch*. http://sciencewatch.com/articles/single-author-papers-waning-share-output-still-providing-tools-progress.

Klein JT (2010) A taxonomy of interdisciplinarity. In R Frodeman (ed.). *The Oxford Handbook of Interdisciplinarity*. Oxford: Oxford University Press, pp. 15–30.

Knorr-Cetina K (1999) *Epistemic Cultures: How the Sciences Make Knowledge*. Cambridge, MA: Harvard University Press.

Latour B (1999) *Pandora's Hope: Essays on the Reality of Science Studies*. London: Harvard University Press.

Latour B and Woolgar S (1986) *Laboratory Life: The Construction of Scientific Facts*. Princeton: Princeton University Press.

Lewis J and Bartlett A (2013) Inscribing a discipline: Tensions in the field of bioinformatics. *New Genetics and Society* 32(3): 243–263.

Lewis J, Bartlett A and Atkinson P (2016) Hidden in the middle: Culture, value and reward in bioinformatics. *Minerva* 54: 471–490.

Lezaun J (2013) Commentary: The escalating politics of 'Big Biology'. *Biosocieties* 8(4): 480–485.

Mackenzie A (2003) Bringing sequences to life: How bioinformatics corporealizes sequence data. *New Genetics and Society* 22(3): 315–332.

MacKenzie DA (1981) *Statistics in Britain: The Social Construction of Scientific Knowledge*. Edinburgh: Edinburgh University Press.

McNally R (2008) Sociomics: CESAGen multidisciplinary workshop on the transformation of knowledge production in the biosciences, and its consequences. *Proteomics* 8: 222–224.

Marijuán PC (2002) Bioinformation: Untangling the networks of life. *Biosystems* 64: 111–118.

Markowetz F (2017) All biology is computational biology. *PLoS Biol* 15(3): 1–4.

Osborne JW and Holland A (2009) What is authorship, and what should it be? A survey of prominent guidelines for determining authorship in scientific publications. *Practical Assessment Research Evaluation* 14: 1–19.

Penders B, Horstman K and Vos R (2008) Walking the line between lab and computation: The moist zone. *Bioscience* 58(8): 747–755.

Penders B, Vos R and Horstman K (2009) A question of style: Method, integrity and the meaning of proper science. *Endeavour* 33(3): 93–98.

Shapin S (1989) The invisible technician. *American Scientist* 77(6): 554–563.

Spengler SJ (2000) Bioinformatics in the information age. *Science* 287(5456): 1221–1223.

Stevens H (2011) On the means of bio-production: Bioinformatics and how to make knowledge in a high-throughput genomics laboratory. *BioSocieties* 6(2): 217–242.

Suárez-Díaz E (2010) Making room for new faces: Evolution, genomics and the growth of bioinformatics. *History and Philosophy of the Life Sciences* 32(1): 65–89.

Sulston J and Ferry G (2002) *The Common Thread: A Story of Science, Politics, Ethics and the Human Genome*. Washington, DC: Joseph Henry Press.

Torgersen H (2009) Fuzzy genes: Epistemic tensions in genomics. *Science as Culture* 18(1): 65–87.

van Baren-Nawrocka J (2013) The bioinformatics of genetic origins: How identities become embedded in the tools and practices of bioinformatics. *Life Science, Society and Policy* 9: 7.

6 On the road

Collecting bloods and stories

Large-scale psychiatric genetics can give the appearance of being a 'data science' driven by high-throughput laboratory processes and statistical manipulation of big datasets. In Chapter 4, we explained how scientific labour is distributed and its productivity intensified to allow biological research to (superficially) retain the appearance of small-scale science. In Chapter 5, we explained that GWAS involve abstracting biological resources from their material context to produce a mass of inscriptions amenable to a statistical style of reasoning. But, of course, this biological data has no reference or purpose beyond its correlation to clinical data. The processes for extracting the 'natural resources' of GWAS are also expertise developed and honed in a *clinical style* of reasoning. As we will see, the labour-intensive practice of collecting 'cases' and then ordering symptoms by comparison and taxonomy is a skill that has been resistant to the extensive rationalization and automation that has otherwise accompanied the increases in the scale of psychiatric genetics.

In this chapter, we discuss the *emotional labour* of fieldworkers collecting phenotypic data and blood samples within the bipolar team at the Centre. We detail the ways in which recent increases in the collection of clinical data in 'Big Biology' involves a series of trade-offs and compromises. What we find is a moral economy of exchange, the scientific value of which is almost always written out of research publications. As the value created by this labour is rarely acknowledged, the skill and labour involved is to some degree 'invisible', concealing the scale of these Big Biology projects. Much like the early-career postdocs, bioinformaticians and technicians we examined in Chapters 4 and 5, fieldworkers are the 'stand-ins' of Big Biology (Lezaun 2013). Although fieldwork is a role literally defined by its physical mobility – as fieldworkers spend much of their time 'on the road' – there are few opportunities to move *within* the structures of the Centre or the consortium, with their career mobility expected to involve a path *away* from and, indeed, *outside* psychiatric genetics research altogether.

Natural resources

The 'natural resources' of psychiatric genetics are the individuals and families with schizophrenia, bipolar disorder and other psychiatric disorders, who are recruited into large research projects. As with any natural resource, human labour must be applied to transform it into something with use value: once people have been enlisted as research participants, scientifically valuable material must be 'extracted' from them. This includes not only biological material, taken in the form of blood samples from which DNA is isolated, but also phenotypic data. Much like Kraepelin's early methods of prognosis (see Chapters 1 and 2), this involves a clinical style of reasoning, collecting detailed life histories of the *course* of illness. Given that GWAS are essentially correlational studies, genotypic data has no value independent of its phenotypic description. Definitions of phenotype are not only an important starting point for genetic research but capturing phenotype variation (phenotypic heterogeneity) is essential to identifying susceptibility variants (Craddock *et al.* 2009). Interviews designed to capture the subtleties of psychiatric conditions are seen as the best way of collecting data that might allow these diagnostic categories to be explored biologically. Leading scientists at the Centre were proud to tell us that before the era of *very* large-scale studies, the Centre had established a reputation for the quality of its clinical data because fieldworkers were intensively trained in psychopathology. But with the introduction of Big Biology, the training of fieldworkers and the definition of fieldwork itself has been increasingly 'rationalized'.

The considerable task of increasing the scale of phenotyping for GWAS has transformed the way that fieldwork is conceptualized and conducted at the Centre. In the days of family or linkage studies, sufficient cases could be collected by a small group of clinicians, but in recent years the move to full-time, dedicated fieldwork teams has intensified the management of data collection. An experienced fieldworker at the Centre described this change in scale over the last decade as follows:

FIELDWORKER 1: When I was on the field team … I think we had 800 people to recruit in five years.

INTERVIEWER: And the new target?

FIELDWORKER 1: Four thousand in about two to three years, so when it was decided to do that, then we had to sit down and go, actually how are we going to speed things up?

This transformation in scale and speed, a corollary of the changes described in Chapter 4, has not only changed the relationship between the fieldworkers and their work but also the relationship between fieldworkers and research participants. Those taking part in the research are not, for the most part, under the *care* of clinicians working at the Centre and, as such, there is no opportunity for fieldworkers to build the kind of rapport found in a healthcare relationship. Instead, research participants are recruited from all across the UK, and fieldworkers collecting data for GWAS must spend a significant proportion of their time 'on the road', spending only a few hours with each participant, extracting from them blood and stories.

Emotional labour

Historically, the clinical style of collecting and interpreting research data in psychiatric genetics has been an activity mostly conducted by clinicians. But since the era of large studies, this task has been increasingly assigned to fieldwork teams who perform the technical labour of drawing blood and collecting case histories from patients and research participants. To do this work effectively, fieldworkers must also engage in 'emotional labour' (Hochschild 1983): putting research participants at ease, asking them to describe some of the most distressing moments in their lives, keeping them on track in a semi-structured[1] interview, and even distracting them as blood is drawn. It involves managing the emotions of the research participants within the fieldwork encounter as well as managing their own emotions; both in presenting a 'face' to research participants and re-setting their emotions between interviews. This work is skilled work, though the necessary labour and expertise is often rendered 'invisible' (Star and Strauss 1999) in many accounts of large-scale psychiatric genetics.

Emotional labour has been studied in a wide variety of contexts, from the empathic labour exemplified by Hochschild's (1983) classic study of airline employees to the antipathetic labour of debt collectors, police officers and security guards (see Ward and McMurray 2016 for a detailed review). Emotional labour has also been the focus of studies in healthcare professions, such as counselling and nursing (see Henderson 2001; Mann 2004; Erickson and Grove 2008; Kessler *et al.* 2015).[2] But the relationship between fieldworkers and research participants – as opposed to patients – is a departure from the norms governing such labour in the healthcare setting. The emotional labour of fieldworkers is different in two significant aspects: it does not take place within a 'care' relationship – the fieldworker offers no diagnosis or promise of treatment – and the relationship between fieldworker and research participant is not (necessarily) a sustained one. That is, the research 'encounter' between fieldworkers and participants is almost always temporary and fleeting.

The emotional management of these research encounters is oriented to the production of material of scientific value, in the form of high-quality data. But the emotional material contained in the life histories of the participants has little or no scientific value in itself. It is a necessary by-product of the process of resource extraction. Writing about pharmacogenomics research on psychiatric patients, Svendsen and Koch (2011) also observe that 'emotional management' takes place within exchange relations that facilitate the production of these materials. They see no moral contradiction between the altruism of research participants and the production of these exchange relations in biological research. However, our focus is not on whether these exchange encounters 'exploit' research participants, but in exploring the 'invisible' labour of these encounters as a feature of the transition to Big Biology.

The elision of emotional labour from 'official' accounts of science is linked to broader notions of 'invisible work'. Since the mid-1980s, this term has been used to describe a variety of (usually gendered) work conducted physically or culturally 'out of sight', ignored or overlooked, and quite often socially marginalized (Shapin 1989; Star and Strauss 1999; Nardi and Engeström 1999; see Hatton 2017 for a theoretical review). In this chapter, we argue that the increasing rationalization of labour in large-scale psychiatric genetics has not spared the emotional labour of fieldworkers, though this labour has proven more resistant to these processes than laboratory work. Fieldwork has not been 'outsourced', but the fieldwork team has become increasingly distinct from the laboratory scientists, moving further away from the circuits of scientific reward and recognition, with little expectation that fieldworkers will pursue a research career in the field. While the relative invisibility of fieldworkers within Big Biology has implications in terms of their opportunities within the career structures of science, we risk missing not only their scientific contributions but also their necessary exposure to stressful and risky working conditions.

A 'natural' division of labour

During our fieldwork at the Centre, the main device for collecting phenotypic data for the bipolar disorder group was the 'semi-structured' interview. Despite its implied flexibility, the interview was actually a 40-page questionnaire that took approximately 90 minutes to complete. It covered topics including the participant's current mental state, the history of their illness and medication, five pages covering symptoms of depression, three on the symptoms of mania/hypomania, nine pages on hallucinations and delusions, as well as sections on perinatal episodes, panic attacks, family history and so on. The interview allowed participants to give detailed descriptions of symptoms, episodes, treatment histories etc., which the fieldworker scored *in situ* according to standardized criteria. The interview was as demanding on the fieldworker as it was on the research participant, not least because the rigorous extraction of information produced distressing accounts of mental illness. Eliciting emotional content from research participants thus required skilled emotional work.

The fieldwork team consisted almost entirely of recent female psychology graduates. This gender imbalance matters in understanding the way in which the emotional labour of fieldwork was tacitly and explicitly conceptualized. A senior scientist at the Centre offered the opinion that young male graduates lacked the 'emotional maturity' to skilfully conduct the interviews. One of the fieldwork managers explained the propensity for hiring women:

> We have noticed this and we have discussed it at length.... We have employed males here in the past. But in answer to your question, yes the majority of psychology students are females. I don't know what the ratio is now, but it's a marked excess of females. The majority of applicants for our jobs are females, but we do get male applicants. And I am conscious of the fact that we shortlist more females as well. And I do think there's a difference in how males and females present themselves on the application forms ... I do think that males are more prone to using 'job application speak' than

women are. And that just puts me off. Because we're looking for somebody with good interpersonal skills. And also when we have employed male interviewers, they haven't been as successful as the female interviewers. Now that could be me making a completely illusionary correlation because we haven't employed that many male interviewers, who knows. But I think they have found it harder.

(Fieldwork manager)

The manager accounts for the excess of female fieldworkers on the basis that male and female candidates present differently in interviews. In the first instance, male applicants fail to meet the criteria of the post because they are 'more prone' to using instrumental language ('job application speak'). The few who are employed are apparently less successful than their female counterparts. In admitting this might be a 'completely illusory correlation', the manager is acknowledging that this gender bias might rest on shaky empirical foundations, and yet the assumption that women are more skilled in emotional labour holds. Consistent with the observations of others (Hochschild 1983; James 1989; Acker 1990; Taylor and Tyler 2000), organizations conducting interactive work and emotional labour are frequently gendered. In many cases, women are expected to excel in the suppression of negative emotional displays and the presentation of positive emotions (Erickson and Ritter 2001).

As far as scientists and research managers were concerned, the recruitment of female fieldworkers was a 'natural' division of labour. The emotional skill required to successfully do fieldwork at the Centre was seen by many as an innate aptitude – unequally distributed between women and men – that could be honed with practice and advice, but not a skill that could be explicitly taught. As the person with responsibility for managing a fieldwork team said:

I'm quite heavily involved in organising the training. [The emotional, interpersonal skills are] something that we think about a lot. And it's difficult because I don't know if you can train that. I think some people have got it, and some people, no matter how much training you give them, are never going to have that certain something that kind of makes them a good interviewer. In the training that I've been involved with I think we have had a session as part of the training called Interview Skills, which is the 'accept a drink', those kind of things.[3] But I think it is hard to teach.

(Fieldwork manager)

Emotional labour, as this fieldworker put it, is 'natural', just something that people do.

I think [fieldworkers] are naturally very warm, very sociable people who naturally put people at ease. So I don't think it's really something that I've ever thought too much about, because it just kind of seems to be a natural part of the process. So I suppose, you know … obviously their facial expressions, they're kind of open and warm, very friendly, and it's not just a case of entering the house and sitting down and saying, right we're going to start here. It's a bit of small talk and it's a lot more casual and involves putting people at ease, making sure they know exactly what they're taking part in. And the way the interview is set out as well is that it starts off [with] very simple questions and then goes into the more possibly emotionally draining stuff, to talk about specific symptoms and things. So I suppose from the interviews I've witnessed, it's not a kind of calculated thing it's just something that people do.

(Fieldworker 2)

To a fieldworker, it seems entirely 'natural' to build rapport with participants before taking them through an 'emotionally draining' process. The naturalness of being 'warm', 'friendly' and 'sociable' elides the fact that this is skilled work that not everyone can perform. An important aspect of this work is to mitigate the potentially negative effects of the interview. Extracting information from research participants can be socially and emotionally demanding for both parties. Much of this labour is conducted 'offsite', on the road, and in the homes of research participants; it leaves few traces in the data produced and is rarely acknowledged in the scientific papers produced by the Centre.[4] Unlike the longer-serving fieldworkers who joined the team before the transition to Big Biology, for the newer fieldworkers, 'fieldwork' was increasingly envisioned as a temporary post for new psychology graduates. Fieldworkers may accrue experience and some prestige from working in a big group, but their prospects for career mobility lie beyond the Centre or outside of psychiatric genetics research more broadly.

Streamlining and standardization

At a public event, one of the senior scientists at the Centre told us that the new batch of fieldworkers were expected to be different to existing members of the field team. The role of the fieldworker, they explained, had been 'streamlined'. Work that required a high level of psychiatric expertise – such as drawing up clinical vignettes from case notes – was the preserve of the more experienced members of the team, some of whom have PhDs and had contributed to scientific publications. For the new fieldworkers, the typical working week was expected to involve conducting six interviews, with four days on the road and one in the office.

This acute division of labour leaves the newer fieldworkers somewhat distant from the research at the Centre. For example, here, a fieldworker discusses the degree to which they follow the wider work of the project:

We don't really. I don't know if it's just because, maybe I haven't shown enough interest. So, well, no [laughs]. Once we've collected the data and handed it on, I mean, that's pretty much it, really. Obviously every year we have a meeting at Christmas, and we'll obviously have teleconference meetings, but we don't really discuss findings in them. But in the meeting at Christmas they might discuss it and tell us about things. But the problem with that is it's genetics and I really just don't understand it at all. So it's just right over my head. But I don't know what it would be like in the future, once the main study's written up. I guess that would, again, be if I was interested in it or not. I guess working on it for a short timeframe, because our contracts are all relatively short, means you don't really always get that involved.

(Fieldworker 3)

This apparent lack of interest in research is lamented by some more experienced members of the field team.

I think one of the things that I find most difficult about the way that we've changed over the years is that we do have these young people who come to work with us who don't have the passion for the research. Yeah, they've got the passion to learn about mental illness and listen to the stories, but they don't have the passion for … well why are we doing this? What's the aim? How is it going to help people? And that I find quite difficult because I want them to be interested.

(Fieldwork manager)

The first account seems to confirm the manager's complaint that fieldworkers 'don't have a passion' for research. Since the move to large-scale biology, the growing division between 'work' and 'research' is consistent with the increasing rationalization of large-scale projects. Where fieldwork was one route to an 'apprenticeship' in psychiatric genetics, it is now merely a 'job of work'. The fact that 'genetics' is cited by the fieldworker as an obstacle to engaging in the wider meaning of the project confirms that knowledge of genetics is not required to conduct good fieldwork. In any case, fieldworkers are not regularly included in group meetings and their contracts are 'relatively short'. Similar to the 'value tensions' (Hackett 2005) we observed in Chapter 5, the social and epistemic organization of Big Biology creates an increasing division between the instrumental and intrinsic values of fieldwork.

A fieldworker is trained to take blood samples and conduct standardized interviews, which are scored as the interview progresses. This assigns a numerical score to each listed symptom. When we observed the training sessions, we asked the trainers about the ways in which the role-play examples, in which senior members of the Centre acted out fieldwork interviews, involved the interviewer 'pressing' the participant, asking a similar question several times. They told us that a fieldworker cannot give a rating of '0' for a symptom if they are unsure that the symptom is completely absent. This technique of pressing must be handled delicately with participants who are reticent and with those who try to help by providing irrelevant detail. The scoring of these interviews is controlled by reliability exercises, as described by one of the senior fieldworkers during the training:

> When you have reliability exercises, these [mood incongruence] are the ones you'll really dread. It feels so hard to judge. But when we do the reliability exercises, these measures come out as very reliable. We all give them very similar scores.... You do sometimes feel you're uncertain. Less so with the people [research participants] we're recruiting now. In the past we recruited people with a wide range of symptoms. Less so now. But you can always put 'uncertain'.
>
> (Fieldworker 2, from fieldnotes)

Again, this points to the 'streamlining' of the fieldwork process. The new fieldworkers were being trained to exercise less 'clinical' judgement by interviewing research participants with a more circumscribed range of symptoms.

The interviews almost always took place in the homes of the research participant, and covered topics that included some of the most distressing times in their lives, such as periods of acute mental ill health, suicide attempts and suicidal ideation, and time spent in psychiatric hospitals. We asked a fieldworker to describe the typical rhythm of their work:

> What I actually do is to interview people who have usually a diagnosis of bipolar disorder and about their experiences and symptoms. That involves the initial contact, ringing them on the phone, screening and checking they meet criteria. And then arranging a time to see them, and then the organization of going to see them as well. You know, obviously [you're] trying to find people in the same area, so it's not like just one person or whatever if it's a long way. And then the interviews themselves take about an hour and a half from start to finish, including asking about the onset and symptoms, life events, everything like that, and then taking their blood. That's it really. And obviously, the follow up, which is storing the blood, and requesting case notes, things like that. And then following up, making sure we get the questionnaires that we need from them. So in a week, the aim is to interview six people. So depending on circumstances sometimes it's six, sometimes it's four, sometimes it's ten. You know, it just really depends on who's available and where they are and everything.
>
> (Fieldworker 3)

This interview, and the fieldwork protocol, was under development while we were conducting our research at the Centre. During our observations of the training, an experienced fieldworker said that there were new sections that were unfamiliar to her. Significantly, efforts were being made to rationalize the interview – to make it more efficient and quicker to complete. One aspect of this was a move to machine-readable questionnaires.[5]

I think the biggest change that happened with our team was when we went from the paper interviews to the interviews that are compatible with the computer.... So then we had to take everything that was contained ... well actually ... we wanted to make the interviews slightly shorter because we wanted to make it a lot more concise, and we had big discussions about maybe if things could be asked differently or removed from the interview altogether and the things we really, really wanted to focus on.

(Fieldworker 2)

Other elements of standardization were designed to reduce or eliminate the messiness of fieldwork. One fieldworker told us that they often left out the section that involved drawing up a chronological 'life chart' because it was simply not practical when in the field. Some fieldworkers were explicit that they felt that the increasing streamlining and standardization was stripping away the engaging, skilled nature of the work. This was understood not only as a subjective loss for the fieldworkers, but involved a trade-off for the project – a reiteration of the tension between scale and quality that we discussed in Chapter 4.

I think the quality of the data that we get isn't as good nowadays. Because as you've probably been told we have reliability exercises where we listen to recordings of interviews. And every so often I'm thinking, oh you needed to have asked more about that. But the interviewer is probably thinking, I've been here for 45 minutes.... So I do think that the richness of the data that we get is poorer these days ... I think yeah the dataset that we're collecting is pretty unique in terms of [the richness of the data]. We also make an effort to try and get their case notes as well to get that data. So it's, yeah, it's a rich dataset compared to others, but compared to the data we were collecting in the olden days.... We were trained differently, I think we had a much deeper understanding of the psychopathology and I think I could ... you know, by the end of it I didn't even need a piece of paper. I could have done it in my sleep I'd done it so many times.... And I think that is different nowadays because the interviewers don't have that depth of knowledge that we had. I think probably they do work through it in more of a formulaic way.

(Fieldwork manager)

The manager recognizes that high-throughput data extraction has its disadvantages. The task of collecting several thousand cases within two or three years means certain sacrifices in quality are necessary. Indeed, the contrast between the 'olden days' and present efforts to rationalize fieldwork suggests there has been an incremental reduction in the clinical style of extracting phenotypic data. Before the era of Big Biology, interviews were longer and informed by a 'much deeper understanding of psychopathology'. Researchers had greater flexibility to score symptoms in the ebb and flow of talk, whereas the new batch of fieldworkers tend to work through the interview in a 'formulaic way'. The clinical style of reasoning, with its tacit knowledge of psychopathology, has been externalized and rationalized in the interview schedule; the interview has become more an instrument streamlined to serve high-throughput processes than to aid clinical reasoning. Nevertheless, fieldworkers are skilled in reliably scoring interviews, drawing blood from participants and, as we will see in the next section, skilled in empathically responding to the emotional demands placed upon the research participants, and the fieldworker, by the interview protocol.

Emotions *at* work

The emotional labour of fieldwork often involves aligning the scientific aims of psychiatric research with the social circumstances of the interview. Sometimes, managing this alignment is complicated by the mood of the participant, their capacity to recall relevant information, or the presence of family members in the home. As the fieldworker explains below, having family members present can both assist and hinder the interview:

> If I've got a person who isn't particularly … either doesn't have much insight into their illness or they don't remember anything, then it can be really useful to have someone else around to give their point of view and to say what they've witnessed or what they've said. Sometimes you can have, you know, maybe a couple there and it can get … the other person can get in the way because they'll keep saying stuff that's either not really that relevant or you've already got that answer and they won't stop nattering on about it and you're like, okay, okay. If it's a case of, say, children or teenage children, who may be a bit more able to understand, it can make … some of the questions are quite difficult, quite personal, and I think, is that going to affect the person's true answer if this kid wasn't here? You know, it's questions of sex drive and stuff. I sometimes just don't ask them if someone else is around. All the psychotic questions, because sometimes they wouldn't want to admit it in front of their kids, just how ill they are. So it can have an effect. I mean, it's not that common that there is someone else. It's normally actually if it's a man you're interviewing it's a wife that's around. It's never really the other way around. And obviously if you're just [interviewing] a woman their kids might be around.
>
> (Fieldworker 3)

The fieldworker's account orients to the complex circumstances of asking questions when others are present. If adults are present they may help to verify information about the participant's illness, but they may also distract the interview process by offering irrelevant information. If children are present, the fieldwork must assess whether their understanding will affect or limit the participants' accounts, or whether it is appropriate to proceed with questions that may elicit distressing information. The fieldworker must effectively 'know the minds of others' to assess the emotional space of the interview.[6]

The technical matrix of questions that comprise the interview protocol is designed to elicit accurate information about the phenomenological components of bipolar disorder – the frequency and quality of episodes, their mood and ideation. Many of the fieldworkers reported that certain sections of the interview asked participants to recall states that also reactivated their corresponding mood. For instance, questions on 'depression' were the most demanding because participants frequently became upset.

> We have like three sections of the interview. We've got depression, mania and psychosis. So I would say, depending on the mood of the person, depression's usually the hardest … because it's like putting themselves back into that mood and saying, oh yeah, this is how I felt, this is how I felt. And I noticed when we were in training – you know, a year and a half ago – there's a tendency when you're asking the depression sections to be like this and then when you're asking the mania ones you start to pick up. But in the depression section, the hardest are about suicide, probably, because it's not like just have you attempted … yes/no … move on…. We then have to push them on it and find out how many times and what they've done and if they intended to actually die or if it was a cry for help and things like that. So I suppose that's one of the tough ones that can cause people to get upset.
>
> (Fieldworker 3)

Performing emotional labour in these circumstances involves displaying a nuanced awareness of the participant's subjectivity, which ranges from building polite rapport to reading and responding to the emotional dynamic of the interview. It also involves eliciting information that contains an emotional residue, a residue which has little or no scientific value to large-scale research. The fieldworker above refers to her training in order to explain that interviewing has different rhythms corresponding to the sections on 'depression, mania and psychosis'. The 'hardest' section – meaning those which are the most distressing for the participant and difficult to manage for the fieldworker – are the questions on depression and suicide. Skilled emotional labour is required to 'push' people into giving detailed information about suicidal ideation and suicide attempts while sensitively managing 'residual' emotions.

Although the interview was an increasingly routinized and standardized instrument, collecting data from different participants is not a task of rote drudgery; there is room for fieldworkers to act with skill and autonomy. They do this by guiding participants to provide the *right kind of* accounts, not just those that the research participant finds interesting, but those relevant to the interview schedule. In these instances, fieldworkers resort to *articulation work*: 'the work that gets things back on track in the face of the unexpected' (Star and Strauss 1999: 10). As Star and Strauss explain, an important feature of articulation work is its *invisibility* to rationalized models of work. In fieldwork, this invisible work operates at the delicate intersection of extracting information efficiently while being sensitive to people's tangential stories:

When people start going off on one and just go off on their own story, I'll listen to an extent because they actually sometimes end up answering other questions without you having to ask them. Otherwise, I can ... you know, if they're in a depression section, they might start talking about some psychosis, so sometimes I can say, oh, you know, I'm just going to stop you there because I'll ask you about that later. If it's completely irrelevant, it is a bit tricky really ... it can be quite hard. You just sort of have to listen and then maybe when you can hear them coming to a break in their story or coming to ... you know, just sort of moving them on without ... hopefully without offending them. Just be, like, oh and also ... you know, maybe just sort of try and find a way to cut in. Or if they sort of hint in any slight way towards another symptom like, oh so have you felt like this then? It is quite hard, generally ... I think that it's harder to cut people off who are nattering on than to make people who aren't talking talk.

(Fieldworker 1)

Other kinds of work which are essential to extracting useful information, but leave no visible trace as 'data', include modulating questions, offering apologies and reassurances, and normalizing participant's responses. In the following account, the fieldworker tries to explain some of the subtleties of interviewing:

So it's like being very subtle about the questions that you ask and the way you ask. Some people are really open about it and some people are a bit more ... obviously you don't really want to ... I think it's all about reading their reaction to the question as well as just writing ... it can't be a set way that you do it. And I suppose if people do get upset, I always just sort of say, thanks very much for being honest about that. Or, if you don't want to talk about it, it's absolutely fine. Or, if you want to take a break, just things like that really. I mean one of the ways, I suppose, is to just normalize it and just say, well you know, it's completely normal for you to feel like this and for you to be upset because of the type of question it is. But I'm sorry, you know, I have to ask it of everybody.

(Fieldworker 3)

Although psychology graduates have no formal training in clinical psychiatry, nor in genetics, their background is not misplaced in settings that require sophisticated awareness of other people's emotional states. For instance, the ability to ask questions indirectly, or to 'read' a participant's reaction to questions, are skills that help to mitigate the emotional intensity of the interview. The subtlety of these techniques are developed through performing the interview a great many times, and while the topics may be intensely personal for each individual research participant, for the fieldworkers they are simply variations on a theme. The fieldworker's skill at performing emotional labour must make it seem that each of these interviews *matter*. However, despite some similarities with emotional work conducted in healthcare settings (see Henderson 2001; Mann 2004;

Erickson and Grove 2008; Kessler *et al.* 2015), we reiterate this is not a 'care' relationship. One of the fieldworkers made this fairly explicit:

> I think the frustrating thing is that as a research team we can't do anything to help and sometimes you hear people's stories and you're really worried about them because its … you're with that person for an hour, an hour and a half, and during that time you're asking them some really personal questions and it's very difficult then to just detach yourself emotionally and go on your way and not feel affected by what you've heard. And there have been instances where what [fieldworkers] have been told has really upset them.… And its I guess it's quite difficult because, apart from the feedback and the discussion of it and trying to kind of get them to offload it in that way, we can't – unless we feel that they are at risk at that moment – we actually can't do anything to help that person, apart from, you know, give them contact details for MDF [Manic Depression Fellowship] Helpline and the Samaritans and things like that. Apart from that we can't do anything and I think that must be really difficult.
>
> (Fieldworker 2)

This topic of concern came up during our observations of the fieldworker training. The trainees were warned that they are likely to hear complaints about their treatment and care, in which case they need to be non-committal in their responses. Trainees were told not to dispute the accounts of the participants, which might damage emotional rapport, but neither should they legitimate their complaints. To do so would upset the relationship between the researchers and the clinical team upon whom the Centre depends for recruitment. The trainer recommended that the fieldworkers respond with stock phrases like, 'that sounds very difficult for you'. The difference in the relationship between researcher and research participant and between healthcare professionals and patient is thrown into sharp relief here. The relationship is, in essence, unilateral, in which emotional skill is applied to the task of extracting material of scientific value.

Drawing the blood is often the final part of a fieldworker's visit, and is one of the final pieces of emotion work that the fieldworker must perform. Needles and blood frighten many people, and so relaxing and distracting research participants becomes the goal.

> I do the blood at the end of the interview once we'd established, you know, rapport and I'd try and make the person as relaxed as possible and normally if I was just about to put the needle we'd, you know, ask a question, just chatting, you know, just chat about what are you doing this afternoon, you know blah blah blah.
>
> (Fieldworker 1)

One fieldworker told us that she also had experience of research participants being reluctant to provide a sample at the conclusion of the interview. Taking blood first therefore removed the anxiety of giving a blood sample from among the many other emotional obstacles at play during the interview:

> Some of the people who were particularly anxious about it, would want you to do it at the beginning of the interview so that they weren't worrying about it. So of course if that's what they wanted then I was happy to do it. I would say for the majority of people if they were on Lithium they would always have their bloods checked every few months anyway so to be honest, it wasn't an issue for quite a lot of people. Although yes, I mean if somebody was anxious … I suppose just to repeat that it would just feel like a sharp scratch, it wouldn't take long and it was just a small amount of blood that we were extracting. Yes, I mean sometimes people even got to that part, completed the interview and then would say, is the blood, you know, is that important? And of course we'd have to stress that in fact it was. Also just letting them know that you've taken hundreds of samples as well. When I finished it was hundreds of samples. And that you were fully trained and competent in what you were doing.
>
> (Fieldworker 4)

These examples of articulation work – distracting and relaxing participants, working up accounts of competence and expertise – are various strategies of keeping the interview on track. In fact, at this critical moment of the interview, emotional labour becomes more urgent because without the blood sample the interview has no scientific value to the Centre. Even the extraction of biological materials relies on the emotional management of the research encounter. In the next section, we consider the ways in which fieldworkers manage their own emotions in the field.

Emotions *as* work

For all the skills that fieldworkers possess, it is almost impossible to imagine being unaffected by participants' stories of mental illness. Indeed, 'being affected' is a key aspect of performing emotional labour, especially in the early phases of learning the role. But as fieldworkers develop as emotional labourers it seems that one of the aspects of their development is the ability to detach themselves emotionally from the interview process. Indeed, many fieldworkers describe a transition in how emotional labour is performed. Hochschild (1979, 1983) refers to 'surface' and 'deep' acting as different ways of managing emotions and feelings. Deep acting involves changing or modifying an emotion in ways that are aligned with the organization and requirements of work, while surface acting involves conforming to display rules by simulating emotions. However, the task is not, as is the case of 'deep acting', to learn how to feel deep, genuine sympathy for the research participants, but rather to learn to perform sympathy without being too deeply moved. Given this, tensions can arise between how workers would *normally* treat participants and how they are *required* to treat them. Hochschild (1983: 90) describes this tension of 'maintaining a difference between feeling and feigning' as 'emotional dissonance'. Especially when interactive work becomes routinized, these tensions can create problems of identity and authenticity for workers (see Leidner 1993; Erickson and Ritter 2001).

To understand the effects of routinization on the field team, we need to establish the way in which fieldworkers account for the management of emotions when they first entered the field. Even the most seasoned fieldworkers we interviewed told stories of their intense initiation into fieldwork:

> Especially at the beginning, I used to come out of interviews ... especially having done the blood as well ... with extra anxiety, so you'd sit in the car and go, did I do alright? Like, are they okay? Did I leave them alright? And you'd feel very apprehensive about having done it right and asking the right questions. Had you left them alright? Yeah, definitely. And it took a long time for me to ... at least six months for me to feel much more confident in knowing what I was doing.
>
> (Fieldworker 5)

Here, the fieldworker is establishing a pattern of feeling immediately after the interviews. Various rhetorical and affective markers convey an intense responsibility for their performance, as well as an implied risk of 'having done it right and asking the right questions'. While a fieldwork interview is not a formal 'care' relationship, this account displays the way in which a fieldworker understands that she has a clear 'duty of care' towards participants. For this fieldworker, emotional labour involves the management of acute, and sometimes involuntary, feelings of responsibility for participants' wellbeing.

But even when sufficient confidence is acquired, many fieldworkers report situational factors that can trigger negative feelings. In the following account, the emotional resolve of a fieldworker with 18 months' experience is still tested in certain circumstances:

> I suppose just where they live, sometimes as well, can make you ... because if you walk up to a house you can see it's very unkempt and, you know, we've seen some of the most bizarre places in this job. You know, I suppose at that point, you would be having to psych yourself up because you'll be like, oh my gosh, do I actually want to go in there?
>
> (Fieldworker 3)

The locations where emotional labour is performed can invoke feelings of danger and risk which, as others have noted, reflects the status of women who are exposed to stressful and vulnerable circumstances (Hochschild 1983; Kessler and McLeod 1984; Mann 2004). Reference to 'having to psych yourself up' before entering premises indicates something similar to the kind of deep acting of summoning a professional persona and preparing oneself to produce *real* feelings (Mann 2004). Nevertheless, the fieldworker's ability to 'read' the situation – most importantly the mood of the research participant – has been honed by practice:

> But generally the actual interview ... interviewing them is pretty much fine until you get in and then it depends on their mood. If they're irritable, then you sort of read it and know how to do the interview or whatever. But otherwise, now it's fine. It's just something that I suppose you learn. At first it would have been a bit scary ... it's only recently that I've got to the stage of doing four interviews a day. Before that, it probably would have almost seemed a bit, you know, too much.
>
> (Fieldworker 3)

Even as fieldwork becomes more routinized, there is still a sense that emotional labour is something that can be done naturally, only learned tacitly by practice, and subsequently difficult to render explicit ('It's just something that I suppose you learn'). While those running fieldworker training offer occasional insights to the trainees into the emotional labour required, by and large it is seen as an aspect of the work resistant to the logics of rationalization. However, for *individual* fieldworkers the skilled processes of emotional labour do, in a sense, become routinized, which allows them to perform their role day after day. Similar to Leidner's (1993) study of fast food and insurance sales workers, there is a sense that routinization of emotional labour has protective effects of limiting personal involvement, thereby avoiding burnout. Of course, the fieldwork experience is more intensely demanding than the momentary interaction of a fast food worker, and fieldworkers also described the way in which acquiring this tolerance is physically and psychologically demanding. Having worked in the field for a year and a half, only now has the fieldworker developed the resilience required to do 'four interviews a day'. Considering these emotional demands, we asked one of the research managers if fieldworkers had access to formal counselling:

> There isn't a formal process, no. I think it is just the team. Yeah, and it was the same in my day. Because it's one of those things that you can't really discuss with anybody outside of the team. So it's ... yeah, I think having that support within the team is important, yeah. Yeah and it was important for me. And I think especially in the early days because as I say, I didn't really know what schizophrenia was.
>
> (Fieldwork manager)

The isolation of the fieldwork team is compounded by the ethical constraints of collecting sensitive data. The labour of managing their own emotions is not only invisible in its interiority, but remains invisible to any formal process. Support is provided through informal processes, such as discussing difficult cases with other members of the research team. The research manager, who was herself a fieldworker with no clinical training in psychiatry, recognizes the importance of 'support within the team'. Speaking from her own experience, fieldworkers who have unrealistic notions of psychiatric illness need to be prepared for how 'completely traumatic' interviews can be.[7]

Others have reported the ways in which emotional labourers distance their emotions in routinized interactions (Hochschild 1983; Leidner 1993; Mann 2004). For instance, in Henderson's (2001) qualitative study of mental health nurses, practitioners describe the benefits of surface acting by performing a prescribed set of responses and patterns that guide them through dynamic encounters. While descriptions of being 'detached' or 'switched off' allow practitioners to apply clinical judgement objectively, they are frequently accompanied by moral accounts of 'genuine' engagement. In our interviews with fieldworkers, we found a similar oscillation between detachment and engagement, the management of which indicates a moral concern about identity and authenticity. In the account below, we asked a fieldworker how she manages the emotional demands of the interviews:

> I'll speak to other members of the research team and I feel like, oh you know, we all do it. We'll be like, oh I heard this really sad story from this woman. And you'll just be like, oh that's a shame. And obviously you feel sad for them but, I suppose, mainly because you see so many different people ... and because they're not someone I know – you just have to like brush it off. I don't know, I am sometimes quite ... I can't think of the word, but I'll see an old person walking down the street and I'll be like, oh God, look at them, and I can't forget it. And I am a bit like that. So sometimes I'll see someone and their case will really move me or just affect ... not affect me but I'll be like, oh God, and you'll always remember that person. But I don't think it would ever really upset me because I'm not personally involved, I suppose, and because I see them once. I guess when you are actually working with someone as a psychologist or as CPN [Community Psychiatric Nurse] or something, when you do see the same person over and over again, you might become more involved and it might affect you more. But I guess because I hear so many different things, meet so many different people and never see them again it just doesn't really bother me much I guess. I don't mean to sound really cold but I guess you have to sort of be like that, otherwise....
>
> (Fieldworker 3)

Referring to the informal processes of support we discussed earlier, the fieldworker describes releasing some of the emotional strain by 'offloading' to other members of the research team. On the one hand, she is sympathetic to the research participants that she interviews, but on the other the fieldworker explains and justifies her detachment from the interviews ('you just have to brush it off'). In fact, the repetitive, day-to-day routinization of emotional labour is supplied as a reason for this detachment ('because I hear so many different things, meet so many different people and never see them again'). In contrast to healthcare relationships, the fact that fieldwork involves a succession of isolated encounters appears to aggravate this tension between 'feeling and feigning' (Hochschild 1983). Fieldworkers clearly find this emotional double-bind difficult to account for.

Many of the experienced fieldworkers reported diminishing affect towards cases which would have been distressing when they were new to the role. For instance, the interview section dealing with suicide is usually difficult for both the interviewer and the participant, but in the account below a fieldworker describes how emotional labour has become a detached engagement:

> Probably when we first started asking that suicide question and you heard people were attempting – I suppose it probably would shock you. You think oh God, this person's had ten suicide attempts or whatever. But I have to say that now it does tend to wash over me, not that at the time obviously I'm kind of like you know, they – I've got my face on and obviously there for them, and ... very rarely now do I come out and go oh, that was like, I mean only when they've been talking too much and you just feel wow, it's like that was long, but actually not. To them they think it is obviously very relevant to their life and they say you've probably never heard this before and I'm going to tell you this, but actually you have heard it before. So I have to say I don't really take it on board now, kind of let it wash over me.
>
> (Fieldworker 5)

Although 'shock' is a normal and expected reaction to hearing people describe suicide attempts, the fieldworker explains her departure from this norm. The fieldworker has developed the skill required to let these stories 'wash over me', while maintaining her capacity to be sympathetic ('I've got my face on and obviously there for them'). This account stresses the disparity in the balance of emotions at play in the fieldwork encounter. Fieldworkers might have to engage in a number of these intimate encounters each day in order to extract material of scientific value (see Cohn 2008 for a discussion on the role of intimate relations in 'making objective facts') and in doing so they develop the emotional skills required to build rapport, maintain a sympathetic attitude, elicit information, while at the same time being resilient to the strains of this labour. For the research participant, the emotions being elicited are, literally, the product of their life stories; while for the research, these are by-products, which 'wash over' the field and are washed out of the data extracted.

On some occasions, however, managing the fieldwork encounter *as an interview* is not possible. Here, the same fieldworker describes how she had to manage one particularly distressing encounter:

> I can think of one really vivid occasion when the lady, I mean in hindsight probably shouldn't have gone to see her on that day. She said she'd been well but I actually turned up and she was really low and had had a really rough ride with her whole life and illness. And the whole interview was

basically her just telling me her whole life story and how awful it was, you know, and it was awful.... She obviously was crying most of the way through it and in the end it just wasn't appropriate for me to actually ask many of the questions at all and I kind of had to just try and wrap it up and say I think we should come back, you know, when it's a better time for you. And that was probably the most emotional one – I think I'm fairly emotionally robust, or what's the word, with people. But that was the only one because you know when you sort of genuinely do feel for people, you think that does actually sound you've had a really shit time. It does sound as though people haven't really been paying you much attention. And she was very distressed currently, so that was quite difficult to listen to. But I've spoken to her, we followed that up recently and she's managed to send us some more information so there are ways of going back and getting bits.

(Fieldworker 5)

Fieldworkers and research participants can have different priorities that may not align in the interview. The fieldworker endeavours to elicit information efficiently according to the rhythms of the interview schedule, while participants may want to tell their 'whole life story'. This presents a problem for fieldworkers, both in terms of the emotional labour of managing the interview, and because relevant information might very well be embedded in the messy content of their life histories in ways that the participant, the fieldworker and the interview schedule struggle to disentangle. In the encounter described above, the 'emotionally robust' fieldworker must concede to genuine sympathy and abandon the interview. When interviews do break down, fieldworkers have the capacity to gather scientifically relevant information at a distance. However, this is to some degree dependent on the 'successful' management of the emotions at play in the face-to-face encounter.

Given the intensity and routinization of research interviews, emotional labour requires some degree of flexibility between drawing on genuine emotion and 'surface acting'. For the most part, the experienced fieldworker continues to feel culturally appropriate emotions *in spite* of routinization. But as we see in this last account, emotional labour is also conditional upon the alignment established with research participants:

Generally, I don't find being sympathetic a problem. It is genuine sympathy as well. I mean, it's generally not put on. Obviously, there are people who are difficult but I think that those kind of people would be the ones that wouldn't care anyway, because if they're very short with you and you feel like you're in a rush and they don't really want you in their house then, yeah, I wouldn't really be able to get much sympathy for them conjured up. But then they probably wouldn't really care because it's like they don't really want you there anyway. So yeah I don't really find it to be too much of a problem.

(Fieldworker 3)

Having established that 'genuine sympathy' is central to fieldwork, the field-worker is preparing an account of circumstances in which emotional labour does *not* involve surface or deep acting. When participants are 'difficult', 'very short' or 'they don't want you in their house', the difficulty of maintaining genuine sympathy for, or particularly effective surface acting towards, participants is justified because participants do not 'care'. The fact that fieldworkers oscillate between accounts of surface acting and genuine felt emotion conveys the flexibility of skilled emotional labour, but it also reveals their moral concerns of maintaining and presenting an authentic identity. Given that research protocols impose routinization on the interactive work of fieldworkers, fieldworkers find themselves accountable for cases where 'real' emotions are simulated or restrained.

Conclusion

Without thousands of hours of skilled labour performed by fieldworkers there would be no large-scale psychiatric genetics. Senior scientists at the Centre took great pride in the quality of their phenotypic data, drawing contrasts between their approach and that of rival laboratories who they saw as having sacrificed detail and nuance in the pursuit of ever bigger sample sizes. In Chapter 8, however, we will see that since our time at the Centre, leading scientists have temporarily bypassed fieldwork to meet the demands for greater scale and greater statistical power. Fieldwork, which involves an irreducible human element, is not amenable to the kind of expansion of scale required to genetically dissect psychiatric conditions. Unlike work within a laboratory style of reasoning, automation is not a serious possibility. Work in the clinical style of reasoning of psychiatric genetics is necessarily labour-intensive and messy. Not only does fieldwork involve some cognitive and intuitive understanding of psychopathology, but it requires emotional labour to extract and transform life histories into stable scientific objects.

The changes in the fieldwork processes that were described to us by field-workers, fieldwork managers and senior scientists are consistent with the logics of Big Biology. The demands to increase the scale of data production have led to scientists adopting a model of increasing rationalization and a more acute division of labour. However, the nature of clinical reasoning, with its demand for emotional skills that are difficult to render explicit, has meant that fieldwork has been more resistant to this model than laboratory processes. The recruitment of mainly young female psychology graduates reflects an apparently 'natural', gendered division of skilled emotional labourers. Under the guise of 'emotional maturity', these women are expected to excel in suppressing their negative emotions while at the same time conveying warmth and sympathy. These skills are deployed in order to extract information of scientific value from research participants. The streamlining and standardization of the interview as a research instrument was seen by some as a trade-off, an increase in quantity with a concomitant decrease in the quality of data. Consistent with post-Fordist regimes of

production, the clinical aspects of fieldwork have become increasingly frag-
mented and instrumental in Big Biology; fieldwork is essentially stripped of clinical reasoning. Fieldworkers are mainly operators of an instrument that requires
skilful emotional management. This may offer a better explanation for why new
fieldworkers are said to lack the 'passion' for research. Indeed, we might expect
the erosion of aspiration from those socialized into the expectations of 'science
as a vocation' rather than merely another job.

Perhaps, the most vividly illustrated effects of increasing scale on fieldwork
are the ways in which fieldworkers themselves account for the rhythms and
intensity of their work. The autonomy and skill of fieldworkers is essentially
invisible to rationalized models of work (Star and Strauss 1999). The articulation
work of 'pressing' and 'keeping' participants on track, the intuitive awareness of
the emotional dynamics of the interview, are situated factors that require emotional management. Fieldworkers must manage, with sensitivity and skill, a challenging alignment between the priorities of extracting information efficiently and
participants wanting to tell their 'whole life stories'. A core aspect of performing
this invisible, emotional labour is reconciling the tension between 'being
affected' by the stories they hear and the routinization of interviews. While fieldwork is not a 'care' relationship, there are instances in which fieldworkers
clearly express a 'duty of care' towards their participants. But as their capacity
to resist the strains of emotional labour increases with experience, fieldworkers
must manage the 'emotional dissonance' (Hochschild 1983) of simulating or
producing feelings of compassion and sympathy towards participants. The ways
in which fieldworkers account for this tension of 'feeling and feigning' highlights their moral concerns of maintaining an authentic identity.

Notes

1 Fieldworkers at the Centre described the interview as 'semi-structured', stressing the
latitude that interviewers had within the schedule. Nevertheless, the interview was
much more tightly structured than those that a qualitative sociologist would describe as
being 'semi-structured'.
2 Most recently, we have witnessed an 'affective turn' in STS in which emotional work
and interactions of affect are the focus of work examining scientific practice (see, for
example, Fitzgerald 2013, 2017; Myers 2008; Pickersgill 2013; Swallow and Hillman
2018).
3 A number of fieldworkers mentioned the importance of accepting the hospitality of
research participants in building rapport at the start of the fieldwork encounter.
4 An illustration of how fieldwork is rendered invisible in scientific outputs can be found
in two GWAS publications (International Schizophrenia Consortium 2009; Psychiatric
GWAS Consortium Bipolar Disorder Working Group 2011). The 2009 paper published
in *Nature* reported 3,322 cases and 3,587 controls, while the 2011 paper published in
Nature Genetics boasted 7,481 cases and 9,250 controls. These studies involved thousands of hours of fieldworkers engaging not only their cognitive and technical skill, but
also their expertise as emotional labourers. This work is often missing from popular
accounts and only tacitly acknowledged in the literature.
5 When we were observing fieldworker training, one of the experienced fieldworkers
described the way in which scored interviews are scanned and 'read' by software.

This reduces mistakes caused by laborious hand-and-eye input, but the fieldworker leading the training also stressed that it reduces the physical labour involved. She described, with the help of MIME, the work of her PhD. This involved a lot of data input leading to wrist aches and back strains. She cautioned that the software introduces its own systematic mistakes when 'reading' the interviews – the software 'loves its sevens' – which demands that the fieldworkers involved adapt the way they write numbers. These changes are a direct result of the scaling up of psychiatric genetics, of the move to Big Biology. As the fieldworker leading the training said, 'Every little minute saved is valuable' as they have 'such a lot of people to collect'.

6 One of the fieldworkers had experience of interviewing research participants in the hospital to which the Centre was attached, and reflected on the way in which the formal setting influenced the interaction:

> It does change the dynamic. I suppose it feels more professional and feels perhaps … yeah, like you say, it's sort of on my turf and they're coming to see me. Probably people maybe aren't quite as relaxed. But it does, yeah, it feels like more a formal interview. But I think, I don't know, I've only ever done a few. But it did feel as though it had gone fairly well. And maybe it makes it, you know, more regimented and you're able to kind of keep to time a bit more and get through what you need to because there's no distractions.

(Fieldworker 5)

7 Recounting her experience of working on a schizophrenia project, the research manager describes being emotionally unprepared for the fieldwork:

> I was young and naive and I think I was thinking oh this is going to be really fascinating, and I don't think I was prepared for how completely traumatic it was going to be. And I had, I think it was four patients to see, so I went for two days, stayed overnight, so I had two one day and two the next, which for me was a concentration of interviews. Yeah, and I found that difficult.

References

Acker J (1990) Hierarchies, jobs, bodies: A theory of gendered organization. *Gender & Society* 4: 139–158.

Cohn S (2008) Making objective facts from intimate relations: The case of neuroscience and its entanglements with volunteers. *History of the Human Sciences* 21(4): 86–103.

Craddock N, Kendler K, Neale M, *et al.* (2009) Dissecting the phenotype in genome-wide association studies of psychiatric illness. *The British Journal of Psychiatry* 195(2): 97–99.

Erickson RJ and Grove WJC (2008) Emotional labor and health care. *Sociology Compass* 2(2): 704–733.

Erickson RJ and Ritter C (2001) Emotional labour, burnout, and inauthenticity: Does gender matter? *Social Psychology Quarterly* 64(2): 146–163.

Fitzgerald D (2013) The affective labour of autism neuroscience: Entangling emotions, thoughts and feelings in a scientific research practice. *Subjectivity* 6: 131–152.

Fitzgerald D (2017) *Tracing Autism: Uncertainty, Ambiguity, and the Affective Labor of Neuroscience*. Seattle: University of Washington Press.

Hackett EJ (2005) Essential tensions: Identity, control and risk in research. *Social Studies of Science* 35(5): 787–826.

Hatton E (2017) Mechanisms of invisibility: Rethinking the concept of invisible work. *Work, Employment and Society* 31(2): 336–351.

Henderson A (2001) Emotional labour and nursing: An under-appreciated aspect of caring work. *Nursing Inquiry* 8(2): 130–138.

Hochschild AR (1979) Emotion work, feeling rules and social structure. *American Journal of Sociology* 85: 551–575.

Hochschild AR (1983) *The Managed Heart: Commercialization of Human Feeling*. Berkeley: University of California Press.

International Schizophrenia Consortium (2009) Support for the involvement of large copy number variants in the pathogenesis of schizophrenia. *Human Molecular Genetics* 18(8): 1497–1503.

James NJ (1989) Emotional labour: Skill and work in the social regulation of feelings. *Sociological Review* 37(1): 15–42.

Kessler I, Heron P and Dopson S (2015) Managing patient emotions as skilled work and being 'one of us'. *Work, Employment and Society* 29(5): 775–791.

Kessler RC and McLeod JC (1984) Sex differences in vulnerability to undesirable life events. *American Sociological Review* 49: 620–631.

Leidner R (1993) *Fast Food, Fast Talk: Service Work and the Routinization of Everyday Life*. Berkeley: University of California Press.

Lezaun J (2013) Commentary: The escalating politics of 'Big Biology'. *Biosocieties* 8(4): 480–485.

Mann S (2004) 'People-work': Emotion management, stress and coping. *British Journal of Guidance & Counselling* 32(2): 205–221.

Myers N (2008) Molecular embodiments and the body-work of modelling in protein crystallography. *Social Studies of Science* 38(2): 163–199.

Nardi B and Engeström Y (1999) A web on the wind: The structure of invisible work. *Computer Supported Cooperative Work* 8: 1–8.

Pickersgill M (2013) The social life of the brain: Neuroscience in society. *Current Sociology* 61(3): 322–340.

Psychiatric GWAS Consortium Bipolar Disorder Working Group (2011) Large-scale genome-wide association analysis of bipolar disorder identifies a new susceptibility locus near ODZ4. *Nature Genetics* 43(10): 977–983.

Shapin S (1989) The invisible technician. *American Scientist* 77(6): 554–563.

Star SL and Strauss A (1999) Layers of silence, arenas of voice: The ecology of visible and invisible work. *Computer Supported Cooperative Work* 8: 9–30.

Svendsen MN and Koch L (2011) In the mood for science: A discussion of emotion management in a pharmacogenomics research encounter in Denmark. *Social Science & Medicine* 72: 781–788.

Swallow J and Hillman A (2018) Fear and anxiety: Affects, emotions and care practices in the memory clinic. *Social Studies of Science* OnlineFirst DOI: 10.1177/0306312718820965.

Taylor S and Tyler M (2000) Emotional labour and sexual difference in the airline industry. *Work, Employment and Society* 14(1): 77–95.

Ward J and McMurray R (2016) *The Dark Side of Emotional Labour*. Abingdon: Routledge.

7 Scientific imaginaries and their publics

Imagining the future plays an essential role in science. Scientific imaginaries are not only the stuff of grant-writing, press releases or strategic planning, but are also ways of aligning research with contemporary culture. In this sense, imaginaries are not trivial social practices but important forms of work. Indeed, Appadurai (1996: 31) argues that 'imagination is now central to all forms of agency, is itself a social fact, and is the key component of the new global order'. This chapter is concerned with the imaginaries of scientists working at the Centre. By examining the intersection of culture and psychiatric genetics, we seek to understand how scientists justify their styles of reasoning through prospective visions of therapeutic hope. We argue that, more so than many other scientific fields, psychiatric genetics needs a public as a key resource for accomplishing their research goals. In recent years, public engagement has become a mechanism for shaping external networks that assist (and on occasion, obstruct) biological research. This chapter reflects on the relationship between Big Biology and public engagement, and the role social science plays in this accord.

The imaginaries of psychiatric genetics

In Chapter 1, we argued that early European psychiatry held fatalistic views of hereditary disease. One of the early drivers of stigma surrounding hereditary mental illness was an entrenched view of therapeutic pessimism. We return to this point here because we argue that contemporary imaginaries of psychiatric genetics represent a distinct break from the past. Although many psychiatrists acknowledge that severe psychosis has poor prognostic outcomes, the belief structure that underpins recent biological research is that psychiatric conditions *are* tractable and thus *potentially* treatable conditions. In this section, we examine two prospective visions in psychiatric genetics that broadly encompass the biological and the clinical.

Scientific imaginaries are prospective statements that assemble 'revolutionary' futures around specific styles of reasoning. At the discourse level, they have a strong justificatory design. Biological imaginaries, in particular, seek to align programmes of biological research with culture in ways that justify the value (and therefore the cost) of research. For instance, Fujimura's (2003) study of genome scientists shows how future imaginaries build relations between biology and culture that work to convince Japanese and Asian publics that new genomics technologies are, or will be, congruent with their values. In psychiatric genetics, biological imaginaries seek to restore *disease* to its rightful place within mental health services:

> I am now a very biological psychiatrist. I think we've gone too far in throwing the biology out of psychiatry ... it's become too social and, you know, it needs to be [biologically] led for severe mental disorders. And I think part of the problem is that the remit of psychiatry has broadened too much and we're expected to deal with a lot minor psychiatric disorders for which a medical model isn't necessarily the right approach. But for things like schizophrenia and bipolar disorder and severe recurrent depression, you know, these are very biological diseases and it's not really appropriate to just think of them in terms of social constructs. And I mean, of course, all diseases are to some extent constructed, but there's something there and it's hard to define. And I get very angry because I think our patients suffer, you know, you can have clever intellectual arguments about it but ultimately there are people out there with severe diseases living dreadful lives who aren't helped by thinking – well if you just treat everyone well and provide social care it will go away. It doesn't go away.
>
> (Centre director of neuropsychiatric genetics)

The director is referring to cultural factors that have led to the 'creeping devaluation of medicine' (Craddock *et al.* 2008: 6) within psychiatric care. As he sees it, the legacy of psychoanalysis, anti-psychiatry and social constructionism have marginalized biomedical models of mental illness. However, a distinction is made between 'minor' and 'severe' psychiatric disorders, with disorders on either side of this boundary warranting not just different kinds of treatment, but potentially entirely different approaches. For minor psychiatric conditions, the director concedes that a medical model may not be the 'right approach', but neither is social care an effective treatment for severe conditions, which he maintains are 'very biological diseases'. From this point of view, a medicalized approach demands that the biological component of a disorder is identified. What makes aspects of this vision plausible is the concession that psychiatric conditions are 'to some extent constructed' (they are 'real' but difficult to define) and that some conditions perhaps should not be medicalized. But a stronger case for justifying biological research is the argument that social care does not make severe diseases 'go away'. Here, a biological imaginary establishes a vision of care in which severe psychiatric disorders justify a biomedical model. This is not simply a vision of the future, but a vision of the cultural and institutional landscape in which a biological approach is justified.

Other biological imaginaries operate on a different scale, concerned not so much with clinical futures but with the validity of research programmes in psychiatric genetics. These also contain a strong justificatory design. In the following account, a biological vision of psychiatric illnesses constitutes a defensive reaction to a critique of GWAS.

> I think genome-wide associations have delivered actually and they have identified genes, not a huge numbers of genes, just a handful of genes which are telling us something about the illness, but more importantly they are telling us about the pathways and the biological systems that are involved. So these are not barn door hits in the genome, they don't rise up to the signals saying these are the big hits so we can say this is a gene. I hate that phrase 'a gene for' ... if you look below the surface then there's going to be a lot of genes which don't hit that level of significance but are still susceptibility genes for the illness, and what's interesting when you look at those they seem to be in the same biological pathways and therefore that's telling us something quite interesting, and these systems might well be involved in the illness, and that is something that we would not have known without genome-wide association studies.

And the hope is to go back to biology?

> Yeah that's the point, that's the purpose of this. We're not stamp collecting. And we're not just trying to get a bunch of significant hits and then just list them and say, hey we've identified X number of genes for schizophrenia, we want to realize why they cause the illness or schizophrenia because I've worked on it for such a long time, but we want to find out why these genes cause the illness. So therefore what is the biology that underlies the illness? Because we know so little about most of these psychiatric illnesses. If we can correlate the functions of these genes that might tell us something about the biological pathways involved, and that might lead to treatments down the line. But it certainly should lead to a better understanding.
>
> (Senior lecturer in molecular biology)

The then senior lecturer of molecular genetics gives a cautious account of the progress made in GWAS. That only a 'handful of genes' were found by 2008 is contrasted with the present situation where statements made with the benefit of GWAS findings are considerably more confident (see Chapter 8 for full discussion of recent progress). The signals from GWAS – even those 'which don't hit that level of significance' to be 'a gene for' – act as signposts for revealing biological pathways and systems that were otherwise unknown before the data-intensive, Big Biology of GWAS. The scientist is cautious to distance these findings from cultural discourses that position gene discovery as an enterprise of simple genetic determinism. The statement 'I hate that phrase "a gene for"' establishes alignment with cultural scepticism regarding a single-gene model. By contrast, a complex landscape is imagined in which 'many genes' cluster around 'interesting' pathways. Prompted by the interviewer about whether these findings will lead to a 'return' to experimental, 'wet lab' biology, the scientist gives a surprisingly defensive account. Gene discovery is not an end in itself ('We're not stamp collecting'), but a means of accessing the biological causes of mental illness. The language is uncertain and conditional, but the scientist justifies biology in terms of future 'treatments down the line' or at least a 'better understanding' of disease. Biological imaginaries are both aspirational and defensive because they operate in a climate hostile to psychiatric medicalization, genetic determinism and, to some degree, Big Science. But they also represent a significant departure from the therapeutic pessimism of past European psychiatry. Biological imaginaries reconfigure the ontology of mental illness as tractable and therefore potentially clinically treatable problems.

As such, biological visions of psychiatric disorders also create futures in which the clinical style of reasoning will be reshaped. Similar to the expectations that circulated on the eve of the HGP, the clinical imaginaries of psychiatric genetics belong to a family of promissory discourses on 'personalized' and 'stratified' medicine (Hood 1993; Sander 2000). Acutely aspirational, clinical imaginaries create futures in which genetic markers orient patients to individualized drug treatment:

> I hope that even before we understand the biology we can use the genetics as an object or marker to try and subdivide or categorize people into groups that are a bit more similar to each other than just their symptoms would predict. That will form the basis for different styles of stratified medicine trials because we know that most of the drugs work in some people but none of the drugs work in all people. It may be that we can do things like that. I would hope that with the development of the sequencing and the enhanced GWAS that we'll get better biological anchors that will help uncover what's fundamentally wrong in groups of people that could be targeted with treatment.
>
> (Professor of neuropsychiatric genetics, schizophrenia)

Given that psychiatric symptoms have not proven to be a reliable basis for prescribing medicines, the hope is that identifying genetic markers that can be used in a clinical setting will lead to more effective drug development. This future vision of pharmacogenomics justifies current research programmes of GWAS and next-generation sequencing that will eventually produce a broad complement of 'biological anchors' to facilitate targeted treatment. A more persuasive, though remote, vision imagines that psychiatric diagnosis will be no different to receiving a medical diagnosis for heart attack.

> In the clinic, I think we will end up ... if you think about other branches of medicine then you have a whole kind of hierarchy of diagnosis. You turn up to the clinic with severe chest pain and short of breath, sweating, thready pulse, the diagnosis is you are having a heart attack. That's the clinical diagnosis. And that's equivalent to your psychosis, you have got schizophrenia, you know. And then beneath that, you do some enzymes and ECG and then

you say, this chest pain is an MI [Myocardial Infarction]. And then beneath that you have got … your blood pressure is high, you are overweight, you don't do enough exercise, smoke like a chimney, and I think psychosis will end up like that. So you will retain your syndromic diagnosis but that will be gradually refined through the clinical process … I think that's the way it will go. So saying, oh schizophrenia or clinical diagnosis are a waste of time in the clinic, I don't think they are. The danger is when researchers, clinical researchers in genetics, biologists say that schizophrenia is a 'thing' and it's different from autism, which is a different 'thing' and bipolar is another … why can't we find a biomarker that will help us distinguish autism from schizophrenia or schizophrenia from bipolar disorder and we never can because there's no clear distinction in the population between them, they merge into each other.

(Centre director of neuropsychiatric genetics)

The director imagines a similar clinical scenario to the one given earlier but offers an optimistically mundane account of clinical diagnosis ('You turn up to the clinic …'). The analogy of *Myocardial Infarction* is an illustration that future clinical practice in psychiatry will no longer simply resemble medicine but will become a genuinely applied medicine. The clinical imaginary is nuanced; it accepts that patients will present with non-specific symptoms 'that will be gradually refined through the clinical process' by identifying relevant risk factors and biomarkers. Not to be confused with an essentialist view that psychiatric categories can be grounded on genes, as if genes were discrete 'things' or natural kinds (Kendler 2006), the current biological imaginary of psychiatric genetics upholds the view that biomarkers are a stable but complex reference to dynamic, biological systems. This vision also aligns with renewed interest in the 'neurodevelopmental hypothesis' (Owen *et al.* 2011), whereby psychiatric disorders are imagined as groups of related and overlapping syndromes, held together by complex genetic and environmental factors.

Scientific imaginaries play an important strategic role in psychiatric genetics. To suggest that they are fantasies or mere imaginations is to misconstrue their purpose and to underestimate their effects. Imaginaries, like expectations and other prospective claims, are future representations which have a *performative* quality. They shape the way society makes sense of science and technology, actively constitute pathways of innovation and 'mobilize, legitimate, and coordinate concrete activities involved in the real-world construction of science and technology' (Konrad *et al.* 2017: 468, also see Borup *et al.* 2006; van Lente 1993). Psychiatric genetics forms part of our contemporary 'regimes of hope' (Moreira and Palladino 2005; Martin *et al.* 2008), capturing distinct ways in which therapeutic optimism is realized. The role of visions in driving biomedical innovation and investment are not only features of 'biocapitalism' (Rajan 2006), but also legitimate and sustain the styles of reasoning that underpin large-scale biological research. Psychiatric genetics *needs* a public to align its scientific imaginaries with culture, to shape the field into which it imagines biology will improve treatment, but it also, more than many other research fields, needs a public to accumulate biological capital in order to accomplish its research goals.

Psychiatric genetics and its publics

Despite the optimistic claims of psychiatric genetics, in contemporary Western culture mental illness threatens to be an escalating and intractable problem. The 'burden' of mental health is now widely reported in the mainstream media through personal narratives, national statistics and economic analyses.[1] In the UK especially, there is an impending sense of crisis as mental health services struggle to accommodate increasing numbers of service users. Over the past decade, an array of programmes, from transnational mental health awareness campaigns such as the European Brain Council's *Year of the Brain*, social enterprises in mental health 'first aid' training, the enrolment of celebrity mental health ambassadors including the royal family, and sensitive portrayals of mental illness in film and on television, to local public engagement initiatives, have provided 'evidence-based' information with the hope of building resilience and reducing the stigma of psychiatric ill-health for individuals and communities. As a result, publics are increasingly well-informed about psychiatric disorders and research, though there remains strong hostility from some service users and providers towards a biomedical model (Craddock *et al.* 2008).

How do scientific imaginaries intervene in a landscape potentially hostile to biomedical psychiatry? Psychiatric genetics imagines that mental illness will be rendered 'diseases like any other' (Read *et al.* 2006). But unlike other fields of biomedicine, psychiatric disorders are difficult to diagnose, and are unlikely to map directly onto biological categories (Burmeister *et al.* 2008; Morgan *et al.* 2008; Green 2014). As we have described in previous chapters, the historical ontology of mental illness is deeply political, not least because governments have a history of misusing and abusing psychiatry and notions of heredity (Propping 2005; Kerr and Shakespeare 2002). That contemporary scientific imaginaries of mental illness are determinedly optimistic amounts to a reversal of psychiatric genetics' controversial history.

The way in which practitioners present a narrative of their discipline is therefore important, with existing popular perceptions of psychiatry and psychiatric genetics ambivalent at best. Smith (2008) argues that few people, apart from psychiatrists, care about the wider practice of psychiatry. Yet they should, he argues, as the 'burden' of mental illness is enormous (Layard 2006). Treating mental illness accounts for 11.7 billion per year of the UK National Health Service budget (Gov.uk 2017), while the cost of work-related mental ill health is estimated to be almost another £35 billion per year (Parsonage and Saini 2017[2]). Although these sorts of statistics are designed to be of compelling interest to the public, making psychiatric ill-health and research a 'democratic' question, Smith's argument goes further; psychiatry needs 'a public' or else it will become further marginalized both within and outside of medicine. Public engagement in psychiatry is presented as a dialogical solution to improving care, reducing stigma and salvaging status (Smith 2008).

Scientists also face the added challenge of genetic stigmatization. Stigma is widely recognized as one of the biggest obstacles to accessing mental healthcare (Sartorius 2007), and efforts to understand and reduce stigma is central to many public programmes (Time to Change[3] 2012). However, there is the fear that the 'geneticization' (Lippman 1991, 1992) of mental illness could in fact reinforce stigma (Rose 1998; Phelan 2002, 2005; Kvaale *et al.* 2013a), reflecting some of the negative discourses of degeneration found in Victorian psychiatry (see Chapters 1 and 2). Yet, while researchers at the Centre speak of public engagement as a means to tackle the stigma of mental illness, they also invoke the 'stigma' that they *themselves* face both as psychiatrists and as geneticists of disorders that have so far proved resistant to genetic dissection (Lewis and Bartlett 2015). Researchers express concerns regarding the standing of psychiatry with medicine, and psychiatric genetics within post-HGP genetics, and the effect this has on their professional identity. The history of psychiatry and genetics has left its mark on the field. Unlike some other branches of genomic medicine, psychiatric genetics has a disappointing history when it comes to 'gene-discovery' (see Chapter 3). And even with the benefits of recent advances in genetics and genomics, psychiatric genetics still struggles to a far greater extent with classifying phenotypes than is the case for genetic studies of 'somatic' illnesses. It is against this backdrop that psychiatric genetics must engage with the public.

In Chapters 4 and 5, we described our ethnographic site as an example of 'Big Biology' – the Centre being a node of production within a broader international consortium. The significant resources required to do large-scale biological research are not limited to specialist networks of scientific expertise and accumulations of technology, but also networks external to science. For those working at the Centre, 'public engagement' includes programmes that work to align its scientific visions with existing cultural values and external professional groups in order to recruit large numbers of research participants. Public engagement is a route to recruiting the raw scientific material of DNA and detailed phenotypes of people with psychiatric disorders. In the next section, we describe the launch of the engagement programme at the Centre in 2009. We reflect on our own involvement in these activities, and consider scientists' accounts of publics and engagement.

Public engagement

'Public engagement' is now a stock phrase used to describe a constellation of activities and initiatives in which science and 'the public' enter constructive or deliberative dialogue.[4] The relationship between science and the general public has been a research concern since (at least) the 1960s, especially in the United States (Bauer *et al.* 2007). However, efforts to promote the public understanding of and engagement with science in the UK received a significant boost following the publication of the Bodmer Report (The Royal Society 1985; Miller 2001). Today, public opinion and public perception are now regarded major 'democratic' influences in shaping science policy, with action in these areas often imagined as work to prevent or mitigate negative public attitudes towards science that result from mistaken, ignorant or unscientific ideas held by 'the public'. Notwithstanding criticisms of the so-called 'deficit model', the Bodmer Report, in the UK at least, led to increasing encouragement for scientific fields to open up to the public (see Lewis and Bartlett 2015).

Since the Report, 'the public' (and their attitudes towards science) has been the subject of intense interest with calls for scientists to engage becoming increasingly louder (Gregory and Miller 1998; House of Lords 2000; Wilsdon and Willis 2004; Bauer *et al.* 2007; Davies 2008; Poliakoff and Webb 2007; Barnett *et al.* 2012). In the UK, funding bodies such as the Medical Research Council (MRC) and the Wellcome Trust encourage scientists to communicate and discuss their work with publics, with such activities commonly described as 'public engagement' (Research Council United Kingdom 2013). But public engagement is no longer simply an abstract civic responsibility; it is increasingly part of the metrics considered when allocating research funding (Pearson 2001). Universities are said to have a 'duty' to communicate with the public and to engage with public groups and non-expert communities (Gregory and Miller 1998). Indeed, the Research Excellence Framework places greater emphasis on the 'impact' of research than its predecessor, the Research Assessment Exercise (Stern Review 2016). While public engagement is not in itself considered 'impact', in many academic departments a common strategy is to invest in public engagement to showcase 'pathways' to impact (Watermeyer 2012).

In the field of genomics, public engagement has been shaped by unique historical circumstances. For instance, the framework known as ELSI (Ethical, Legal and Social Implications) was the brainchild of scientists, for whom the downstream consequences of the HGP was intended to be a 'responsible' public relations exercise (Watson 2000). Between 3 and 5 per cent[5] of the annual HGP budget was set aside to fund ELSI projects with the expectation that such programmes would smooth the path, preventing social and ethical issues from becoming controversial public issues[6] (see Meslin 1997; Roberts 2001; Fisher 2005). The development of ELSI in the United States (Jasanoff 2007) and ELSA (Ethical, Legal and Social Aspects) in Europe (Hilgartner *et al.* 2016) took place in light of specific concerns surrounding the role of 'science' in causing industrial pollution and environmental damage, particularly through the use of insecticides and pesticides in the United States (Carson 1962, see also Gregory and Miller 1998) and the cases of nuclear power (Wynne 1992) and Bovine Spongiform Encephalopathy (BSE, or 'Mad Cow Disease') in the UK (Jasanoff 2007; Collins 2014). Over the last 15 or so years, much of this work has been outsourced to social scientists. As Balmer *et al.* (2015: 4) state: 'social scientists are often positioned as being responsible for the identification and remediation of potential negative downstream consequences of science'. In what follows, we reflect on our own position as sociologists working on public engagement programmes alongside (and for) scientists. We too have not escaped the expansionary logics of Big Biology.

Aligning and facilitating visions

In Chapter 4, we explained that the Centre was established in its current form after securing a large operational grant in 2009. Given that funders now insist on public engagement as a component of biomedical research, a proportion of funding was allocated to developing an 'innovative and creative' public engagement programme. In fact, parts of the grant application were written by social scientists, including one of the authors (Arribas-Ayllon). In August of that year, Lewis was employed on a five-year contract to co-lead the engagement programme and to conduct social science research.[7] The following ethnographic observations and interview data are the result of combining participatory research with the role of leading and coordinating public engagement activities at the Centre.

The public engagement programme was a novel arrangement designed not only with the purpose of representing science but also *intervening* in cultural norms about science. As a sociologist, Lewis was absorbed into the Centre's networks of expertise, acting as an intermediary for scientists and an instigator and engineer of public events. This kind of position is not unusual in multidisciplinary environments where social scientists find themselves working on scientific projects as an adjunct to scientific research centres, especially in the biomedical sciences (Balmer *et al.* 2015). Under these circumstances, the sensibilities of the sociologist are put to work to align and facilitate other people's visions. These visions have a strategic design of mitigating public imaginations of crude reductionism or simple determinism; rebuilding the status of genomic psychiatry as a 'flexible' (but 'hard') science; foregrounding political and social risks to articulate cultural sensitivity; creating mobile ontologies of susceptibility and resilience; and distancing psychiatry from past abuses. Ethical reflections of genetic risk and susceptibility create a kind of 'somatic individuality' (Novas and Rose 2000), in which self-knowledge and self-management are pathways to a better future of treatment and care. Working alongside scientists, the sociologist in these endeavours is often positioned to find ways of aligning these visions of hope with broader cultural values. They too (wittingly or unwittingly) become part of the Big Biology machine.

The engagement programme included a repertoire of public initiatives, many developed and organized by Lewis, including film and discussion events (Lewis *et al.* 2017), school debates and art exhibitions (Lewis and Thomas 2017; Bevan-Jones *et al.* 2017), which supplemented the ongoing research of Arribas-Ayllon and Bartlett.[8] At a very early stage, these ideas were met with some resistance. It was not uncommon to hear phrases such as 'not in front of the children' and 'don't scare the horses' from senior scientists who had experienced negative, even hostile, responses at public events from what they characterized as the anti-psychiatry brigade (see Lewis and Thomas 2017). On one occasion, Lewis was told that a senior scientist nearly had a 'heart attack' when he heard of a proposed event involving visual artists.[9] While post-ELSI research may provide opportunities for various forms of collaborative arrangements between scientists and social scientists (Balmer *et al.* 2015), organizing these events highlight the power struggles involved in aligning the visions of different epistemic cultures. Alongside leading and coordinating these programmes, Lewis also conducted research interviews at the Centre. In the next section, we explore the ways in which scientists account for publics and engagement.

Scientists' accounts of publics and engagement

Literature on the public understanding of science tells us, of course, that 'the public' is not a homogenous group but positioned heterogeneously in relation to science (Renn 2006; Wynne 1995). Scientists at the Centre prioritize different publics, ranging from 'the general public', 'research participants' or 'patients', 'medical professionals' to 'policy-makers' (see Lewis and Bartlett 2015 for a detailed discussion). They also have a variety of ways of talking about public engagement. Some of these accounts are more sophisticated than others. Consider the following accounts from two senior scientists:

> As time's gone on we've had various bits of publicity in relation to the research, some of it in relation to findings that we had or targets that we've tried to set in recruitment, so that's been through things like radio or TV or newspapers stuff like this. We've set up, more recently over the last few years, websites again in order to provide information as well as to enable people to volunteer for research and particularly for the recruitment that we've been having most recently for bipolar studies. We've deliberately tried to engage with the public more, sort of directly about the research.
>
> (Professor of psychiatric genetics, schizophrenia)

And:

> Unless there's a level of public engagement, you can't possibly transfer the findings into ways of actually changing behaviour and treatment and services, that's one thing. The second thing is that patients need hope and you know communicating the fact that there's research going on is a way of instilling hope and the fact that this problem is being taken seriously and there's effort going into it and people are thinking about it. So there's that, and also I think that people have a basic right to know what they can about themselves and what they're experiencing so that, you know, it sort of makes sense, I think those are the main reasons. Also I guess there's a practical reason too, that in order to get funding and resources for research you need to be explaining why it's needed and making a case for it.
>
> (Professor of psychiatric genetics, bipolar disorder)

Though both accounts imply a deficit approach to science communication, they articulate starkly different versions of publics and engagement. In the first account, the professor gives a historical overview of different approaches to involving 'the public'. The framing of 'various bits of publicity' implies a loosely constructed campaign of science communication involving standard media outlets. Scientists themselves appear to be absent in this process; the work could just as easily be outsourced to press officers or public relations personnel. The function of this 'engagement' is explicitly oriented to recruiting participants into biological research. The development of 'websites' suggests perhaps a more dynamic, multimodal approach of information-giving to 'enable people to volunteer for research' at the Centre.

In the second account, public engagement is described as an integral part of the process of 'transfer' through which scientific research is 'actually changing behaviour and treatment and services'. Though this 'transfer' still implies a unilateral approach aligned with impact agendas, it also resonates with the performative role of scientific imaginaries shaping the way society makes sense of science and technology. Reference to 'patients' and 'instilling hope' align with 'regimes of hope' (Moreira and Palladino 2005) that characterize the outward-facing discourses of genomic medicine. The claim that recipients have a 'right to know what they can about themselves' is also persuasive, suggesting that research reveals ontologies of personhood that may lead to better understandings and treatments of mental illness. Lastly, the scientist understands that, notwithstanding these reasons, public engagement serves a practical function within contemporary systems of scientific governance, with funders requiring concrete explanations of the ways in which publics will benefit from the biomedical research that they support.

Read together, the accounts represent contrasting views of public engagement. In the first, one might be forgiven for reading into the extract that 'directly' engaging publics is tolerated as a necessary inconvenience, whereas the second offers a clear explanation of engagement as a process by which relations with publics can be managed and through which successful biomedical research can be realized. The tendency for more and more scientists at the Centre to think (and act) according to the latter may partly explain why the Centre has been successful in vastly scaling up the number of research participants recruited into projects in recent years. While this evolution falls well short of the kind of dialogical and deliberative engagement that some would hope for, a more nuanced and thoughtful approach to both 'publics' and 'engagement' appears to have been an effective way of coupling communities of hope with therapeutic optimism.

When it comes to questions about the function of public engagement, a common refrain among scientists is the need to communicate the 'complexity' of the genetics of psychiatric disorders. This is crucial given that lay perceptions of genetics are often dominated by essentialism and determinism (Nelkin and Lindee 1995), though others report more diverse perceptions of disease causation (Condit 1999; Parrott *et al.* 2003; Chilibeck *et al.* 2010). But rather than focusing on the knowledge deficits of the general public, affected families are seen by scientists as allies in communicating the genetic underpinnings of mental illness:

My experience of talking about genetics is that people understand probably more. I mean there's quite a lot of hostility towards genetics from other psychiatrists but when you talk to patients they all know it runs in families. I mean it's bloody obvious ... I mean they might have very naive views about the complexity and so on but they know it runs in families. And I do think generally speaking people do view biological explanations as being less stigmatizing. I think there are a lot of families who still find it hard to get away from the idea that people with say schizophrenia need to pull themselves together and if they were only more motivated, you know, things would be better or why don't they go and get a job.... Actually I had a patient who we discovered fairly late on in his illness had an arteriovenous malformation and schizophrenia and there had been a lot of conflict between him and his father and his brother. His brother and his father both worked in the family business and thought that he was lazy and feckless and so on. And their attitude to him changed dramatically when they discovered that there was this organic thing that they could somehow pin the illness on.

(Centre director of neuropsychiatric genetics)

Drawing on his own clinical experience, the director claims that affected families are more receptive to genetic explanations of mental illness than is the case for the wider profession of psychiatry. Families may not fully comprehend the complexity of genetic risk but their inter-generational knowledge and experience lends itself to understanding that mental illness 'runs in families'. This alignment of views between patients (or research participants) and geneticists, and the apparent misalignment between scientists and psychiatrists, is also identified in Turney and Turner's (2000) study of schizophrenia. More than any of the other interest groups that they interviewed, patients 'seem to share some features of the geneticists' outlook' (2000: 18). It seems that public understandings of *heredity* among affected families are a stable reference for sharing scientific visions although, as Turney and Turner caution, while these visions share some similarities they are 'worlds away' from each other. Not all patients may see or understand new genetic information as having any immediate personal relevance.

The director's clinical experience also establishes a basis for generalization: biological explanations will de-stigmatize psychiatric conditions. Indeed, this is a core vision of psychiatric genetics. The logics of therapeutic optimism insist that revealing the material ontologies of disease will absolve the individual of personal responsibility and blame. This runs directly counter to claims that genetic categories are essentializing and thus *necessarily* stigmatizing (Nelkin and Lindee 1995). Evidence in the literature to support either of these claims is mixed (Phelan 2002, 2005; Kvaale *et al.* 2013a, 2013b). But an account of biological explanations being 'less stigmatizing' is plausible when contrasted with moral statements of schizophrenia being a personal failure to manage oneself responsibly. The director's narrative concerning a patient offers evidential support to the claim that families undergo attitudinal change when schizophrenia is attributed to an 'organic thing'.[10] Scientists' visions not only create biological futures in which hope can be aligned with downstream therapies, but they also create social futures in which biological categories are decoupled from moral discourses of blame and responsibility.

As a machinery for producing scientific imaginaries, public engagement also has a political design. Biological psychiatry must win the 'hearts and minds' of mental health groups, charitable organizations, mental health professionals, academic colleagues from a range of medical and biological disciplines, and 'expert', activist patients. In recent years, a public-facing institute annexed to the Centre, which we call *Public Mental Health*, was established partly with a view to recruiting participants to research projects but also to foster closer partnerships with mental health services and third sector organizations. Public engagement at the Centre is an opportunity to soften and smooth the terrain over which psychiatric genetics seeks to travel.

> I am very keen to persuade people that psychiatric disorders are tractable to scientific approaches.... Severe psychiatric disorders are disorders of the brain that can be approached by genetics and neurosciences and that is the way to develop new treatments ... I see this really about trying to get across to people an understanding of what we do because I don't think people have any idea of what we do and what the possibilities are.... A lot of people have preconceptions about psychiatric disorders and that makes it interesting as well as difficult, and that compared with other types of disease there is a political dimension to this. These preconceptions are, I think, often unconsciously politically motivated and so one often encounters preconceptions and hostility because this idea of social causation of psychiatric disorders has become so prevalent, and is held by a lot of people who work in mental health, particularly nurses and social workers and so on, often by one's academic colleagues that one tends to be fighting against the whole time.
>
> (Professor working on schizophrenia)

Scientists' visions of engagement are politically oriented to shaping networks external to science. Others have also noticed that large-scale biology is concerned with 'an amplification of the political reflexivity of the scientific enterprise' (Lezaun 2013: 480). Public engagement is viewed by scientists as a means to mitigate resistance to biological research by presenting psychiatric disorders as conditions of complex biology rather than 'politically motivated' manifestations of 'social causation'. Big Biology needs a public not only for legitimacy and support but to recruit human resources to provide the 'capital' for the expansion and intensification of its research efforts (see Chapter 6). The imaginaries of psychiatric genetics are, as much as anything else, *instrumental* visions, the distinctive function of which is to obtain access to networks of patient groups by converting their gatekeepers through regimes of hope.

Cinderella science

Notwithstanding its therapeutic aspirations, psychiatric genetics must contend with its own marginal status vis-à-vis other genetic disciplines. When scientists speak of the challenges of delivering a successful public engagement programme, they often describe the stigma of their profession as being intertwined with the stigma of mental illness.

> If we want to promote this agenda then we have to carry people with us. They have to support it. I want to do it [public engagement] because I think psychiatry is a marginalized speciality within medicine and I think that is bad for people with psychiatric disorders. I think people with psychiatric disorders are marginalized in society.... The road to hell is paved with good intentions and this is a very good example of that. People's attempts to treat psychiatric disorders as being distinct and different has backfired massively and it's one of the reasons why we have such appallingly bad psychiatric services and that stigma continues.
>
> (Centre director of neuropsychiatric genetics)

Whether psychiatry is discredited because those they treat already carry the burden of a 'spoiled' identity (Goffman 1963), or because the reputation of the speciality is tarnished by history, the director's point is that the marginalization of psychiatry (especially biological psychiatry) is 'bad for people with psychiatric disorders'. From the margins of medicine, a bleak vision of psychiatric services unfolds. Under the 'dividing practices' (Foucault 1982) of the dominant social model, mental illness is defined and treated according to symptoms rather than its underlying biology. Failure to objectify illnesses as complex traits has led to poor services and, concomitantly, entrenched stigma. In a society in which biological approaches to mental health are marginalized, scientists are less optimistic about the prospects of treatment and care.

In addition to biological psychiatry being marginalized within psychiatry, psychiatry has an inferior status in relation to general medicine. For instance, it is well-known that medical students view psychiatry as less attractive than other career options because, among other things, it lacks prestige and scientific rigour (Eagle and Marcos 1980; Feifel *et al.* 1999; Malhi *et al.* 2002; DeMello and Deshpande 2015). The processes that mark psychiatry as a 'spoiled' profession seem to occur before and during the socialization of medical students. Below, the professor recounts the realization during his medical training that psychiatry was considered an inferior speciality:

> I was always interested in doing psychiatry in spite of [what] the tutors used to us say if you don't pull your socks up you'll end up a psychiatrist, so I realized that it wasn't necessarily the most prestigious of the medical disciplines but I always wanted to do it.
>
> (Professor working on schizophrenia)

The techniques of 'degradation' employed by teaching staff imply that psychiatry is a failed medical identity. Trainee medics are socialized to regard psychiatry as a poor relation to other branches of medicine, one that lacks the integrity, materiality and success of specialities dealing with somatic illnesses. Once a profession acquires a spoiled identity, the personal characteristics of its members are marked as inferior or even (see below) 'weird'. Senior scientists told us stories of how medical colleagues reacted with surprise when they discovered that they had chosen psychiatry as a career path.

> It really is a joke when you are a medical student. You know, I mean, people really put you off it. I think there is stigma. At medical school you get it and then afterwards, you know, people say but you weren't one of the weird ones.
> (Professor working on attention deficit hyperactivity disorder)

Fitzgerald (2017) tells a similar story about psychology in understanding brain disorders like autism. Before cognitive neuroscience came to the rescue of a flailing 'soft' psychology, Fitzgerald's respondents narrated similar biographies about the perceived stigma of studying 'mental' phenomena. But while psychology, like psychiatry, has been positioned historically at the margins of medicine for being too soft, it appears that psychiatric genetics is regarded with suspicion by psychiatrists precisely *because* of its scientism.

> It's a big problem for psychiatry and more particularly for patients. So there's a general issue which is that in UK psychiatry for quite a long time there's been a terrible nihilism about anything scientific. You know, and partly that's understandable because lots of times people have come up with some finding and it's either not been replicated or it's not fed through to any impact on changing what you do with patients.... And so because of the way the UK psychiatric service is run ... they're not set up in a scientific sort of way, they're fairly de-medicalized and it's just kind of easier for people to kind of think oh well, you know, there is no science in this and nothing that gets published is actually worth knowing about ... so that's a general thing. And then there's a specific thing which is I think quite a lot of people who are in psychiatry have a scepticism about biological in general, and genetic in particular, explanations of illness and they just have a sort of idealistic or theoretical philosophical abhorrence of it. Not all of them but a proportion of people ... I mean don't get me wrong, there'll be plenty of psychiatrists out there who will have a perfectly balanced eclectic view of you know, social and psychological factors are important and biological factors too and you know that's all fine. But in terms of what your average jobbing psychiatrist would think, they wouldn't be keeping up to date with the fact that there's stuff going on.... Whereas in the States it'll be completely different ... there's always been more excitement about science anyway and there's always been more sort of expectation that psychiatrists

would kind of know what was going on in neuroscience because it's probably going to have an influence on the way they practise psychiatry at some
point. But that's not what's been ingrained in British psychiatry.

(Professor working on bipolar disorder)

A common justification for public engagement is to counter the widespread
rejection of, and even 'philosophical abhorrence' towards, biological research
among the UK psychiatry community. The fact that these counter-imaginaries of
scepticism and hostility are culturally specific implies that forces external to
science are seen as a hindrance to improving psychiatric services in the UK. The
professor concedes that poor replication and minimal translation of past genetic
research findings sustains this scepticism, but presents this as an unbalanced
view of science and attributes it not to past failures but to the 'de-medicalized'
framework of psychiatric services. Again, patients are seen to be losing out
because the 'average jobbing psychiatrist' is ignorant of recent developments in
genetics. The contrast of cultural imaginaries is effective in advancing the view
that American psychiatry is progressive and hopeful, while UK psychiatry is
backward and ideological.

Scientists paint a picture in which psychiatric genetics is stuck in an awkward
position of 'damned if you do, and damned if you don't'. On the one hand, psychiatric genetics is derided by the medical sciences for being too 'soft', while on
the other hand it is scorned by psychiatry for being too 'hard'. Public engagement seeks to transform psychiatric genetics into a *Cinderella science*, a previously neglected speciality, the achievements and importance of which are
coming to light after a long period of obscurity. Scientists speak of futures in
which progress is perpetually around the corner, always on the horizon. They
point to the success stories of other disciplines, particularly branches of biomedicine such as cancer genetics, in order to support the claim that large-scale
biology will legitimate psychiatric genetics as a 'hard' science. Big Biology will
not only reveal the biological basis of psychiatry, but it will also lift the 'stigma'
from psychiatry and in doing so attract a new generation of talented scientists:

> Brain research in the future. I think it's going to be one of the areas of growth
> and that message needs to be got over to people who are really genuinely in
> that position of making the decision with what they do with the rest of their
> lives. It's usually towards the end of an undergraduate degree that you think
> where do I go now, and what we need to do is attract the really good scien-
> tists into thinking about, well maybe brain research and not cancer.

(Professor working on Alzheimer's disease)

Analogies to disease

Scientists at the Centre often refer to psychiatric conditions as 'diseases like any
other' (Read *et al.* 2006). Indeed, analogies are powerful heuristic devices for
mobilizing scientific imaginaries. Diseases such as cancer or diabetes provide a

familiar, and successful, reference point, allowing scientists to avoid the task of explaining complex genetics from first principles. Analogies combine biological and clinical imaginaries to invoke medical futures in which progress in psychiatric genetics is tied to existing stories of success.

> Forty, fifty years ago, cancer was regarded as an incurable condition that was very stigmatized, people didn't talk about it. When I was a medical student on the ward, you never told someone they had cancer.... You said well, you've got a bit of a growth or you've got a neo-plastic disorder. And people often wouldn't be told that they were going to die, that they were terminal. And people would never use the word and were ashamed of it. What happened is, in spite of that [researchers] had this sort of war on cancer, money was put into research big time and it became the norm for every single patient, pretty much, with cancer, to be in a drug trial of some sort, or part of research. That improved the care because it attracted smart people into wanting to do it. Smart people want to do things that are exciting, in a way that they can make a difference.... It raised the profile and people started to talk about [it], and now you've got to the situation where cancer's much less stigmatized and also that there are plenty of new treatments around. And this is where we are now in mental illness. It would make a great difference though, if we were doing research in clinics.... Look at Alzheimer's. Alzheimer's is much less stigmatized than dementia used to be and that's because it has a name, but also because it has pathology, it has some potential treatment, it has some genetics. That hasn't made it more stigmatized, it's much less stigmatized.... If we could do the same for schizophrenia or bipolar disorder and depression, that's what we want.
>
> (Centre director of neuropsychiatric genetics)

Take an incurable, stigmatized disease like cancer – previously unmentionable to patients and disavowed by society. Now, imagine investing huge resources at the level of basic science, enlisting patients into drug trials, which in turn attracts talented research scientists and eventually improves clinical outcomes. The public imagination of 'cancer' transforms from an incurable condition into a medically tractable problem, 'solved' by attracting investment, recruiting expertise and enrolling patient involvement. These are presented as the ingredients of a medical success story. The director then asks us to imagine that a similar process can take place in relation to mental illness, highlighting that the crucial, missing ingredient is 'doing research in the clinic'. By connecting a medical history to an imagined future, analogies establish a precedent that difficult biomedical problems are 'doable' (Fujimura 1987), that therapeutic optimism is reasonable, and that social stigma is reversible. Retrospective imaginaries of 'cancer' are powerful devices for enrolling prospective research participants into regimes of hope.

According to the thought styles of genomic science, pathology is now a foundation for therapeutic optimism: 'Alzheimer's is much less stigmatized than dementia used to be … because it has a pathology, it has some potential treatment, [and] it has some genetics.' For biological psychiatry, this amounts to a curious historical reversal of the therapeutic pessimism of early hereditarian discourses on degeneration and 'tainted blood' (see Chapters 1 and 2). Unlike the vagaries of 'pathological heredity' in the nineteenth century, contemporary discourses of *genomic pathology* are complex, mobile and amenable to intervention. By drawing out the parallels between psychiatric disorders and other clinical conditions, it is possible to supplant therapeutic pessimism with optimism. To imagine that mental illness 'has a pathology … it has some genetics' is rendered more acceptable when the same substrate of intervention is linked to stories of success.

When pressed on the relationship between biology and stigma, it was clear that not all analogies lead to medical success or scientific hope. In fact, much like the biology they describe, stigma itself is a complex issue. Consider the following two accounts:

> There's that type of stigma, they are rotten to the core, or their parents were rotten to the core, and stuff like that. And I suppose it is imagined that a greater understanding, you know, that these are not necessarily disorders of personal [circumstances] could in principle reduce stigma. However there's also stigma and prejudice against people who have biological illnesses that are fully understood…. Actually I don't believe that a reduction in stigma necessarily follows from a greater understanding of cause…. We know the causes of AIDS, we know the causes of venereal diseases…. At the core of all this, it's true that a greater understanding does not necessarily abolish stigma, and I'm not convinced it will increase it, but it just does not follow it will reduce it.
>
> (Professor working on schizophrenia)

And:

> There is some granularity in it. I think dementias now are less stigmatized than they were, so that's an example. I think that milder disorders are probably less stigmatized than severe disorders, although stigma's a subtle thing and … one of the problems we have in psychiatry is there's this very broad spectrum and that's changed over the last 30, 40 years. The remit of psychiatry has broadened into much milder sets of conditions that are treated more by GPs and, at that end of the spectrum, social and environmental factors play increasingly important roles. But actually, I think things like stress-related disorders, I think those are quite stigmatizing, at least in some circles. Because people are seen to be weak vessels who can't hack it with the rest who can take stress and … stigma is very subtle and I think it comes back to this idea that … environmental and social explanations are less stigmatizing. I think that's wrong because that starts to approach the view that, well, actually, it's your fault you've got it. You should be stronger, or it's

your lifestyle that's led you into this. I think … stigma is everywhere and it is subtle and different in different bits of psychiatry. I think overdose-type behaviour, personality disorders are very stigmatized, particularly within the caring professions. They're the patients that you really don't want to have.

(Centre director of neuropsychiatric genetics)

In these accounts, the professors are wrangling with their awareness that presumed benefits of public understanding may run up against existing attitudes and presumptions. By implication, they acknowledge criticism of the deficit model: while greater public knowledge of psychiatric genetics may reduce stigma, this knowledge may also be incorporated into existing understandings of mental illness, responsibility, danger, etc. Counter-analogies (the first professor suggests AIDS and 'venereal disease') provide examples in which he sees increased biological knowledge not necessarily leading to the reduction of stigma. This leads to a more conditional account in which biological explanations of disease may not 'abolish' stigma, but nor will they increase stigma to the extent that social and personal explanations do. The professor in the second extract is forced to concede the 'subtlety' of the problem, that stigma is 'everywhere' and works through a range of processes, but that nevertheless stigma can be attenuated through public engagement with psychiatric genetics.

Although these analogies enrol visions that mental illnesses are medically tractable and treatable, they, like metaphors in general, lack the resources to explain different and unequal cases. For instance, understanding 'genetics' in the laboratory means something different to understanding genetics on the street. Communicating complexity and moving away from a simple 'gene for' trope is therefore a primary message that scientists at the Centre want to get across to publics. When engaging different audiences, senior scientists use a 'mobile army of metaphors, metonyms, and anthropomorphisms' (Nietzsche 1954), many of which recruit a presumed equivalence to other conditions to communicate abstract notions of 'genetic contribution'.

You cannot readily explain these things in ten seconds, or two sentences. So it is a huge challenge…. When I try and do it, I kind of resort to analogies that people maybe understand a bit clearer in their own life, which people [might grasp] slightly better – concepts like risk of heart disease where not everyone who doesn't exercise dies of a heart attack next week. And then not everyone who does exercise stays immune from heart attacks. People … they don't necessarily understand it very well, but, I mean, there are a lot of analogies and that's how I tend to do it. But it's pretty difficult to get people to understand it, or for me to be able to persuade people [to support the research] or for me to be able to communicate it, I do acknowledge that.

(Professor working on schizophrenia)

The scientist admits that analogies are imperfect devices, but their strengths are oriented to engaging the public's existing understandings of science.

Counter-imaginaries of determinism, fatalism, reductionism and authoritarianism are the existing (and persistent) cultural materials that scientists have to accommodate in their attempts to inform and engage. These obstacles are not limited to the distant 'general' public; as one senior scientist told us, 'some people [in psychiatry] have a visceral hatred of genetics and genetic testing'. A key problem is seen to be the difficultly of shifting public understandings of genetics from a deterministic to a probabilistic style of thinking (Rose 2013). Drawing out the parallels between mental illness and more familiar (and less 'moralized') diseases are techniques by which counter-imaginaries are circumvented and attractive futures are created in which therapeutic hope can be imagined and realized.

Conclusion

Psychiatric genetics is a field that draws heavily on promissory discourses of therapeutic hope and optimism to persuade a diversity of publics that mental illnesses are biologically tractable and medically treatable conditions. But the field is also uniquely positioned as marginal to psychiatry, inferior to other medical fields, less successful than other genetic programmes, and culturally, politically and even scientifically controversial. The recent transformation of psychiatric genetics into large-scale biology has enabled scientists to invest in public engagement programmes, the purposes of which exceed standard narratives of 'accountability' to publics. Psychiatric genetics *needs* a public, not only for investment and 'democratic' support, but also to access the material resources required to sustain its scale of production. It needs a public in order to access research participants and to persuade gatekeepers and professional communities that genetic research offers hopeful futures for complex problems. Our own sense, as sociologists internal and adjacent to these programmes, is that a large part of 'public engagement' in psychiatric genetics is the work of creating scientific imaginaries, which have the function of shaping and reorienting the domain to which it seeks access. As is the case in the distributed management of biological resources internal to Big Biology, psychiatric genetics seeks to engineer relations external to science by acting on networks that facilitate (and on occasion obstruct) its progress. To circumvent the counter-imaginaries hostile to psychiatry *and* genetics (and there are many), scientists view public engagement as a means of building on what 'the public already know'. Public engagement is social engineering, which entails negotiating and realigning existing understandings of science with contemporary regimes of hope.

Notes

1 Today, it is common to refer to the 'burden of disease' in national and global statistics. However, the language of 'burden' also has sinister connotations. Among medical practitioners and eugenicists in the early twentieth century (especially in Germany), references to 'burden' conjured images of the unproductive lives of the

mentally ill and handicapped – the so-called 'human ballast' who were a moral burden and economic cost to the fit and healthy (Weindling 1989).

2 This is broken down as (1) sickness absence = £10.6 billion, (2) staff turnover = £3.1 billion, and (3) reduced productivity at work = £21.2 billion (Parsonage and Saini 2017).

3 Since the Time for Change campaign began in 2008, it is said to have 'improved' the attitudes of 3.4 million people towards mental health.

4 It is also often used to lend an air of dialogue to old-fashioned public education and marketing programmes.

5 Funding for ELSA research is difficult to generalize given the unique way it was structured (Hilgartner *et al.* 2016). That said, funding allocated to ELSA type projects by the EU for research is said to amount to *circa* 2 per cent of that designated for Life Science research (CORDIS 2001).

6 It is important to be clear that ELSI programmes were not intended to prevent social and ethical issues from arising in themselves, but to prevent such issues from becoming obstacles to genetics and genomics as 'public' issues (and to some extent to prevent scientists making things into 'public issues' by sheer clumsiness). For example, ELSI was not meant to in itself work to further health equalities, but to perform a kind of public relations for personalized medicine, smoothing the path from laboratory to clinic even in the face of its effect on health inequalities. ELSI was never going to prohibitively shape genetic and genomics research.

7 In addition to organizing public engagement events, Lewis also conducted research on public understanding of science and public engagement. Organizing events for the Centre often involved lengthy negotiations with scientists to justify resources and establish meaningful alignments with different practitioners and publics. As such, the challenging nature of this role often raised lingering doubts about maintaining critical distance and a coherent 'social science' identity.

8 Arribas-Ayllon has regularly presented on the social and ethical dimensions of psychiatric genetics research at the Centre's Winter and Summer schools organized to attract the next generation of researchers. Arribas-Ayllon and Bartlett have also contributed to public events organized by the Centre, as well as to staff 'away days' that were arranged to build capacity and foster solidarity within the Centre.

9 The art exhibitions also required some cajoling. Centre members were keen to distance psychiatric genetics from some of the 'soft' practices of psychiatry. For some, there was a concern that aligning science with a soft arts approach would undermine the 'hard' science image they were seeking to present.

10 Whether families do or do not undergo an attitudinal change towards extrapolating the views of families with mental illness to the wider public is not without problems.

References

Appadurai A (1996) *Modernity at Large: Cultural Dimensions of Globalization*. Minneapolis: University of Minnesota Press.

Balmer A, Calvert J, Marris C, *et al.* (2015) Taking roles in interdisciplinary collaborations: Reflections on working in post-ELSI spaces in the UK synthetic biology community. *Science and Technology Studies* 28(3): 3–25.

Barnett J, Burningham K, Walker G, *et al.* (2012) Imagined publics and engagement around renewable energy technologies in the UK. *Public Understanding of Science* 21(1): 36–50.

Bauer MW, Allum N and Miller S (2007) What can we learn from 25 years of PUS survey research? Liberating and expanding the agenda. *Public Understanding of Science* 16(1): 79–95.

Borup M, Brown N, Konrad K, *et al.* (2006) The sociology of expectations in science and technology. *Technology Analysis & Strategic Management* 18(3): 285–298.

Burmeister M, McInnis MG and Zöllner S (2008) Psychiatric genetics: Progress amid controversy. *Nature Reviews Genetics* 9: 527–540.

Carson RL (1962) *Silent Spring*. Boston: Houghton Mifflin.

Chilibeck G, Lock M and Sehdev M (2010) Postgenomics, uncertain futures, and the familiarization of susceptibility genes. *Social Science & Medicine* 72(11): 1768–1775.

Collins H (2014) *Are We All Scientific Experts Now?* Cambridge: Polity Press.

Condit CM (1999) How the public understands genetics: Non-deterministic and non-discriminatory interpretations of the 'blueprint' metaphor. *Public Understanding of Science* 8: 169–180.

CORDIS (2001) ELSA – Ethical, Legal and Social Aspects (29 January). http://cordis.europa.eu/elsa-fp4/ [accessed 20 June 2017].

Craddock N, Antebi D, Attenburrow MJ, *et al.* (2008) Wake-up call for British psychiatry. *British Journal of Psychiatry* 193(1): 6–9.

Davies S (2008) Constructing communication: Talking to scientists about talking to the public. *Science Communication* 29(4): 413–434.

DeMello JP and Deshpande SP (2015) Career satisfaction of psychiatrists. *Psychiatric Services* 62(9): 1013–1018.

Eagle PF and Marcos LR (1980) Factors in medical students' choice of psychiatry. *The American Journal of Psychiatry* 137(4): 423–427.

Feifel D, Moutier CY and Swerdlow NR (1999) Attitudes towards psychiatry as a prospective career among students entering medical school. *American Journal of Psychiatry* 156(9): 1397–1402.

Fisher E (2005) Lessons learned from the Ethical, Legal and Social Implications program (ELSI): Planning societal implications research for the National Nanotechnology Program. *Technology in Society* 27(3): 321–328.

Fitzgerald D (2017) *Tracing Autism: Uncertainty, Ambiguity, and the Affective Labor of Neuroscience*. Seattle: University of Washington Press.

Foucault M (1982) The subject and power. *Critical Inquiry* 8(4): 777–795.

Fujimura JH (1987) Constructing 'doable' problems in cancer research: Articulating alignment. *Social Studies of Science* 17(2): 257–293.

Fujimura JH (2003) Future imaginaries: Genome scientists as sociocultural entrepreneurs. In AH Goodman, D Heath and MS Lindee (eds). *Genetic Nature/Culture: Anthropology and Science between the Two-Culture Divide*. Berkeley: University of California Press, pp. 176–199.

Goffman E (1963) *Stigma: Notes on the Management of Spoiled Identity*. Englewood Cliffs: Prentice Hall.

Gov.uk (2017) Prime Minister reveals plans to transform mental health support. www.gov.uk/government/news/prime-minister-unveils-plans-to-transform-mental-health-support [accessed 20 September 2017].

Green H (2014) Classification in psychiatry: Inevitable but not insurmountable. *Social Theory & Health* 12(4): 361–375.

Gregory J and Miller S (1998) *Science in Public: Communication, Culture and Credibility*. New York: Plenum.

Hilgartner S, Prainsack B and Hurlbut JB (2016) Ethics as governance in genomics and beyond. In U Felt, R Fouche, CA Miller and L Smith-Doerr (eds). *The Handbook of Science and Technology Studies*. Cambridge, MA: MIT Press, pp. 823–852.

Hood L (1993) Biology and medicine in the twenty first century. In DJ Kevles and L Hood (eds). *The Code of Codes: Scientific and Social Issues in the Human Genome Project*. Cambridge, MA: Harvard University Press, pp. 136–163.

House of Lords (2000) *Science and Society 3rd Report*. London: HMSO.

Jasanoff S (2007) *Designs on Nature: Science and Democracy in Europe and the United States*. Princeton: Princeton University Press.

Jones RB, Thomas J, Lewis J, *et al*. (2017) Translation: From bench to brain – using the visual arts and metaphors to engage and educate. *Research for All* 1(2): 265–283.

Kendler KS (2006) Reflections on the relationship between psychiatric genetics and psychiatric nosology. *American Journal of Psychiatry* 163: 1138–1146.

Kerr A and Shakespeare T (2002) *Genetics Politics: From Eugenics to Genome*. Cheltenham: New Clarion Press.

Konrad K, van Lente H, Groves C, *et al*. (2017) Performing and governing the future in science and technology. In U Felt, R Fouche, CA Miller and L Smith-Doerr (eds). *The Handbook of Science and Technology Studies 4th Edition*. Cambridge, MA: MIT Press, pp. 465–493.

Kvaale EP, Gottdiener WH and Haslam N (2013a) Biogenetic explanations and stigma: A meta-analytic review of associations among laypeople. *Social Science & Medicine* 96: 95–103.

Kvaale EP, Haslam N and Gottdiener W (2013b) The 'side effects' of medicalization: A meta-analytic review of how biogenetic explanations affect stigma. *Clinical Psychology Review* 33(6): 782–794.

Layard R (2006) The case for psychological treatment centres. *BMJ* 332: 1030–1032.

Lewis J and Bartlett A (2015) How UK psychiatric geneticists understand and talk about engaging the public. *New Genetics and Society* 34(1): 89–111.

Lewis J, Bisson S, Swaden-Lewis K, *et al*. (2017) Cardiff sciSCREEN: A model for using film screenings to engage publics in University research. *Research for All* 1(1): 106–120.

Lewis J and Thomas J (2017) From trading zones to buffer zones: Art and metaphor in the communication of psychiatric genetics to publics. In L Reyes-Galindo and T Duarte (eds). *Intercultural Communication and Science and Technology Studies*. Basingstoke: Palgrave Macmillan, pp. 175–206.

Lezaun J (2013) Commentary: The escalating politics of 'Big Biology'. *Biosocieties* 8(4): 480–485.

Lippman A (1991) Prenatal genetic testing and screening: Constructing needs and reinforcing inequities. *American Journal of Law and Medicine* 17(1–2): 15–50.

Lippman A (1992) Led (astray) by genetic maps: The cartography of the human genome and health care. *Social Science & Medicine* 35(12): 1469–1476.

Malhi GS, Parker GB, Parker K, *et al*. (2002) Shrinking away from psychiatry? A survey of Australian medical students' interest in psychiatry. *Australian & New Zealand Journal of Psychiatry* 36(3): 416–423.

Martin P, Brown N and Turner A (2008) Capitalizing hope: The commercial development of umbilical cord blood stem cell banking. *New Genetics and Society* 27(2): 127–143.

Meslin EM (1997) Ethical, legal and social implications of research in psychiatric genetics: Thoughts from the ELSI research program at the US National Human Genome Research Institute. *American Journal of Medical Genetics* 74: 6.

Miller S (2001) Public understanding of science at the crossroads. *Public Understanding of Science* 10(1): 115–120.

Moreira T and Palladino P (2005) Between truth and hope: Parkinson's disease, neuro-transplantation and the production of 'self'. *History of the Human Sciences* 18(3): 55–82.

Morgan C, McKenzie K and Fearon P (eds) (2008) *Society and Psychosis*. Cambridge: Cambridge University Press.

Nelkin D and Lindee MS (1995) *The DNA Mystique: The Gene as a Cultural Icon.* New York: WH Freeman.

Nietzsche N (1954) *The Portable Nietzsche*. Translated by W Kaufman. New York: Viking Press.

Novas C and Rose N (2000) Genetic risk and the birth of the somatic individual. *Economy and Society* 29(4): 485–513.

Owen MJ, O'Donovan MC, Thapar A, *et al.* (2011) Neurodevelopmental hypothesis of schizophrenia. *British Journal of Psychiatry* 198(3): 173–175.

Parrott RL, Silk KJ and Condit C (2003) Diversity in lay perceptions of the sources of human traits: Genes, environments, and personal behaviours. *Social Science & Medicine* 56(5): 1099–1109.

Parsonage M and Saini G (2017) *Mental Health at Work: The Business Case Ten Years On*. London: Centre for Mental Health.

Pearson G (2001) The participation of scientists in public understanding of science activities: The policy and practice of the U.K. research councils. *Public Understanding of Science* 10(1): 121–137.

Phelan JC (2002) Genetic bases of mental illness: A cure for stigma? *Trends in Neurosciences* 25(8): 430–431.

Phelan JC (2005) Geneticization of deviant behavior and consequences for stigma: The case of mental illness. *Journal of Health and Behavior* 46(4): 307–322.

Poliakoff E and Webb TL (2007) What factors predict scientists' intentions to participate in public engagement of science activities? *Science Communication* 29(2): 242–263.

Propping P (2005) The biography of psychiatric genetics: From early achievements to historical burden, from an anxious society to critical geneticists. *American Journal of Medical Genetics Part B* (Neuropsychiatric Genetics) 136B(1): 2–7.

Rajan KS (2006) *Biocapital: The Constitution of Postgenomic Life*. Durham, NC: Duke Press.

Read J, Haslam N, Sayce L, *et al.* (2006) Prejudice and schizophrenia: A review of the 'mental illness is an illness like any other approach'. *Acta Psychiatrica Scandinavica* 114(5): 303–318.

Renn O (2006) Risk communication: Consumers between information and irritation. *Journal of Risk Research* 9(8): 883–849.

Research Council United Kingdom (2013) Concordant for engaging the public with research.   www.rcuk.ac.uk/documents/scisoc/ConcordatforEngagingthePublicwith-Research.pdf [accessed 2 September 2013].

Roberts L (2001) Controversial from the start. *Science* 291(5507): 1182–1188.

Rose N (1998) Governing risky individuals: The role of psychiatry in new regimes of control. *Psychiatry, Psychology and Law* 3(2): 177–196.

Rose N (2013) The human sciences in a biological age. *Theory, Culture & Society* 30(1): 3–34.

The Royal Society (1985) *The Public Understanding of Science*. London: Royal Society.

Sander C (2000) Genomic medicine and the future of health care. *Science* 287(5460): 1977–1978.

Sartorius N (2007) Stigma and mental health. *Lancet* 370(9590): 810–811.

Smith MJ (2008) Public psychiatry: A neglected professional role? *Advances in Psychiatric Treatment* 14: 339–346.

Stern Review (2016) *Research Excellence Framework (REF) Review: Building on Success and Learning from Experience*. www.gov.uk/government/publications/research-excellence-framework-review [accessed 2 September 2013].

Time to Change (2012) *A Milestone Year: A Year of Tackling Stigma in the Words of the People Who Made it Happen*. Annual Report 2012/2013. www.time-to-change.org.uk/sites/default/files/Time%20to%20Change%20Annual%20Report%202012–13.pdf [accessed 2 September 2013].

Turney J and Turner J (2000) Predictive medicine, genetics and schizophrenia. *New Genetics and Society* 19(1): 5–22.

Van Lente H (1993) *Promising Technology: The Dynamics of Expectations in Technological Developments*. PhD dissertation, University of Twente.

Watermeyer R (2012) From engagement to impact? Articulating the public value of academic research. *Tertiary Education and Management* 18(2): 115–130.

Watson J (2000) *A Passion for DNA: Genes, Genomes and Society*. Cold Spring Harbor: Cold Spring Harbor Press.

Weindling PJ (1989) *Health, Race and German Politics between National Unification and Nazism, 1870–1945*. Cambridge: Cambridge University Press.

Wilsdon J and Willis R (2004) *See-Through Science: Why Public Engagement Needs to Move Upstream*. London: DEMOS.

Wynne B (1992) Uncertainty and environmental learning: Reconceiving science and policy in the preventive paradigm. *Global Environmental Change* 2(2): 111–127.

Wynne B (1995) The public understanding of science. In S Jasanoff, GE Markle, JC Petersen and T Pinch (eds). *The Handbook of Science and Technology Studies*. Thousand Oaks: Sage, pp. 361–388.

8 Big Biology then and now

The trouble with GWAS

Not long after we began our ethnographic study in 2008, we started to realize that GWAS were in trouble. As we have described in previous chapters, the adoption of GWAS as the gold standard of gene-identification led to a significant reorganization of the field; from small-scale studies of family pedigrees to the international consortia required to conduct and manage large-scale population studies. The expectation was that this approach would reveal the 'genetic architecture' of complex human diseases. Though scientists have been inclined to make promises about gene discovery, in Chapter 3 we explored how psychiatric genetics had adopted a cautious narrative of moderated optimism. In this respect, it would be remiss to suggest that psychiatric genetics entered the 'genomics revolution' making false or unrealistic promises. Nevertheless, promises were made to secure the substantial resources required to fund the first wave of GWAS. The first GWAS results in psychiatric genetics were published in 2007 (Wellcome Trust Case Control Consortium 2007). By 2008, signs began to appear that not only psychiatric GWAS, but GWAS in general, were failing to deliver findings equal to their investment and scale.

Heavy publicity in the media might have cast the impression that GWAS were an overwhelming success. The reporting of new risk genes for diabetes, lupus and cardiac disease anticipated the long-awaited era of personalized medicine (Macarthur 2008). However, early indications that GWAS were in trouble became evident when *Nature Genetics* published three GWAS findings on height (Gudbjartsson *et al.* 2008; Lettre *et al.* 2008; Weedon *et al.* 2008). Height is an interesting benchmark against which to measure the success of genetic studies as it is highly heritable ($\approx$80%) and easy to measure. The combined studies comprising 65,000 participants and 400,000 SNPs identified 20, 10 and 21 SNPs respectively, accounting for 2.9 per cent, 2.0 per cent and 3.7 per cent of the total variation in height. Eight of these SNPs were identified in two studies and only two were found in all three (see Turkheimer 2012 for a critical review of these studies). Visscher's (2008) commentary in the same issue claimed that these studies were proof of principle that GWAS were techniques capable of detecting robust associations. The small effect sizes for a handful of SNPs were not, as those outside the field might think, discouraging findings. Rather, they pointed the way forward, with Visscher urging that 'very large samples sizes' were required. To reach adequate power, future studies would need 'to create consortia of research groups and even consortia of consortia' (2008: 490). In the face of such meagre results, the answer has always been more statistical power.

Of course, scientists were never blind to the limitations of GWAS. As early as 2005, some had warned about the high rate of false positives, the bias of population stratification (mixing different ethnic subgroups), and the occurrence of technical artefacts resulting from, for example, genotyping cases and controls on separate days or on separate plates (Hirschhorn and Daly 2005). But after 2008, a new lexicon of doubt had crept into the scientific community. In Chapter 3, we argued that scientists would routinely cite heritability estimates of twin and adoption studies to stabilize claims that genetic factors are substantially implicated in psychiatric disorders. However, by 2008, estimations of heritability were being used to *criticize* the relatively poor yield from GWAS. The expression 'missing heritability' highlighted the disparity between heritability estimates and the combined genetic variance identified by GWAS results (Mayer 2008; Manolio *et al.* 2009). Only 5 per cent of the heritability of height was accounted for, while bipolar disorder, a condition estimated at 80–90 per cent heritability, had identified only one signal with a very slight odds ratio (WTCCC 2007). By highlighting the small effect sizes of common variants, the missing heritability problem had struck at the heart of the 'common disease, common variant hypothesis'.

The missing heritability problem had become a runaway argument generating an array of explanations ranging from genetic risk being the combined effect of *all* genes in the background to the role of genes being severely overestimated (Turkheimer 2012; Joseph 2012). An example of how this argument exploits scepticism is illustrated in a perspective piece in *Molecular Psychiatry*, a main outlet for publishing GWAS results for psychiatric disorders:

When asked at a recent schizophrenia congress to estimate how much of the heritability could be accounted for by known genes the chairman of the genome-wide association studies schizophrenia committee estimated between 1 and 2%. If psychosis is 80–90% heritable some genes are undoubtedly missing. If not detectable in populations of 5,000 or more they are certainly small. Some workers suggest that they may be numbered in hundreds if not thousands. There comes a point at which the genetic skeptic can be pardoned the suggestion that if the genes are so small and so multiple, what they are hardly matters, the dividing line between polygenes and no genes is of little practical consequence. Have we reached this point?
(Crow 2011: 362)

Crow is not being so provocative as to claim that genes play no role in psychiatry but rather that other lines of investigation are overlooked because the field has become preoccupied with GWAS. 'Missing heritability' is used as leverage in the argument to consider other kinds of chromosomal and epigenetic variation that evade detection by linkage and association studies.

A key article that sought to stabilize GWAS was incidentally one of the first articles to give the missing heritability thesis serious scientific consideration. Published in *Nature* and authored by some of the most prominent genetic researchers in medicine (including Francis Collins), the Manolio *et al.* (2009) paper provided an important reference point for genetics research. The authors concede that 'the identification of genetic variants contributing to these "complex diseases" has been slow and arduous' and refer to missing heritability as the 'dark matter' of genome-wide association (2009: 748). The paper proposes various strategies for locating heritability, including detection of rare variants which are not sufficiently captured by genotyping arrays, detection of structural variations such as Copy Number Variations (CNVs), the expansion into non-European populations, the application of whole-genome sequencing, and, of course, the old argument of increasing sample sizes. In attempting to contain the problem they conclude that finding the 'dark matter' of GWAS is not an end in itself but a means to an end. The goal is to understand the underlying biology and aetiology of complex disease. Though this should provide a route to disease prediction in the long term, the scientific value of GWAS is to understand the 'true functionality' of variants associated with disease.

Rather than containing the problem of missing heritability, the perceived failure of GWAS had reinforced earlier claims of 'genohype' (Holtzman 1999). Social scientists had already begun to critically reflect on the role of hyperbole and promise in creating new economies of biological capital (Rose and Novas 2005; Rajan 2006; Fortun 2008). Others argued in favour of deflating the 'genomic bubble' given its disappointing findings and its poor clinical utility (Evans *et al.* 2011). More radical critics drew on 'geneticization' (Lippman 1991, 1992) style arguments, claiming that the paradigm of genetic determinism had failed. For instance, Latham and Wilson (2010) concluded that '[t]he dearth of disease causing genes is without question a scientific discovery of tremendous value' (para. 17). Turning the missing heritability thesis on its head, they argued that invocations of 'dark matter' is a 'process of special pleading', which obfuscates the issue that GWAS have failed. The stalwart critic of psychiatric genetics, Jay Joseph (2012), observed that 'missing heritability' provides a ready-made excuse for the continuing failure of behavioural and psychiatric genetics.[1]

By 2010, it became evident that having revealed far fewer gene-associations than their medical colleagues, psychiatric disorders were particularly resistant to GWAS. The conviction among researchers was that complex neuropsychiatric disorders required massive sample sizes of 8,000 to 20,000 cases to detect strong signals of gene-association (Psychiatric GWAS Consortium Coordinating Committee 2009). On the one hand, the missing heritability argument justified the forming of 'consortia of consortia' to generate larger sample sizes, on the other hand the disappointing results of GWAS suggested that psychiatric genetics was approaching a 'null field' (Joseph 2012). John Ioannidis (2005: 700) describes a null field as an area of research with 'absolutely no yield of true scientific information'. In his much-cited paper, 'Why most published research findings are false' (2005), he applies a series of power calculations to show that discovery-oriented research with massive testing is one of the worst offenders of producing spurious findings. By implication, GWAS are characterized as programmes with very low 'positive predictive values' where 'highly significant effects may actually be more likely to be signs of large bias' (2005: 700). Joseph (2012) borrows the null field argument to show that a different conclusion can be reached about the findings of psychiatric genetics: there are no genes (missing or otherwise) for psychiatric disorders. The 'missing heritability' of neuropsychiatric disorders is confirmation of a flawed scientific programme – a field that refuses to accept that it has long occupied a null field.

Joseph's (2012) argument is interesting not because we take seriously the claim that psychiatric genetics is a pseudoscience but because the controversy of GWAS and missing heritability reveals the ways in which a scientific community seeks to *authenticate* its styles of reasoning (Hacking 1992). The means by which scientists collectively defend their methods say more about the durability of psychiatric genetics than do speculations on its intrinsic validity. That psychiatric genetics was approaching a null field coincides with events we witnessed in 2010 when the 'special pleading' of missing heritability engendered a unique display of solidarity. In the next section, we describe how the field rallied to protect its core methodology.

Don't give up on GWAS

The World Congress of Psychiatric Genetics held in Athens in 2010 had a different tone to previous meetings. GWAS were clearly the priority. There were fewer papers discussing mouse models, epidemiology and traditional molecular genetics, and more focusing on large-scale genomics: the different classes of variants, their presence and absence, and the biological pathways they implied. The 'pathway' metaphor in genetics (see Armstrong 2017 for an interesting discussion) allowed researchers to infer progress by extrapolating modest findings to show genes clustering in regions of biological interest (e.g. autoimmunity, neurotransmission, neurogenesis, etc.). Conceptually, it 'mapped' (Lakoff and Johnson 1980) one domain onto another: the mathematical onto biological, the statistical association onto functional systems. The many slides where we observed this relationship were indeed persuasive; the pathway metaphor had the rhetorical effect of suggesting 'clues' for the way forward, salvaging the validity of GWAS while also raising expectations. But if we had to single out a metaphor that dominated the conference it was the troubling language of *structure*, the immense difficulty of understanding the 'genetic architecture' of common disease. Confirming our previous observations, the ability to see this structure was confounded by the 'extreme complexity' of polygenicity, heterogeneity, epistasis, etc. In fact, one session concluded with the speaker stating: 'we have no clue what nature is doing'.

Another reason the conference had a different tone to previous conferences that we had attended was because the problem of 'missing heritability' was very much in the foreground. There was a litany of references in various sessions to 'dark matter', 'gene deserts' and unknown 'culprits', and a whole symposium dedicated to 'finding (some of) the lost heritability in psychiatry'. Here, we witnessed a strangely ambivalent display of working up complexity as impenetrably messy and confounding on the one hand, and hopeful optimism that larger sample sizes will deliver real progress on the other. Images of icebergs and film noir scenes were used to illustrate 'the case of missing heritability'. In the plenary sessions, there was a sense that we were observing a community that had little alternative but to defend their only method for genetically dissecting common disease. Speakers frequently mentioned the huge progress that had been made, often contrasting their findings with how little they knew ten years earlier. But there was also a sense that psychiatric genetics was a 'waiting game', waiting for the next technological breakthrough to increase resolution. The consensus was that complexity justified delays in discovery but the problem was *tractable*; it was still a 'doable problem' (Fujimura 1996). Heritability was not 'missing' as so much as 'hiding' behind the poverty of statistical power.

The final day of the conference presented a summary of the findings of various disorder groups. A professor from Cambridge gave the plenary lecture, showcasing his GWAS work on Type 1 diabetes. A common strategy at these meetings is to invite plenary speakers working on non-psychiatric medical diseases where more progress with GWAS has been made (see Chapter 7). No doubt, the raft of gene-associations for diabetes was intended to inspire the audience, showing that GWAS can tell a coherent biological story of pathways connecting genetics to immunology. The summaries from the neuropsychiatric disorder groups that followed were modest by comparison, though the discovery of new GWAS signals for schizophrenia and Alzheimer's disease were hailed as a success. The next section focuses on the final session of the conference titled 'Where do we go from here?'

Where do we go from here?

After each of the disorder groups had reported their findings, ten people (including Patrick Sullivan, the lead investigator of the Psychiatric Genomics Consortium, and Nick Craddock, the president of the International Society of Psychiatric Genetics) assembled on the stage. For all intents and purposes, the panel represented the 'core set' (Collins 1981) of investigators in psychiatric genetics. The ensuing discussion was surprisingly frank and dynamic. It became apparent that there was an anti-GWAS camp of 'Mendelian' geneticists and neuroscientists who believed that SNP-based genotyping was an un-informative research programme – a dead end. David Curtis, regarded by some as a maverick within the community, conceded that GWAS were only 'partially evil', having aired his concerns in previous meetings that the community's preoccupation with GWAS had marginalized other approaches. He expressed concern that GWAS were a wasteful use of resources since current microarray chips were missing at least half the common variation in the samples. He wondered whether the next phase of GWAS would have to re-genotype all the samples using next-generation chips. Members of the panel explained that re-genotyping and replication would cost at least 50 million dollars and, given the current funding environment, investigators would have to be smarter about designing platforms using a combination of cheaper and more expensive chips to increase coverage for a list of candidate genes. Whilst there was a desire to re-genotype samples with better chips, many of the panellists agreed that larger sample sizes were a higher priority.

As the discussion continued, it became evident that the future of GWAS in psychiatric genetics was not straightforward. The magnitude of the funding problem the community faced was addressed by the following question from the audience:

> I just have one question, we have heard that sample size does matter. I mean, we've heard that all along but we hear it even more now. Outside this room, in the press you can still read GWAS has failed, and so now we have only a limited amount of resources. How do you see the field proceeding? We know we need larger sample sizes, maybe better phenotyped sample sizes. On the other hand we also want sequencing and pathway analysis. So, given the funding restrictions, how should we proceed, how much effort should we allocate to this and that approach … taking into account the current funding situation?

The question poses an interesting problem because scientific consensus to increase sample sizes is contrasted with press statements claiming that 'GWAS has failed'. How do we prove that GWAS works with 'a limited amount of resources'? To put it another way: in a climate of increased scepticism and reduced funding, how do researchers prove that psychiatric genetics is not a null field? Alluding to the problem of 'missing heritability', the panel unanimously agreed that the way forward was to convince the National Institutes of Health to fund projects that 'fill in the genetic architecture' by addressing both rare and common variation and continuing to expand sample sizes. The defensive statement from one American panellist 'that genetics is not done, genetics has not failed' was an admission that psychiatric genetics was indeed at risk of null status. The way forward was to move beyond statistical association to the more secure ground of 'figuring out biology', to understand how variants impact on brain structure and function. Neuroscience will rescue genetics when new imaging technologies detect how these variants affect brain architecture. Again, the reference to 'pathways' is integral to stabilizing a narrative of future success.

Having accepted that 'missing gaps' in GWAS needed to be filled, a pivotal moment occurred when a member of the audience broke from the technical aspects of the discussion to reflect more earnestly on the community's position:

> I would like to challenge the comment that we should be cautious at this point. I would like to advocate exactly the opposite. I think we should be

triumphant, I think we should be getting out there and saying, hey look, this works, everybody said it wouldn't work five years ago look at what we have done, look at what we've seen this morning. Spectacular progress in schizophrenia, in Alzheimer's in particular. And there is no reason why it can't work for the other diseases as well. We just need the numbers and this is not a time for turning away saying this hasn't worked. This is the time to be actually really forcing and doing a lot more of it. And that includes obviously, a lot more money for GWAS of samples already there, not mucking around with 20K chips, perhaps in doing 1 million or 5 million chips on the whole lot. And of course in five or ten years we hope to be sequencing the whole lot. But on top of that, based on our calculations, it's clear that we actually need more samples, so we need to keep funding the large cohort studies to get these numbers up. Now we know it works, and I think there will be collective enthusiasm of this group, we could all probably go home before the end of the evening and write down a number of ideas as to how you could get those samples. And I think we really need to be making that point very forcefully and triumphantly so the policy makers hear this [inaudible] and getting walked over by the people that say oh well, if we haven't produced anything we all need to do sequencing [applause].

The excerpt speaks for itself. The main point to take from this 'charismatic' account is the issue of timing: 'now is not a time for turning away saying this [GWAS] hasn't worked'. Progress in schizophrenia and Alzheimer's disease, and the prediction of power calculations, are grounds for statistical optimism, which indicate a need for more samples rather than deviating to new methods or technologies. The speaker advocates taking a forceful approach of extolling the 'triumphant' success of recent findings and pressuring 'policy-makers' to continue funding GWAS. The applause from the audience confirms the statement's success, after which the discussion takes a more collective turn. Patrick Sullivan, the energetic broker of international consortia, announced that he was drafting a letter:

A colleague of mine, who shall go unnamed, said that the different NIH's have personalities, okay so like [inaudible] Switzerland, they're logical and rigid and careful and controlled. Whereas [inaudible] is a little more like an unnamed Italian Island if you get my drift. And the other part of this is that the funding decisions that control us, they tend to be difficult to predict, and they tend on occasion to be driven by forces which are kind of at odds with the field, or with the mainstream opinion. And I don't know why that exactly happens but I think you could demonstrate that it is the case. And so something that [a colleague] suggested to me a couple of days ago and we were talking about it yesterday was in fact the possibility of writing a letter. And writing a letter which basically states that really now is not the time to abandon GWAS, when in fact it is working. What we need to do is to do more and do it carefully and do it comprehensibly and get some hard hits, hard clues ... that can actually drive the next generation of innovation and discovery. And so, in talking about this and talking to a number of you I am actually drafting a letter, and with lots of people who agree with the concept, we can get a number of the PIs to sign it we can actually try and get it published somewhere relatively influential. I don't think, you know, jumping to just exome sequencing, which apparently is the indication now, I think methylation is really important, and I think that should be on our list because there are a bunch of reasons for it. But I think GWAS is working, and exactly at the time it is working and beginning to deliver is not the time to do pathway measures as opposed to reinforcing them. Because we are told that doing what you want to do, which is actually GWASing all these people is simply not going to fly from a money perspective. So it is a tricky time but I think as a group, I think we've been a little, I don't know, maybe historically it has been different, but we don't throw our weight around. We don't try and influence things in a collective way and we are going to give a shot to do that.

For a group of scientists to lobby funders *collectively* in such a public way in order to protect their core methodology is unusual. A characteristic of 'Big Biology' is that scientists are much more at the direct mercy of funders who take a more active role in deciding on the definition of 'excellence' of the field. The locus of judgment shifts from the core set of a community to funding bodies and politicians.

Our observations of the Athens congress in 2010 provide a backstory of an unprecedented letter published the following year in *Molecular Psychiatry*. Signed by 96 authors, the letter titled 'Don't give up on GWAS' sets out the case that GWAS cannot be declared null until sample sizes are sufficiently large. The authors argue that findings for schizophrenia are no worse than other medical conditions using the same approach. They also anticipate that: 'With sample sizes four times larger than those currently available, 30–60 more loci might be identified for schizophrenia and bipolar disorder.' The letter concludes by urging 'the major funding bodies worldwide to continue to support GWAS as a major investigative tool for uncovering hard leads about the fundamental biology of psychiatric diseases' (Sullivan *et al.* 2012a: 2).

What's in a letter?

How do we make sense of this letter-writing strategy? When the excellence of Big Biology is decided by funders, politicians and press statements, the methods of stabilizing science changes. It is not enough for a scientific community to puzzle-solve through a framework of 'normal science' (Kuhn 1962). Arguably, Big Biology operates within a regime of 'extraordinarily normal' science (Bartlett 2008) in the sense that solving scientific problems at the level of 'gene discovery' is not one of scientific creativity but of assembling a large-scale infrastructure for increasing the outputs of normal science. Given the cost and investment of genotyping larger sample sizes, the quality assurance of scientific outputs belongs to an extended community, in which case writing a letter co-signed by its core set is a collective act of intervening in the political landscape of large-scale research. As with the statements on 'complexity' we reviewed in Chapter 3, the stability of Big Biology is reliant on the production of rhetorical statements in the public domain as well as testing the truth or falsehood of their styles of reasoning. In this type of 'extraordinarily normal' regime of large-scale biology, the letter asks its informed readers: who is better positioned to decide on the excellence of science, the scientists or the funders?

GWAS have continued to be a well-funded component of psychiatric genetics. If a single letter was directly responsible for maintaining funding for GWAS then that would have been a remarkable story. However, in a recent interview, the director of the Centre offered a different explanation:

> I think what saved [GWAS] was the fact that a lot of samples had been collected and quite a lot of money came from philanthropic sources in the Broad Institute, and this really was Ed Scolnick who was one of the people who set up the Stanley Centre in Broad which is the mental health bit of it. And he is a very energetic guy, with a lot of connections, and he raised a lot of money and so the samples have been collected by various academic groups and the Broad were able to fund the genotyping in a lot of instances ... we had samples of genotypes with the Wellcome Trust Case Control Consortium and other local groups ... but really the big increase in sample numbers came from the Broad.
>
> (Centre director of neuropsychiatric genetics)

The Stanley Centre at the Broad Institute was established in 2007 after receiving a $100 million donation from the philanthropists Ted and Vada Stanley.[2] The director, Edward Scolnick, allocated this and other donations to assembling the world's largest collection of DNA samples in psychiatric research. By offering genotyping services worldwide in exchange for access to data, the Broad Institute effectively 'subsidized' the field. The provision of 'free' genotyping allowed individual laboratories to continue GWAS, but at the cost of giving the Broad Institute prior access to data all over world. To remain competitive, smaller laboratories were drawn into a regime of consortium-based data sharing; that is, to fund a proportion of the genotyping in order to retain *ownership* of their data. The timely injection of philanthropic funds transformed the field of psychiatric genetics by establishing the Broad Institute as the dominant group (along with DECODE genetics in Iceland) while also forcing smaller groups to create consortia to compete with these large groups. Perhaps it is no coincidence that the PGC formed at the same time – not only for altruistic reasons of sharing and increasing samples – but to maintain the survival of their own programmes.

As far as the director was concerned, the letter was an act of catharsis rather than successful lobbying in the public sphere:

I don't know whether it worked, I don't recall us getting loads of money as a result of it to be honest, it maybe made people feel better huh. Our own funding efforts were ... we always included both studies of common and rare variants in our work, and we did some of the earliest GWAS in this area, so the Medical Research Council was reasonably supportive actually. I think in the UK we have had a very effective champion in genomics ... establishing the Sanger Institute and the big groups were working on things like diabetes and hypertension and so on, you know, they were producing data. And I think it was less hard to persuade the MRC that this was a good idea than our American colleagues who had more trouble persuading NIMH.

It seems a combination of factors were responsible for saving psychiatric GWAS. There was the persistence of the scientific community that larger samples sizes would indeed resolve the problem of missing heritability. In order to meet this challenge, a community that was accustomed to rivalry and competition was forced into a situation of forming consortium-based data sharing. But there were also unusual, even exceptional, events such as charitable gifts from wealthy philanthropists that essentially 'bailed out' the field. The latter established the Broad Institute as a nexus within a global network of GWAS. Their 'gift' of genotyping in exchange for access to other laboratories' data gave rise to the formation of competing consortia. Smaller laboratories unable to meet the expense of large-scale genotyping, and yet reluctant to concede ownership of their data to the dominant groups, formed their own networks in order to exploit the economies of scale. If 2010 was a precarious time for psychiatric GWAS, by 2012, the further growth of consortium-based GWAS had meant that psychiatric genetics had escaped the null field.

* * *

The Athens congress had signalled the end of the first phase of our fieldwork. We continued to maintain our links with senior scientists at the Centre who had come to regard us as useful members of their network, inviting us to teach 'ethics' on their summer school programmes, and to organize public engagement events to propagate their message (see Chapter 7). After all, this was the price of admission. We were always mindful that social science was viewed as the 'handmaiden' of the life sciences, an expedient tool to measure the public's pulse[3] and to soothe concerns. Occasionally, we challenged this view by joking that the scientists were the 'rats' of our study. Their puzzled reaction confirmed a sometimes opaque understanding of our research. But we recognize that the scientists we spoke to and observed generously gave their time. Indeed, collegiality and trust were the hallmarks of our odd relationship. In the next section, we give an account of how the Centre has fared since the revival of GWAS. We also revisit Joseph's (2012) provocative claim – which has not gone away – that psychiatric genetics is a 'null field'.

Inside the 'Death Star'

Davies *et al.* (2013: 394) use an interesting turn of phrase to define the changing landscape of large-scale biological research. What they call the 'diminishing outside' of Big Biology describes a kind of inevitable accretion by which 'there is less and less scope to be left outside its logics and research, for scientists and perhaps for social scientists too'. Back in 2007, those researchers working outside the PGC might have considered the growth of consortium-based collaboration as an unwelcome totality. But when we re-entered the field in 2017, we found that most, if not all, gene-discovery programmes were now consortium-based. The issue was no longer about forming collaborations to maintain the survival of individual research programmes but of maintaining survival *inside* the logics and scope of Big Biology.

Consortium-based collaboration

Since 2007, there had been an acceleration in the sharing of biological resources. Consortium-based collaboration had been so successful that the PGC trebled in global coverage, from 19 to 60 countries. In terms of the increasing power and scale of psychiatric GWAS, one of the consortium managers described the cumulative increase in sample size as follows: 'the kind of trajectory would be 2007 (3,000), 2011 (9,000), 2014 (30,000), 2017 (70,000)'. The 'diminishing outside' reached the limit at which there is no 'outside' of any great significance. Almost all attempts to understand the human genetics of psychiatric disorders are GWAS-based, and almost all GWAS are consortium-based. As we returned to the field, we found that Big Biology was bigger than ever.

In Chapter 4, we explained how large-scale collaboration was experienced as an uncomfortable arrangement, a compromise in which scientists and individual laboratories were forced to move beyond their circle of trusted collaborators. Reflecting on this period, a senior manager of the PGC described it as a 'dance of enemies' because exchanging data with hitherto rival groups 'was not a mode of activity that people were used to'. So, what had changed when we re-entered the field?

> I think people are much more comfortable in GWAS terms in collaboration because they pretty much know that there's no hope of them finding anything themselves. So I think that's why it's easy.
>
> (Professor of neuropsychiatric genetics, schizophrenia)

The so-called 'muscle game' of sharing common variants in 2008 has been replaced by a kind of 'wary interdependence' (Hackett 2005) of exchanging data on rare variants.

> People are a bit cagier at the moment about sharing the rare variant data, but that will build up. And in part it's because, to generate the rare variant data

is, at the moment, economically so substantial that there are huge power imbalances, certain centres get hundreds of millions of pounds and they have the potential to really just suck up the work of everyone who has spent decades accumulating and interviewing patients. So one view is you're trying to steal our work. Another view is, well, they have the ability to do that bit of the work and you have the ability to do that bit of the work and you've got to get together. And that will happen. I'm sure it will happen, but I think it's a bit dicier with the rare variant stuff at the moment.

(Professor of neuropsychiatric genetics, schizophrenia)

Despite its stated egalitarian values, the Consortium continued to be an assembly of unequals. Smaller laboratories sitting on high-quality phenotypic data may not have the expertise or the resources necessary to secure funding to genotype and analyse their own samples. By contrast, the larger laboratories with significant capital are able to maintain their position by securing large grants. Capital accumulates. In the above account from a manager of the PGC, we can hear the ambivalence of the field; the contrasting voices of those who protest that the inherent 'power imbalances' result in work being 'stolen' from smaller groups, and those who justify these arrangements in terms of scientific necessity, presenting the contributions of larger groups not as expropriation but as making use of their 'ability' to add value to the collective accomplishment. At least from the point of view of a manager of the PGC, there is a sense of optimism that in the end, a Big Biology built from a federation of laboratories will prevail as the accepted organizational model.

A similar account was given to us by a professor who is more intensively involved in the day-to-day work of molecular genetics. In the following extract, he reflects on the way in which the field had changed as GWAS became Big Biology:

We were going through a huge period of flux, so we were going from being small, independent groups, so we were the [Centre], and there was the Boston group etc., and we were probably competitors, starting to work together ... and the PGC was seen as, for want of a better analogy, the Death Star, taking all the samples and taking all the money.... But we've had to do it to survive, we've had to adapt, and I think we're doing it quite well, and we've had to think proactively to adapt and be pretty determined to do it and I'm pretty pleased with the way we've done this, and we've looked for opportunities, and I think the optimistic way to look at this is to say, we now have foundations in which we can do laboratory work, and which I think is exciting actually for researchers, if they see it that way, that's good. They might see it in a completely different way.

(Professor in molecular biology)

The pattern of accretion, whereby smaller groups are absorbed into the PGC, is likened to the 'Death Star', which suggests that Big Biology is not a preferred arrangement for the community. Complaints about large-scale science trampling the excellence of small-scale biology are not new. Weinberg (1961) raised similar concerns that, by 'invading' universities and dominating funding, 'Big Science' constrained diversity. Here, there is a similar sense of inevitability that individual laboratories cannot 'survive' outside the Consortium, but for those working inside, the PGC provides the stability for a laboratory style of reasoning to continue doing meaningful biological work.

Doing biology

As described in Chapter 4, when we spent time in the field between 2008 and 2010 we heard complaints that consortium-based GWAS was eroding the excellence of experimental, laboratory biology at the Centre. A significant problem was the 'frustrating' reliance on outsourcing. While outsourcing reduced the costs of genotyping and removed much of the skilled work at the bench, it also played a role in the displacement of a laboratory style of reasoning:

> The problem in 2010 we had is that a lot of the data was being sent away and there was less work to do in the laboratory. I think, over the last five or six years we've seen that as a bit of a problem here, so a large proportion of the genotyping now is being done here, and a lot of the sequencing work is being done here, which is great because it gives us first look at the data ... if we can do the work in-house it keeps our laboratory running, it keeps people employed and keeps our expertise.
>
> (Professor in molecular genetics)

Bringing genotyping back 'in-house' has been a significant development for the Centre, which involved hard negotiations with Illumina, the company that supplies the technology. By 2012, the Centre was at risk of 'losing the laboratory' unless Illumina cut their prices for the UK. Illumina agreed, and this enabled the Centre to genotype 20,000 samples at a low cost, which retained laboratory expertise and their potential to 'go back to biology' once GWAS, a programme built on a statistical style of reasoning, had run its course. The professor describes this 'mixed economy' combining outsourcing and in-house genotyping/sequencing as the 'more difficult option'; the easier option for most laboratories is to 'outsource everything', even at the risk of losing expertise and reputation. Certainly, in-house genotyping and sequencing means that the Centre can contribute to the PGC *after* they have had the 'first look' at the data: 'so we can contribute data to the PGC *when we want* and that actually gives us a bit more control, but we have to be active'. Being 'active' implies independently seeking local solutions to maintain a competitive advantage within the collective.

Being inside the Consortium gives members equal access to aggregated data, the major benefit of which is to develop innovative projects for investigating the biology of GWAS signals. This creates internal competition between groups because everybody in the Consortium can see the data, meaning that funding to extract value from it is highly competitive. However, as you would expect, it is not the case that funding is awarded to laboratories with the best ideas; the size of the group often determines the distribution of success:

> Ironically the better funded laboratories are the more successful because they tend to put the better applications together and funders like that. So you can have a rogue researcher in some obscure university and it'd be very difficult for them to get high level funding, they could get small funding, but I think if you're coming from a large institution with a track record and you're asking for several million pounds' worth, I think you're more likely to get funding.
>
> (Professor in molecular genetics)

The analysis of GWAS data requires that biologists work closely with bioinformaticians. The mass of 'primary inscriptions' (see Chapter 5) produced by genotyping thousands of samples at thousands of points on the genome requires the perspective of scientists comfortable working in a statistical style of reasoning. Even asking biologically relevant questions of the great mass of data produced by GWAS – in order to produce 'secondary inscriptions' that can be used to make knowledge claims – requires that the researcher is at ease with this style of reasoning.

Not all of this expertise need be 'imported', with attempts to develop the bioinformatic repertoire of biologists. As the professor of molecular genetics said of the training programme at the Centre:

> typically they [biologists] need to learn coding and, so what we are helping them do is set up training programmes that they can actually integrate their data, and that allows them to do some basic analysis of their data and that gives them ownership.

In Chapter 5, we described the way in which 'ownership' of data, and access to the reward system of science, was an issue in collaborations between biologists and bioinformaticians. Training biologists in the rudimentary principles of a statistical style of reasoning might defuse some of the tensions generated by these collaborations by developing a degree of individual interdisciplinarity (Calvert 2010).

However, leading scientists within the Centre are pessimistic that individual interdisciplinarity could replace a reliance on bioinformaticians. The scale of data is so vast and the skills required to produce robust secondary inscriptions so sophisticated that bioinformaticians will remain the custodians of Consortium data:

> I would argue that [being in the Consortium] helps people who are more biostatistical than it does people who are more laboratory based. So it's more of a tool really for the biostatisticians and the biomathematicians rather than the laboratory.
>
> (Professor of molecular genetics)

The manager of a consortium put it this way:

> Simply put, we could easily, if we had the money, quadruple the number of biostatisticians and informaticians and we still wouldn't be able to do everything that we want to do. If you've got a computer sitting in the Netherlands with all the data … and we're barely even scratching the phenotype-genotype correlations and so on … I mean, we have nothing like enough … all scientists say they've never got enough. But we cannot do everything that we would like to do.
>
> (Professor of neuropsychiatric genetics, schizophrenia)

Although there is a tendency for bioinformaticians to be seen by their biological colleagues as fulfilling 'technical' roles (see Chapter 5), this devaluation of their scientific contribution is at odds with their epistemic centrality. Producing value from GWAS data requires an ensemble of mathematical, statistical and computational expertise, which is now routinely embedded in processes of laboratory work. The reality that the trading zones between the 'wet' and the 'dry' lab – between laboratory and statistical styles of reasoning – are inevitably 'moist' (Penders *et al.* 2008) seems to be a constitutive feature of extracting value from big data in contemporary bioscience.

By the time of our re-entry to the field, another accomplishment of 'being inside the Consortium' had become clear. 'Mega-analyses'[4] have replicated overlapping regions of gene-association across separate studies (Schizophrenia Psychiatric GWAS Consortium 2011; Psychiatric GWAS Consortium Bipolar Disorder Working Group 2011), and strengthened signals of previously modest associations (Sullivan *et al.* 2012b). The growing accumulation of samples has increased the community's confidence in the data, allowing follow-up studies to investigate their biological function:

> now we have data that is much more confident, so where it's changed I would say over the last seven years or so is that, whereas the laboratory staff were starting to think about, what on earth are we going to do, because everything is now going to consortia and is being outsourced, that is still the case, but now we have data that is giving us high confidence in results, which means that we can now use that as a backbone for designing experiments that need to be validated in the laboratory. So if a particular biological process was implicated we could look at that in the laboratory, so it allows biologists to design experiments, which are based on very good foundations.
>
> (Professor in molecular genetics)

Doing biology within the laboratory style of reasoning was making a return to the Centre. The results of various meta- and mega-analyses of GWAS identified regions implicated in biochemical pathways that had not been identified seven years previously. New methods in molecular biology had become available for the investigation of regions in which susceptibility genes are thought to lie; these included: exploring gene-expression pathways involving messenger RNA and proteins, using gene-editing technologies such as CRISPR to infer function of gene mutations, and, more recently, the use of human-induced pluripotent stem cells (iPSCs) to model disease in brain cells.

We should bear in mind that the professor trained in molecular genetics gives a 'survivalist' account of maintaining the relevance of experimental laboratory research. Speaking to other senior scientists, it was not at all clear that 'doing biology' had a secure place at the Centre.

> It's a big issue and the balance of personnel that we employ is very, very different now to what it was like ten years ago [2007–2008]. Predominately, just off the top of my head, ten years ago, most people that we would have employed in our grants would have been postdocs doing molecular … you know, actual laboratory techniques with some fairly rudimentary statistical ability. Now it's mainly people who don't work in the laboratory who've got much better statistical and informatics ability. And a real challenge is, because you can't not have laboratory people, if you want a laboratory postdoc as opposed to a technician, you really want that postdoc to be able to do some of the more advanced analytic skills. Actually finding people like that is a real challenge, and it's something that we have not successfully met yet.

So how much is there for a biologist to do in the Centre?

> Well, there's a lot of experimental design still required for sequencing and understanding the sequencing and sort of tweaking things … but you still need to target … because you can't afford to do the whole genome in terms of sequencing on everyone, you do the big studies and, at the moment, then we still have to say, okay, we don't have absolute proof for anything after we've sequenced 2,000 or 3,000 people, but we've got kind of suggestive stuff for maybe 100 genes, so we're going to target them…. So you still need that type of input, but the number of very skilled postdoc level people that you need to do that, as opposed to the people who know how to run the laboratory analysis that are in the box, they would be the technicians. You need more of the technicians, fewer of the pure laboratory postdocs, and then more of the analytic postdocs.
>
> (Professor of neuropsychiatric genetics, schizophrenia)

This account of the 'balance of personnel' gives a picture of the changing division of labour at the Centre. Between the technicians who can run the genotyping and sequencing 'in the box' and the statistical postdocs who run bespoke analyses, there are few laboratory postdocs who can ask informed, biologically relevant questions upon which experiments can be designed *and* who are also comfortable working in a statistical style of reasoning. In other words, there are very few postdocs who possess the individual interdisciplinarity to straddle both laboratory and statistical styles of reasoning.

So far, we have seen that 'being inside the Consortium' enjoins an ambivalent arrangement of collective altruism and enlightened self-interest. The sharing of data within the PGC has increased the community's confidence of getting back to 'doing biology', but at the same time the economic logics of Big Biology and the efficiencies of outsourcing had threatened to strip the smaller laboratories of biological expertise, resulting in a shortage of skills to validate results experimentally. However, on our return to the field we found that the ambitions of scientists at the Centre of doing biology (see Chapter 4) were being realized, thanks in part to the changing economics of genotyping and, later, sequencing.

Large-scale phenotyping

Consortium-based GWAS had been relatively successful in powering studies that, during our time in the field, were beginning to generate meaningful signals (Schizophrenia Working Group of the Psychiatric Genomics Consortium 2014). However, while genotyping very large samples is a particular technical and organizational challenge, increasing the scale of phenotyping presents quite different problems. As described in Chapter 6, the clinical style of reasoning required to extract rich phenotypic data from research participants is resistant to automation and expansion. Given the increase in sample sizes by the time we re-entered the field, how has the Centre managed to sustain such output? The answer was surprisingly simple:

> PROFESSOR: In order to get the GWAS numbers, I think it took [director of the Centre] maybe ten years, maybe longer, to collect the first 1,000 samples, and then we moved into almost zero phenotyping and got 15,000 in the next couple of years, which gives you power to detect things but it reduces your power to then understand the consequences.
>
> RESEARCHER: Zero phenotyping?
>
> PROFESSOR: No, we were just relying on the fact that these people had schizophrenia because someone was giving them a drug treatment used for treatment-resistant schizophrenia. This means that the person's been in contact with the services for quite a long time, so it's not that someone has just, on a one-off whim, said they've got schizophrenia, but people have consistently said this person's got schizophrenia.
>
> (Professor of neuropsychiatric genetics, schizophrenia)

Previously, researchers at the Centre had been wary of relying on clinical diagnoses alone when recruiting participants, not only because of a belief that psychiatric diagnoses might well lump together phenotypically and genetically distinct disorders, but also because psychiatric disorders are notorious for misdiagnosis. However, phenotyping 15,000 samples would have been simply impossible in the existing funding climate. A researcher at the Centre had suggested the novel approach of sampling a segment of the patient population taking clozap-ine. Collaboration with Novartis (the manufacturer of a proprietary form of cloz-apine) brokered access to blood samples for a Schizophrenia GWAS, the results of which indicated that the method of ascertainment was valid: patient popula-tions taking clozapine were genetically similar to those receiving a 'research' diagnosis. But given the Centre's clinical reputation for, and pride in, the quality of their phenotypic data, the radical departure of this new approach was greeted with scepticism from the PGC:

> I have to say our colleagues in the consortium were sceptical. But now you can look to see how genetically similar is this sample that [our colleague] collected to the samples that people have gone in minute detail in and have found that they are very genetically similar.... And actually, this is a bit trumpet-blowing, but I think my colleagues in the psychiatric genomics con-sortium would agree because I've heard them stand up and say that, actu-ally, us throwing in this big sample had collectively transformed the fate of schizophrenia GWAS from 20 or 30 little findings to 60, 70, 80 ... and people started going, shit, this really does work, it is about sample sizes.
>
> (Professor of neuropsychiatric genetics, schizophrenia)

The consortium manager plays down concerns that accessing research particip-ants based on medication-type was an unprincipled way of boosting sample sizes. As another colleague put it, 'diluting the quality of the phenotype ... was controversial' because members of the PGC believed that people should be diag-nosed 'properly'. The logics of scale had continued to maintain the tension that we had seen in 2010 between quality and quantity of phenotypic data. The pre-vailing logic is that larger sample size increases the yield of genotype-phenotype correlations which, in turn, attracts more funding. The downside is that, with finite resources, this often has the effect of reducing the 'quality' of the data. The teasing apart of the presumed heterogeneity of established clinical diagnoses, to which scientists at the Centre had hoped their high-quality phenotyping would be the key, was a problem deferred until the 'next phase studies', which would involve 'going back to the old approach'.[5]

Mobility and immobility

In Chapters 4 and 5, we identified the ways in which GWAS had limited the mobility of early and mid-career researchers. The intensification of the manage-ment of biological resources privileges the mobility of samples and data, creat-ing new arrangements of labour in which many scientific workers are contrastingly immobile and *in situ*. For instance, Lezaun (2013: 483) borrowed the concept of the 'stand-in' from Boltanksi and Chaipello (2007) to describe the way in which those at work in Big Biology are unable to 'enhance their own ver-satility and mobility'. The relative immobility of early career researchers and the limited symbolic rewards of middle authorship is a characteristic of scientific life for a substantial proportion of workers; the products of their work are obviously mobile, but their creative contribution is rendered invisible and they are thus prevented from accumulating the kind of symbolic capital to which they had been socialized to expect. So, what has changed since 2010?

Overall, access to Consortium data has increased the 'raw' number of authors, many of whom make limited or specialized contributions to each individual paper. Minor symbolic rewards are widely distributed throughout the PGC, while major rewards – material and symbolic – accrue exclusively to the larger groups: 'people who make the major contributions are getting incredibly successful through this, but they deserve it as well, because they've put a lot of work into this' (Professor in molecular biology). According to the professor, the prospects of early-career researchers accruing transferable reward and scientific capital at the Centre are 'more difficult than ever'. Even to secure a junior faculty position, the required standard of publications is so high that a succession of middle authorship papers is not considered a viable route for promotion.

> You can use it [middle authorship] for your own research exercise framework return, but generally no, you need to be demonstrating that you made a major contribution to that work. So that is very difficult. It's a catch-22 isn't it? If you have a researcher who is part of a big team, and I have seen this happen, very good researchers who are part of really big research teams, so they're part of the cast of Ben Hur, they've done a lot of work, but at the end of the day they're a middle author … they think they've got these great publications, they apply for faculty positions and they really are shot down by other researchers who then look at it very critically and say, well they have another researcher here who has got their own first author publications. That is a real concern I think for people coming through, you need to get into the big groups, but in the big groups you're more likely to be the middle author.
>
> (Professor in molecular biology)

Again, the problem is that the relative invisibility of individual contributions to collaborative work is incommensurate with the standards of visibility required to demonstrate individual excellence. The problem does not lie with the individual but with the distributed nature of collaborative networks, and the systems of valuation that reward 'major contribution' by authorship position. The Centre is in an anomic state: the systems of reward and recognition that functioned in a small(er) science setting are a poor fit for the new arrangements of Big Biology. The permutations of accruing reward are therefore difficult to negotiate for the early-career researcher. They could join a 'smaller group' where they stand a greater chance of improving authorship position but are less likely to be published in high-ranking journals. Alternatively, they could join the 'bigger groups' where they stand a better chance of being published in journals such as *Science* or *Nature*, but in which they are limited to the middling recognition of middle authorship. The professor describes the choices facing the early-career researcher as a 'gamble':

A lot of people will go for the big group of course, and the big name, and I've seen a lot of people fail that way, it's also worked for other people as well. If they're able to manoeuvre themselves into a very good position then that's good ... but I have seen it backfire on people.

(Professor in molecular biology)

The kinds of 'sociological ambivalence' identified in Hackett's (2005) study of scientists also apply to early-career scientists at the Centre. Promising postdocs attracted to the reputational status of a 'big group' risk becoming 'fractional scientists' (Beaver 2001) because they are structurally prevented from accumulating *visible, transferable* symbolic capital. Some can 'manoeuvre themselves' into better positions by making novel or significant contributions, but the tendency of the reward system of Big Science is to pull early-career researchers into the liminal space of middle authorship. Failure to attain sufficient velocity to escape obscurity within the big group is considered a normal trajectory at the Centre; only a few become permanent members.

Turnover of graduate students, postdocs and technicians is common for research laboratories with postdocs joining labs for periods ranging from one to five years (Hackett 2005). Hackett found that research groups are continually changing but, nevertheless, are more-or-less stable. At the Centre, the pattern of turnover was high, in part, because junior researchers are unable to accrue sufficient rewards for promotion. As is well-known, it is easier to attain promotion by moving to a different institution, and so research staff tend leave the Centre after two or three years. One of the molecular biology postdocs we interviewed in Chapter 4 left the Centre after ten years. Despite having middle authorship on several high-ranking publications, he currently works as a 'senior research associate' at another university. Mobility, of a sort, is limited – a sideways move, across space but not 'up' a career ladder. At the Centre, at least, an inherent tension of large-scale biology is that for all it does to produce successful science, there is a continual attrition of expertise as a consequence of the poor opportunities for junior members to accumulate sufficient symbolic capital. The senior scientists we interviewed recognized this problem and described the adoption of a managerial model of succession planning – duplicating and sharing expertise – to ensure that essential skills are retained even if staff are not.

If immobility is a characteristic of those engaged in the day-to-day 'labours' of Big Biology, the same cannot be said for those who occupy senior positions at the Centre. Among those we interviewed in 2010, the senior lecturers are now professors, some of whom have been offered 'personal chairs' for their work on psychiatry, while the others have been rewarded by the British honours system. The ability to accumulate scientific and symbolic capital necessarily lies outside the work of laboratory production; being a result much more of securing funding, developing a public profile and securing access to samples. With respect to the latter, the psychiatrists occupy a key position within the 'coalition of expertise'. Feeding the nodes of laboratory production requires a special kind of mobility –

brokering access to psychiatric health services and patient groups from which research participants are recruited, launching campaigns to boost public interest in medical research, and persuading competing laboratories to share their samples. For those who have visibility in the network and beyond, senior scientists face a separate set of pressures and contradictions.

Identity

Fujimura (1996) and Hackett (2005) describe two sides of a problem that now confronts the continuity of research programmes at the Centre. Fujimura (1996) describes the way in which scientific 'bandwagons' create expanding fields in which an increasing number of groups are investigating the same problems. In Fujimura's study, the molecular biologist Robert Weinberg complains that these bandwagons make future experimental plans 'impossible' because other groups are 'constantly leap-frogging ahead you' (1996: 229). Hackett (2005: 818) identifies a tension in the dynamics of 'cooperative competition' where there is a need for laboratories to sustain independent identities by assembling a 'distinctive ensemble of research technologies'. The Centre faced a similar set of tensions. As the Consortium expanded and organized itself around particular tractable problems, it became more difficult to establish a unique identity while still riding the 'bandwagon' and so justifying future programmes of research. The director alluded to these tensions while reflecting on the Centre's success:

> Well we have managed to stay on the wave ... I mean we were involved in quite a few of the consortia and the fact that [name] led the PGC study, was extremely helpful for us and I was involved in co-leading one of the earlier sequencing studies, so we have continued to do large GWAS and we have got another one that we are trying to get published at the moment where we have found [a number of] new loci and we have got some interesting findings about the evolution of schizophrenia, and we have been doing a lot of rare variant work and you know, we published some big papers in good journals on CNVs and the biology that that is tapping in to, we have published a paper in *Nature* on sequencing and exome sequencing in trios and de novo mutations, so we have managed to sort of stay there or thereabouts.... But you always have to be thinking about what it is that you offer that is if not unique, then at least sufficiently distinct that people will fund you. I mean no one will fund you to do stuff that has already been done better elsewhere. So I think we built our success on seeing the need to collect very large samples before most other people did, putting together a strong statistical bioinformatics team to support the work and working across disorders, which has been very useful and interesting. So it's that sort of combination of things I suppose but there are going to be changes coming up now in the sense that the Centre runs only to 2019.
>
> (Centre director of neuropsychiatric genetics)

Private donations and international consortia have literally 'saved' psychiatric genetics from becoming an anarchic archipelago of competing laboratories using under-powered research methodologies. Perhaps Joseph's diagnosis of psychiatric genetics as a 'null field' might have become the reality had the field not formed a 'bandwagon' around GWAS. The federation of the PGC created an infrastructure that, by harnessing the ensemble of expertise and research technologies in many locales and creating a centralized data repository, rendered tractable the problems of psychiatric genetics. The director attributes their active involvement in these collective organizations as being a large part of their success. Investing in research programmes that focused on both common and rare variants also helped to maintain their competitive advantage. But there is a sense that in order to 'stay on the wave' in a crowded field requires continuous, strategic reflection regarding their own identity. Ensembles of research technologies must be sufficiently distinctive from, and yet connected to, existing streams of inquiry. According to Hackett (2005: 791), in science, the 'quest for identity is perilous' because it involves developing a capacity not only for research but also for evaluating the research prospects of 'an unfolding and uncertain future'. At the time we re-entered the field, the Centre had funding for just the next few years. Speaking to us as that time, the director conceded they would have to 'reinvent themselves', perhaps by carving-off existing programmes, to be picked up by other institutes, and creating a new unit concentrating on the *application* of genomics. He predicted that the future of GWAS itself was secure, as funding was ring-fenced within specific grants. For example, large-scale genotyping and sequencing would continue to feed the bioinformatic pipelines for biology, epidemiology and, more ambitiously, drug-discovery.

The challenge of sustaining an identity occurs alongside the ever-present concern of competing with larger groups. The director's concern is not so much, 'what should we do next?' but, 'how do we fund what we want to do?' The cost of large-scale research as well as the unequal distribution of resources between groups means that there is little room for error when answering these questions. Compared to the Broad Institute which has access to vast resources, the ability to maintain a distinct, notable identity within the field is a central concern for the director:

> We don't have a big group, what's more difficult is … what's happening is more and more data are accumulating not just genomics data but the kind of functional genomics data, that you can use to try and understand the biology. A big challenge is how do you get the biology out of a GWAS signal and that's the next big challenge for the field and there will be lots of naysayers and the usual sort of rending of shirts and wailing and gnashing of teeth, but those data are available. And what's clear is that, I mean, although the Broad and Stanley Centre were able to fund through their philanthropy, they bailed the field out [but] we can't get enough money to do an adequately powered sequencing experiment. So we can get money from the MRC to do

6,000 people, we have also sent a load of our other samples to the Broad for sequencing, so our only hope is that we can combine those.

(Centre director of neuropsychiatric genetics)

Getting 'the biology out of a GWAS signal' is challenging because GWAS are a statistical approach to identifying genetic variants that *might* be of interest in understanding the biology of disease. Genotype-phenotype correlations at the population level may not explain the expression of a gene at the molecular level, nor explain how common variants affect disease risk. Furthermore, the small effects of common variants are difficult to detect in biological experiments. Thus, the next phase of extracting functional biology from GWAS results will involve large-scale whole-genome sequencing studies. The director's biblical reference to the lamentations of 'naysayers' anticipates the chorus of doubt from the Big Science sceptics. The 'only hope' of staying in the game is to find local funding to do in-house sequencing and to outsource the rest to the Broad. The dynamics of large-scale biology are such that in order to sustain an identity, even successful groups such as the Centre must accept a somewhat subordinate role – must bend the knee, so to speak – to their large competitors.

Conclusion

To return to Joseph's claim about 'null fields', none of the senior scientists involved in our research were troubled by the idea that psychiatric genetics would collapse under the weight of 'false' information in the near future. As we described in the Introduction of this book, psychiatric genetics is a discipline that has accomplished a measure of stability and durability by virtue of its styles of scientific reasoning. The field had assembled its own domain of 'tractability' – a problem-field that is economically, politically, and technically difficult to solve but is essentially 'doable'. But in ways that are distinct from Fujimura's (1996) story of co-construction, psychiatric genetics is a story of collaborative networks both inside the laboratory and inside large-scale consortia. The rise of consortia had assembled an infrastructure that not only 'authenticated' GWAS as a research programme, but made it and its successor programme – next-generation sequencing – a 'productive' domain of biological research.

One of the reasons why the 'genetic architecture' metaphor is so alluring for the field is because GWAS have acquired the stability to identify regions of bio-logical interest and, in the process, have implicated previously unknown bio-chemical pathways in disease causation. For example, the 108 loci associated with schizophrenia (Schizophrenia Working Group of the Psychiatric Genomics Consortium 2014) may not have found all the 'missing heritability', but it has vindicated the claim made by the community that GWAS can produce 'biologi-cal insights' when adequately powered by 'very large sample sizes'. By 2017, some of the heritability for schizophrenia has been found in common and rare variants. Of course, sceptics of Big Science could argue that the common vari-ants are artefacts of a statistical style of reasoning, while more radical critics will continue to question the very idea of a relationship between genes and psychiatric disorders – at least the idea that such a relationship could be teased apart in any useful way. Those arguments are outside the concerns of this book. Our interest has been in showing the way in which the scalar politics of psychiatric genetics – a process by which it has become 'Big Biology' – has changed the social and epistemic organization of a single institution, serving as an exemplar of changes in the post-HGP life sciences.

The distributed nature of large-scale biological research is accompanied by an expansive logic of networking, circulation and exchange. The global assemblage of psychiatric genetics oscillates along a dynamic continuum of cooperation–competition, as power imbalances between competing groups and the long-standing reward structure of science play against the necessities of scale required to render tractable the problems of psychiatric genetics. To extract signals of biological value from GWAS requires an intensification of production that includes amassing, sharing and analysing massive data resources, which has transformed the thought styles of psychiatric genetics. It is no longer the case that a facility is judged primarily by the quality of its 'laboratory'. The fact that laboratories needed to be 'saved' in order to retain biological expertise suggests that a laboratory style of reasoning was in the process of being displaced in large-scale psychiatric genetics. Instead, as we see from the accounts provided to us by senior scientists at the Centre, it makes more sense to extol the quality of one's 'bioinformatics team', in which a statistical style of reasoning is applied to the task of turning the bare primary inscriptions of GWAS into the kind of secondary inscriptions that are 'actionable' when, as these scientists hope, the science 'returns' to the molecular biology laboratory.

As for the 'labours' of Big Biology, the intensification of the management of biological resources and the distributed nature of expertise and collaborative work have sharpened the tensions between quality and quantity, visibility and invisibility, mobility and immobility. The depreciation in the value of scientific work in a field where 'authorship' is shared so thinly is certainly a feature of the structural inability to accumulate symbolic capital among junior researchers. This is in stark contrast to the spectacular visibility of those who control the nodes of scientific production. The leading scientists are opinion leaders in the field who supply these nodes not only with samples, but also with funding and public approval. But for the senior scientists who plan programmes, lead consortia and justify research programmes in the face of claims that they have failed, 'visibility' is achieved at the price of tangling with the contradictions of sustaining 'identities of scale' or 'identities *in spite* of scale' in a resource-hungry and highly competitive environment.

In 2010, the director of the Centre hoped that one day they might return to a lost golden age of small-scale biology: comfortable, honourable and concrete. As we write this book in 2018, this golden age is still to be restored. It seems that psychiatric genetics has created a domain in which the complexity of its problems is only rendered tractable by imagining even greater scale. Big(er) Biology is here to stay:

You have got to balance being a participant in large things ... no one funds a participant. You have got to show what added value your group is bringing and I think we have managed to do that. Will it go on? There is no sign of it stopping at the moment, perhaps as we move into the biology it will become maybe smaller scale again but I suspect the lessons we are learning is that you need Big Science for big problems.

(Centre director of neuropsychiatric genetics)

Notes

1 Citing one example from behavioural genetics, Joseph (2012) shows the way in which the reporting of negative GWAS findings for personality traits are explained in terms of 'missing heritability'. Rather than accepting the null hypothesis that perhaps 'no such genes exist', the researchers conclude that gene prediction for personality traits will require 'newer technologies ... novel statistical approaches combined with larger samples and meta-analyses' (Verweij *et al.* 2010 cited in Joseph 2012: 67). Like the pattern of scientific accounting we observed in Chapter 3, the invocation of 'missing heritability' forms part of a new rhetorical strategy for locating hope perpetually on the horizon.
2 In 2014, the Stanley Centre received a further $650 million for biomedical research on psychiatric conditions – one of the largest private donations ever given for scientific research (Zimmer and Carey 2014). No doubt, this extraordinary gift has shored up the Broad Institute's hegemonic position as the epicentre of psychiatric genetics research.
3 Other social scientists have expressed similar ambivalence towards their 'collaborative' role of working with life scientists (Calvert and Martin 2009).
4 Mega-analyses are different to meta-analyses: the former combines individual-level genotype and phenotype data from all subjects in each study, while the latter combines 'summary results' across multiple studies.
5 As we were in the final stages of editing this book we were told that the collection of phenotypic and genotypic data at the Centre had changed, and not back to the 'old approach'. Rather than automating or rationalizing the labour involved, it is 'externalized'. Potential participants are sent a pack through the post and are asked to visit their GP who will draw a blood sample and send it to the Centre. The phenotypic 'narrative' is now mostly done online with participants asked to complete an online form. The removal of direct human interaction and the move to impersonal data collection has been accompanied by heightened concerns on the part of mental health service users that their information will not be ethically managed.

References

Armstrong D (2017) Molecularisation and metaphor. *Sociology of Health and Illness* 39(7): 1195–1205.
Bartlett A (2008) *Accomplishing Sequencing the Human Genome*. PhD Thesis, Cardiff University.
Beaver DD (2001) Reflections on scientific collaborations (and its study): Past, present and future – feature report. *Scientometrics* 52(3): 365–377.
Boltanski L and Chiapello E (2007) *The New Spirit of Capitalism*. London: Verso.
Calvert J (2010) Systems biology, interdisciplinarity and disciplinary identity. In JN Parker, N Vermeulen and B Penders (eds). *Collaboration in the New Life Sciences*. Farnham: Ashgate, pp. 201–219.

Calvert J and Martin P (2009) The role of social scientists in synthetic biology. *EMBO Reports* 10: 201–204.

Collins H (1981) The place of the 'core set' in modern science: Social contingency with methodological propriety in science. *History of Science*: xix.

Crow T (2011) The missing genes: What happened to the heritability of psychiatric disorders? *Molecular Psychiatry* 16: 362–364.

Davies G, Frow E and Leonelli S (2013) Introduction: Bigger, faster, better? Rhetorics and practices of large-scale research in contemporary biology. *Biosocieties* 8: 386–396.

Evans JP, Meslin EM, Marteau TM, *et al.* (2011) Deflating the genomic bubble. *Science* 331 (6019): 861–862.

Fortun M (2008) *Promising Genomics: Iceland and deCODE Genetics in a World of Speculation*. Berkeley: University of California Press.

Fujimura J (1996) *Crafting Science*. Cambridge, MA: Harvard University Press.

Gudbjartsson DF, Walters DF, Thorleifsson HS, *et al.* (2008) Many sequence variants affecting diversity of adult human height. *Nature Genetics* 40: 609–615.

Hackett EJ (2005) Essential tensions: Identity, control and risk in research. *Social Studies of Science* 35(5): 787–826.

Hacking I (1992) 'Style' for historians and philosophers. *Studies in the History and Philosophy of Science* 23(1): 1–20.

Hirschhorn JN and Daly MJ (2005) Genome-wide association studies for common diseases and complex traits. *Nature Genetics* 6: 95–108.

Holtzman NA (1999) Are genetic tests adequately regulated? *Science* 286(5439): 409.

Ioannidis J (2005) Why most published research findings are false. *PLoS Medicine* 2: 696–701.

Joseph J (2012) The 'missing heritability' of psychiatric disorders: Elusive genes or nonexistent genes? *Journal of Applied Developmental Science* 16(2): 65–83.

Kuhn TS (1962) *The Structure of Scientific Revolutions*. Chicago: University of Chicago Press.

Lakoff G and Johnson M (1980) *Metaphors We Live By*. Chicago: University of Chicago Press.

Latham J and Wilson A (2010) *The Great DNA Data Deficit: Are Genes for Disease a Mirage? The Bioscience Research Project.* http://independentsciencenews.org/health/the-great-dna-data-deficit/ [accessed 16 August 2017].

Lettre G, Jackson AU, Gieger C, *et al.* (2008) Identification of ten loci associated with height highlights new biological pathways in human growth. *Nature Genetics* 5: 584–591.

Lezaun J (2013) Commentary: The escalating politics of 'Big Biology'. *Biosocieties* 8(4): 480–485.

Lippman A (1991) Prenatal genetic testing and screening: Constructing needs and reinforcing inequities. *American Journal of Law and Medicine* 17(1–2): 15–50.

Lippman A (1992) Led (astray) by genetic maps: The cartography of the human genome and health care. *Social Science & Medicine* 35(12): 1469–1476.

Macarthur D (2008) Why do genome scans fail? www.wired.com/2008/09/why-do-genome-wide-scans-fail/ [accessed 16 August 2017].

Manolio TA, Collins FS, Cox NJ, *et al.* (2009) Finding the missing heritability of complex diseases. *Nature* 461: 747–753.

Mayer B (2008) The case of missing heritability. *Nature* 456: 18–21.

Penders B, Horstman K and Vos R (2008) Walking the line between lab and computation: The moist zone. *Bioscience* 58(8): 747–755.

Psychiatric GWAS Consortium Bipolar Disorder Working Group (2011) Large-scale genome-wide association analysis of bipolar disorder identifies a new susceptibility locus near ODZ4. *Nature Genetics* 43: 977–983.

Psychiatric GWAS Consortium Coordinating Committee (2009) Genome Wide Association Studies: History, rationale, and prospects for psychiatric disorders. *American Journal of Psychiatry* 166: 540–556.

Rajan KS (2006) *Biocapital: The Constitution of Postgenomic Life*. Durham, NC: Duke Press.

Rose N and Novas C (2005) Biological citizenship. In A Ong and S Collier (eds). *Global Assemblages: Technology, Politics and Ethics as Anthropological Problems*. Malden: Blackwell Publishing, pp. 439–463.

Schizophrenia Psychiatric GWAS Consortium (2011) Genome-wide association study identifies five new schizophrenia loci. *Nature Genetics* 43: 969–976.

Schizophrenia Working Group of the Psychiatric Genomics Consortium (2014) Biological insights from 108 schizophrenia-associated genetic loci. *Nature* 511: 421–427.

Sullivan P, *et al.* (2012a) Don't give up on GWAS. *Molecular Psychiatry* 17: 2–3.

Sullivan PF, Daly MJ and O'Donovan M (2012b) Genetic architecture of psychiatric disorders: The emerging picture and its implications. *Nature Genetics* 13: 537–551.

Turkheimer E (2012) Genome Wide Association Studies of behavior are social science. *Philosophy of Behavioral Biology* 282: 43–64.

Visscher PM (2008) Sizing up human height variation. *Nature Genetics* 40: 489–490.

Weedon MN, Lango H, Lindgren CM, *et al.* (2008) Genome-wide association analysis identifies 20 loci that influence adult height. *Nature Genetics* 40: 575–583.

Weinberg AM (1961) Impact of large-scale science on the United States. *Science* 134(3473): 161–164.

Wellcome Trust Case Control Consortium. (2007). Genomewide association study of 14,000 cases of seven common diseases and 3,000 shared controls. *Nature* 447: 661–678.

Zimmer C and Carey B (2014) Spark for a stagnant search: A $650 million donation for psychiatric research. www.nytimes.com/2014/07/22/science/650-million-psychiatric-research.html [accessed 16 August 2017].

Conclusion
Big Biology and scientific revolutions

In conclusion, we return to the book's opening claim that psychiatric genetics is 'Big Biology'. This statement serves to frame and align the ways in which changes in the epistemic and social organization of a particular scientific community exemplify broader manifestations of scale in post-HGP life science research. Here, 'scale' involves more than simply a quantitative increase in the size and speed of production. As others have noted (Davies *et al.* 2013), emerging forms of Big Biology have diverse characteristics, which are not all encapsulated by shifts in the scale of research. There are also qualitative changes in the epistemic and social organization of scientific work. The existing literature on 'Big Science' offers some basis for comparison, though importantly large-scale biology does not necessarily conform to its dimensions of visibility and centralization. A key feature of our ethnographic site was the *intensification of production through the distributed management of resources*. Key components of production were offloaded to inscription machines, outsourced to service laboratories or carved-off to less visible research practices that included a wide variety of expertise. The laboratories we visited were frankly unremarkable at first appearances because many of their essential processes were automated, miniaturized and externalized.

Indeed, exteriority is a central feature of the high-throughput laboratory. Big Biology appears 'ordinary' when connected to a *network*. The 'federation' of cooperating and competing laboratories that became the PGC had formed around the technical necessity of combining biological samples and creating economies of scale to spread the costs of genotyping many thousands of cases and controls. The field re-formed around a predominantly statistical style of generating power to detect robust 'associations' of genotype and phenotype. The PGC created a 'circle of trust' on a scale that scientists had been previously unaccustomed. Before the era of consortia, trust was a contingent affair influenced by mutual benefit and interpersonal factors, but the PGC institutionalized trust, distributing it more widely (and more thinly), to ensure the centralization and standardization of data to which all groups could have access. In principle, no particular group would have priority over another group's data, but in reality the larger laboratories with greater scientific capital were better positioned to exploit the collective accomplishment. Despite these power imbalances, the PGC has prevailed not only because it balances collective altruism with enlightened self-interest, but because most laboratories had recognized there was no viable alternative. Any hope of finding the genetic components of psychiatric disorders will be a collective accomplishment.

It is true the HGP produced an infrastructure that enabled psychiatric genetics to re-enter the discovery phase, but it was the consortium-based GWAS which 'saved' the field from the fate of persisting with underpowered studies. In the early days of GWAS, when research was faltering under the criticisms of 'null fields' and 'missing heritability', it was the contributions of charismatic leaders, energetic brokers, local funders and charitable billionaires who supplied the money and the political infrastructure to reorganize the field into large-scale consortia. The birth of the PGC transformed the conditions for exchanging data in a competitive field by assembling an international network around a 'doable' problem (Fujimura 1996). With sample sizes increasing substantially from a modest 3,000 cases in GWAS reported in 2003 to 70,000 cases in the next phase of studies, it seems that a politics of scale was deployed to deliver 'meaningful' biology. Consider the 'biological insights' from a schizophrenia GWAS conducted around the time we were in the field. The study of roughly 37,000 cases and 113,000 controls identified associations strongly involved in immune functions and the expressions of neurons in multiple cortical regions. Only by amassing large samples through international consortia can biology claim enrichment of genes converging on plausible pathways expressed in the brain; only then can it claim 'entirely new insights into aetiology', such as molecules implicated in existing anti-psychotic drugs, or those involved in synaptic plasticity (Schizophrenia Working Group of the Psychiatric Genomics Consortium 2014).

But for all its scale and reorganization, the recent achievements of 'Big' psychiatric genetics have been far less than revolutionary. This is in contrast with the transformational view of genetics that was fashionable among bioethicists and social scientists during the HGP. For instance, in their report on 'mental disorders and genetics', the Nuffield Council on Bioethics (1998) gave priority to Lippman's (1991, 1992) concept of 'geneticization'. Reflecting the sentiments of those who responded to the Working Party's consultation, geneticization established a framework for thinking that scientific and technological development is the vanguard of an onerous revolution, not just, for instance, in healthcare, but in the way in which we conceive of ourselves, our bodies and so on. And yet, in the two decades since its publication, the geneticization revolution has yet to take place: one could argue that for all the advances that have been made within psychiatric genetics there have been no scientific discoveries with the revolutionary potential to warrant such ethical and social concerns.

We accept that transformation is an emergent property of twenty-first-century bioscience, but the scale and reach of the effects of post-HGP genetics and genomics must be considered alongside careful histories of scientific practice and empirical studies of their domain of production. Only then would we see that ideas of genetic 'essentialism' (on which notions of geneticization are derived) had collapsed in the field of psychiatric genetics long before the completion of the HGP (Kendler 2006). Of course, transformational accounts of science are often alluring, but our research points to little that might suggest that molecular genetics and genomics has transformed, or is close to transforming, clinical and biological psychiatry. If anything, our story, which places these narratives of transformation in the context of history and practice, shows that this transformational potential is limited by the sheer complexity of its own objects. Psychiatric genetics has become 'Big Biology' precisely because the clinical and genetic *heterogeneity* of psychiatric disorders are resistant to revolutionary discoveries.

Taking a 'styles' approach to the history of psychiatric genetics introduces another kind of epistemological 'handbrake' on narratives of revolution. Hacking's (1992) 'styles of reasoning' offer a more precise tool for differentiating science in terms of its conditions of possibility, which are characterized by their stability and duration. In Chapters 1 and 2, we showed that psychiatric genetics crystallized from the interplay of *clinical*, *statistical* and *laboratory* styles of reasoning in the early twentieth century. The birth of psychiatric genetics in Germany marked the point at which a science of heredity crossed the 'threshold of scientificity' (Foucault 1972) – an event that coincided with new standards of testing the truth and falsity of Mendelian patterns of segregation. Rüdin's family study of schizophrenia was the first large-scale study of a stable, clinical disorder selected for its endogenous factors and its chronology of symptoms. However, schizophrenia was an object that both united and divided the field of psychiatric genetics. A Mendelian model contained the contradiction that relatives of schizophrenia patients carried features of heterogeneity that did not fit clear Mendelian categories. It was this heterogeneity that led to an emerging division between those who applied a statistical style of reasoning on twin (and later adoption) samples and those who applied a laboratory (molecular) style of reasoning on family pedigrees.

From the 1920s to the 1970s, during which a statistical style of reasoning prevailed, psychiatric genetics was dogged by controversy and criticism. Moderate critics were constructive, seeking to retain but also improve the central methodology, while radical critics denounced the whole research programme as being the product of determinist ideology. A pattern of these radical critiques was to show that, by its own standards of reasoning, psychiatric genetics was merely a facade of scientificity because it could not distinguish its positive claims from its eugenic assumptions. It is certainly the case that many of the Munich-trained researchers held eugenic beliefs, but it does not necessarily follow that psychiatric genetics lacked scientificity *because* of its eugenic origins, nor is there sufficient evidence that it lacked scientificity according to its own standards of objectivity. We point out that twin and adoption studies have not remained constant, but have evolved in relation to criticism, resulting in incremental improvements in methodological design. What has remained relatively constant though is the epistemic uncertainty of genetic heterogeneity. We suggest that rather than being an intractable problem, heterogeneity is a source of productivity. By the 1960s, belief in polygenic inheritance consolidated heterogeneity – even when studies focused on a single major locus it was understood in the context of a polygenic background of multiple genes, incomplete penetrance and non-genetic factors. The emergence of this 'enlightened' discourse of geneticization (Hedgecoe 2001) has more in common with the stability of styles of reasoning than a so-called shift in Kuhnian paradigms (Hacking 1985).

By the time we reach the 'event' of GWAS explored in the ethnographic chapters of this book, the heterogeneity of psychiatric conditions are recast as *tractable* problems. The possibilities of automating the detection of 'diallelic polymorphisms' (Risch and Merikangas 1996) allowed the field to reimagine the scale of its research problems. The accounts of 'complexity' we discussed in Chapter 3 are not merely ontological descriptions of an elusive phenomenon but performative statements of a cautious, flexible and responsible science. The rhetoric of complexity acts on a broader field of expectations by marshalling scientific and political capital and building hope that research problems are, in fact, tractable to increases in scale and multidisciplinary reorganization.

The availability of high-throughput technologies revitalized research programmes, establishing new techniques for testing the 'common disease-common allele' model proposed by Gottesman in the 1980s. The epistemic organization of GWAS can be thought of as the re-integration of laboratory and statistical styles of reasoning in which laboratory techniques of gene-finding are co-dependent on robust testing of statistical correlations. GWAS are examples of 'extraordinarily normal' science in the sense that solving problems does not involve scientific creativity or new standards of reasoning. They are an infrastructure for collecting and exchanging large samples to which clinical, statistical, and laboratory reasoning are applied, presupposing that many psychiatric disorders are continuous polygenic traits. Rather than coherent entities sharing a one-to-one correspondence with genetic variants, psychiatric conditions are quantitative traits with real molecular properties (Kendler 2015). And because there is no 'gene for' this or that condition, criticisms of these programmes for their essentialism and determinism are misdirected. Accounts of the 'geneticization' of disease fail to account for the perpetual postponement of revolution, while practices of *molecularization* reveal a complex biological architecture, only tractable to large-scale, multidisciplinary collaborative research.

The ongoing molecularization of psychiatric disorders is, according to some, 'flattening' the space between personhood and biology (Rose 2007). The engines of genotyping and sequencing in biological psychiatry are remapping the psychological space of mental pathology, and filling this space with many new objects for further biological and psychopharmaceutical studies. Psychiatric disease has become an informational and mechanistic biology amenable to neurochemical intervention and clinical risk management. And yet, for all the hope of delivering therapeutic targets, predictions of novel drug efficacy, improved calculations of polygenic risk and of clearer diagnostic boundaries, not one of these expectations has yet been realized in the clinic. As we write, psychiatric genetics remains in a perpetual state of attempting to close the gap between genomic findings and genetically informed, clinically valid diagnostic testing, classification and treatment. But to say that anchoring our clinical understanding of psychiatric disorders in genomics appears to be epistemically futile is far less interesting than addressing the sociological question of how the field has stabilized in the face of relatively modest achievements (see Chapters 3 and 8).

In our contemporary regimes of hope, psychiatric genetics has assembled a domain of tractability by harnessing networks and resources around a predominantly statistical style of scientific reasoning. Current discourses of promise in psychiatric genetics offer enough flexibility to anticipate and accommodate delays in discovery and clinical translation by strategically foregrounding strong and moderate versions of 'complexity', by enrolling metaphors to describe the frustrating 'plasticity' of phenotypic traits, and by highlighting the small but aggregate effects of common variants. In any case, there is profit to be made by promising future discoveries to a pharmaceutical industry, for which new, effective treatments for mental ill-health could be extremely valuable (Rose 2007). Despite lingering doubts (see Chapter 8), these genomic futures are far from exhausted and continue to mobilize resources in support of large-scale research programmes. To borrow a phrase from Weinberg (1961: 161), it seems that 'Big Science is here to stay'.

Some commentators are suspicious of this reorganization of the biosciences. The 'expansionary logics' and 'diminishing outside' of Big Biology implies a kind of intrusive totality (see Davies *et al.* 2013; Lezaun 2013). These observations apply to our own field work insofar as the PGC was likened to the 'Death Star', which, for its own survival, was sucking up 'all the samples and all the money'. But our focus has been to understand Big Biology from the point of view of its local heterogeneity, in terms of the internal contradictions it generates for its members *inside* these networks of production. Based on the observations and interviews collected over nearly a decade, we have seen how consortium-based GWAS have produced tensions that are reminiscent of other 'Big Sciences' and symptomatic of the transition to large-scale data-driven biology.

How does the politics of scale impress upon its practitioners? Consortium-based GWAS have introduced a new level of discomfort. Many scientists were frank when articulating their frustration of 'rapid transitions', 'collaborating with enemies' and 'outsourcing everything'; while others were positive that adapting to collaborative networks of exchange was the only way for the field to progress. Over the course of our observations and analysis, several 'value tensions' (Hackett 2005) have come into view, some of which are endemic to science and others particular to Big Biology. The most distinctive tension is the dynamic of competitive-collaboration by which groups are forced to move beyond their circle of trusted collaborators. Tensions in collaboration arise because the distribution of rewards are asymmetrical: one group's initiative is seen as 'stealing' work by another. Over the years, the tensions of balancing group-specific recognition with scientific communalism have been moderated by 'federal' coordinating committees. But what binds the community is acceptance, perhaps resignation, that no solitary group can do successful discovery science outside consortia.

During our visits at the Centre, we witnessed the epistemic reorganization of the laboratories. The craft-skills of molecular biology were no longer central to the thought styles of psychiatric genetics. Laboratory work had been displaced by the statistical reasoning of data-driven biology, which required new kinds of expertise. Indeed, one of the molecular biologists we interviewed, now a consortium manager, confessed to being no longer capable of conducting a laboratory experiment – 'I can't do the statistics anymore'. Forces external to the Centre have contributed to this reorganization – the automation and miniaturization of laboratory processes, the outsourcing of biological resources to commercial laboratories, and the economies of scale that intensify collaboration and competition. Scientists occupy hybrid positions of expertise within networks of information, particularly those capable of developing methods and tools for extracting value from annotated data. New relationships have emerged in so-called 'trading zones' (Galison 1999) where the mixing of 'wet' and 'dry' styles are arranged in research projects (Penders *et al.* 2008). Rather than dissolving jurisdictions, multidisciplinary networks expose tensions in epistemic cultures that re-inscribe boundaries between scientists and technicians, some of whom are hidden away as service providers.

Other tensions endemic to consortium-based GWAS arise from the unintended effects of outsourcing. Outsourcing is a condition of entry into consortia through which smaller laboratories collaborate and compete with larger groups. Divesting work to other groups allows smaller laboratories to do high-throughput genotyping and sequencing, but it also increases tensions in the values and norms of science. The tensions we observed at the Centre between quality and quantity and between intrinsic and instrumental value were typical of the pressures of managing and sustaining large-scale collaborative research. In this case, the effect of reducing costs and increasing genotyping displaced molecular biologists to activities of coding and programming that, by their own admission, contain little intrinsic value. A similar tension occurs in large-scale phenotyping, where the quality of information is reduced to augment the quantity of samples. Even the relationship between biologists and bioinformaticians can be characterized by (mis-)attributions of intrinsic and instrumental value. Though bioinformaticians are key to the network, they are often (mis-) recognized as instrumental technicians and thus prevented from enhancing their own intrinsic value.

More so than 'small science', the value tensions endemic to Big Biology oscillate around the mobility and visibility of actors in large networks. Consider the postdoc who cannot lead on a project because it deviates from the group's core activities, or the bioinformatician 'who sits down and analyses other people's data'; the fieldworker whose emotional labour is invisible to others in the network, or the junior researcher who cannot escape the orbit of middle authorship. They are all figures of immobility. In a 'connectionist world' of network-based organization, immobility has become the new inequality (Boltanksi and Chiapello 2007). Those who are the least mobile are the 'stand-ins' of Big Biology: the actor who must remain *in situ* while other people and other things circulate. Visibility and mobility are complementary dimensions by which actors 'enhance their own versatility' (Lezaun 2013: 483). But in large-scale networks, to be seen, recognized and valued is more difficult when each actor is adding value 'incrementally' along a chain of inscriptions. Extracting raw materials from research participants or providing tools to 'help' others see and navigate biology are merely *services* that enhance the mobility of others. Conversely, scientists who broker collaboration, lead on grants, write papers and impute biology are certainly figures who move and increase their value.

These tensions of mobility and visibility are aggravated by a value system developed within the social organization of small science that cannot distribute rewards in a way suited to large-scale collaborative research. Middle authors, for example, are assigned token positions on papers, preventing them from accumulating the intrinsic value of leading on grants or publications. In collaborative networks of research, reward systems privilege the excellence of any biology done, often favouring senior biologists and psychiatrists who routinely occupy key authorship positions. Junior researchers, PhD students, postdocs and bioinformaticians all play a factor in production but their contributions have no intrinsic worth, only the instrumental value of moving processes down a chain of inscriptions. It makes less sense to say that these actors are 'excluded' because their participation is essential; more precisely, they are 'exploited in the sense that the role they play as a factor of production does not receive the acknowledgement it merits' (Boltanksi and Chiapello 2007: 363).

A key theme that runs through our observations of the Centre is the ways in which immobility appears to be a necessary condition for scaling-up biological research. Big Biology is a network-based organization that privileges the technical and charismatic expertise of those who control, supply and move beyond the nodes of production. Their visibility and mobility is spectacular insofar as their achievements and promotions outstrip those who cannot enterprise themselves *in situ*. Where large-scale research is governed by the intensification of production, the interconnectivity of networks are simply more effective regimes of exploitation.

A central question we have asked in this book then is how does a controversial science of psychiatric genetics acquire the prestige and stability of 'Big Biology'? What has made it so durable? This, for us, is a more interesting question than framing the transformational aspects of genomics in terms of 'revolution' or 'geneticization'. The fact that psychiatric genetics cannot tame its own complex ontologies implies that determinism and essentialism are not the most interesting lines of critical inquiry. Others may want to focus on how psychiatric genetics forms part of our contemporary regimes of hope, the molecular targets of which create new relations of biological value and exchange. The fact that no obvious developments in drug discovery have come to pass suggest that the vitality of mental illness has not yet acquired the stability for capitalization. Rather than pondering what genomics may or may not have achieved in this domain, we have found more purchase in critically exploring the local conditions of knowledge production. The labours of 'Big Biology' say more about the contradictions of collaborative, multidisciplinary research, the impermanence of stability, and the immobility of those who cannot maximize their value in large-scale networks of biological research.

References

Boltanski L and Chiapello E (2007) *The New Spirit of Capitalism*. London: Verso.

Davies G, Frow E and Leonelli S (2013) Introduction: Bigger, faster, better? Rhetorics and practices of large-scale research in contemporary biology. *Biosocieties* 8: 386–396.

Foucault M (1972) *The Archaeology of Knowledge*. London: Tavistock.

Fujimura J (1996) *Crafting Science*. Cambridge, MA: Harvard University Press.

Galison P (1999) Trading zones: Coordinating action and belief. In M Biagioli (ed.). *The Science Studies Reader*. New York: Routledge, pp. 137–160.

Hackett EJ (2005) Essential tensions: Identity, control and risk in research. *Social Studies of Science* 35(5): 787–826.

Hacking I (1985) Styles of scientific reasoning. In J Rajchman and C West (eds). *Post-Analytic Philosophy*. New York: Columbia University Press, pp. 145–165.

Hacking I (1992) 'Style' for historians and philosophers. *Studies in the History and Philosophy of Science* 23(1): 1–20.

Hedgecoe A (2001) Schizophrenia and the narrative of enlightened geneticization. *Social Studies of Science* 31(6): 875–911.

Kendler KS (2006) Reflections on the relationship between psychiatric genetics and psychiatric nosology. *American Journal of Psychiatry* 163: 1138–1146.

Kendler KS (2015) A joint history of the nature of genetic variation and the nature of schizophrenia. *Molecular Psychiatry* 20(1): 77–83.

Lezaun J (2013) Commentary: The escalating politics of 'Big Biology'. *Biosocieties* 8(4): 480–485.

Lippman A (1991) Prenatal genetic testing and screening: Constructing needs and reinforcing inequities. *American Journal of Law and Medicine* 17(1–2): 15–50.

Lippman A (1992) Led (astray) by genetic maps: The cartography of the human genome and health care. *Social Science & Medicine* 35: 1469–1476.

Nuffield Council on Bioethics (1998) *Mental Disorders and Genetics: The Ethical Context*. London: Nuffield Council on Bioethics.

Penders B, Horstman K and Vos R (2008) Walking the line between lab and computation: The moist zone. *Bioscience* 58(8): 747–755.

Risch N and Merikangas K (1996) The future of genetics studies of complex human diseases. *Science* 273: 1516–1517.

Rose N (2007) *The Politics of Life Itself: Biomedicine, Power, and Subjectivity in the Twenty-First Century*. Princeton: Princeton University Press.

Schizophrenia Working Group of the Psychiatric Genomics Consortium (2014) Biological insights from 108 schizophrenia-associated genetic loci. *Nature* 511: 421–427.

Weinberg AM (1961) Impact of large-scale science on the United States. *Science* 134(3473): 161–164.

Index

Page numbers in **bold** denote tables.

230   *Index*

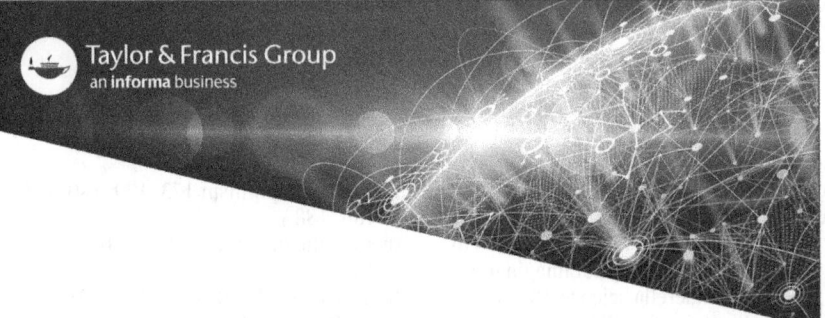
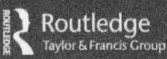
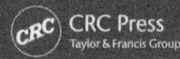